Atlas of
Cardiac Surgical Techniques

Atlas of
Cardiac Surgical Techniques
A Volume in the Surgical Techniques Atlas Series

Editors

Frank W. Sellke, MD

Chief of Cardiothoracic Surgery and Karl E. Karlson and Gloria A. Karlson Professor of Cardiothoracic Surgery
Alpert School of Medicine of Brown University, Rhode Island Hospital, and The Miriam Hospital
Co-Director of the Lifespan Heart Center
Providence, Rhode Island
Visiting Professor of Surgery
Harvard Medical School
Boston, Massachusetts

Marc Ruel, MD, MPH, FRCSC

Associate Professor of Surgery, Cellular and Molecular Medicine, and Epidemiology
Cardiac Surgery Research Chair
University of Ottawa Heart Institute
Ottawa, Ontario
Canada

Series Editors

Courtney M. Townsend, Jr., MD

Professor and John Woods Harris Distinguished Chairman
Department of Surgery
The University of Texas Medical Branch
Galveston, Texas

B. Mark Evers, MD

Professor and Robertson-Poth Distinguished Chair in General Surgery
Department of Surgery
Director of UTMB Comprehensive Cancer Center
The University of Texas Medical Branch
Galveston, Texas

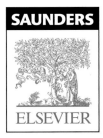

SAUNDERS

ELSEVIER

SAUNDERS
ELSEVIER

1600 John F. Kennedy Blvd.
Ste 1800
Philadelphia, PA 19103-2899

ATLAS OF CARDIAC SURGICAL TECHNIQUES ISBN: 978-1-4160-4065-1

Notice

Knowledge and best practice in this field are constantly changing. As new research and experience broaden our knowledge, changes in practice, treatment, and drug therapy may become necessary or appropriate. Readers are advised to check the most current information provided (i) on procedures featured or (ii) by the manufacturer of each product to be administered, to verify the recommended dose or formula, the method and duration of administration, and contraindications. It is the responsibility of the practitioner, relying on their own experience and knowledge of the patient, to make diagnoses, to determine dosages and the best treatment for each individual patient, and to take all appropriate safety precautions. To the fullest extent of the law, neither the Publisher nor the Authors assumes any liability for any injury and/or damage to persons or property arising out of or related to any use of the material contained in this book.

The Publisher

Library of Congress Cataloging-in-Publication Data
Atlas of cardiac surgical techniques / editors, Frank Sellke, Marc Ruel.—1st ed.
    p. ; cm.—(Surgical techniques atlas series)
  Includes bibliographical references.
  ISBN 978-1-4160-4065-1
  1. Heart—Surgery—Atlases. I. Sellke, Frank W. II. Ruel, Marc. III. Series.
  [DNLM: 1. Cardiac Surgical Procedures—Atlases. 2. Cardiovascular Diseases—surgery—Atlases.
WG 17 A88147 2010]
  RD598.A925 2010
  617.4'12—dc22

2008046857

Acquisitions Editor: Judith Fletcher
Developmental Editor: Kristina Oberle
Publishing Services Manager: Tina Rebane
Project Manager: Amy Norwitz
Design Direction: Steven Stave

Printed in China

Last digit is the print number: 9 8 7 6 5 4 3 2 1

To Amy, to Catherine, and to our patients,
who make the relentless efforts more than worthwhile

CONTRIBUTORS

Arvind K. Agnihotri, MD
Assistant Professor of Surgery, Harvard Medical
    School, Massachusetts General Hospital, Boston,
    Massachusetts
Postinfarction Ventricular Septal Defect

Craig J. Baker, MD
Assistant Professor of Surgery; Vice Chair of Surgical
    Education, Cardiovascular Thoracic Institute,
    University of Southern California Keck School of
    Medicine, Los Angeles, California
Ross Procedure

Joseph E. Bavaria, MD
Brooke Roberts-William M. Measey Professor of
    Surgery; Vice Chief of Division of Cardiovascular
    Surgery; Director of Thoracic Aortic Surgery
    Program, University of Pennsylvania School of
    Medicine, Hospital of the University of
    Pennsylvania, Philadelphia, Pennsylvania
*Thoracic Endovascular Aortic Repair for Descending Thoracic Aortic
    and Aortic Arch Aneurysms*

Munir Boodhwani, MD, MMSc
Clinical Associate, University of Ottawa Heart
    Institute, Ottawa, Ontario, Canada
Incisions for Cardiac Surgery

William T. Brinkman, MD
Cardiovascular Surgeon, The Heart Hospital
    Baylor Plano, Baylor University Medical Center,
    Dallas, Texas
*Thoracic Endovascular Aortic Repair for Descending Thoracic Aortic
    and Aortic Arch Aneurysms*

Vincent Chan, MD
Chief Resident, Division of Cardiac Surgery,
    University of Ottawa Heart Institute Ottawa,
    Ontario, Canada
Minimally Invasive Cardiac Surgical Coronary Artery Bypass Grafting

Michael A. Coady, MD, MPH
Associate Professor of Surgery, Brown University
    School of Medicine, Providence, Rhode Island
Type A Aortic Dissections

Lawrence H. Cohn, MD
Professor of Cardiac Surgery, Harvard Medical School;
    Cardiac Surgeon-in-Chief Emeritus, Brigham and
    Women's Hospital, Boston, Massachusetts
Repair of the Myxomatous Degenerated Mitral Valve

William E. Cohn, MD
Associate Professor, Baylor College of Medicine;
    Director of Minimally Invasive Surgical Technology,
    The Texas Heart Institute at St. Luke's Episcopal
    Hospital, Houston, Texas
Percutaneous Mitral Valve Repair Techniques
Pulsatile and Axial Ventricular Support

Joseph S. Coselli, MD
Professor and Cullen Foundation Endowed Chair,
    Division of Cardiothoracic Surgery, Baylor College
    of Medicine; Chief of Adult Cardiac Surgery, The
    Texas Heart Institute at St. Luke's Episcopal
    Hospital, Houston, Texas
Thoracoabdominal Aneurysms

Tirone E. David, MD
Professor, University of Toronto; Head of Division of
    Cardiac Surgery, Toronto General Hospital, Toronto,
    Ontario, Canada
Aortic Valve–Sparing Operations

John R. Doty, MD
Clinical Associate Professor of Surgery, University of
    Utah; Staff Surgeon, Intermountain Medical Center,
    Salt Lake City, Utah
Aortic Root Enlargement Techniques

Amir K. Durrani, MD
Categorical Resident, Department of Internal
    Medicine, Yale University School of Medicine, New
    Haven, Connecticut
*Minimally Invasive Mitral Valve Replacement: Partial Sternotomy
    Approach*

Volkmar Falk, PhD
Professor, University of Leipzig; Heart Surgeon, Heart
    Center of Leipzig, Leipzig, Germany
Robotic Coronary Artery Bypass Grafting

Lynn M. Fedoruk, MD, FRCSC
Clinical Instructor, University of British Columbia, Vancouver, British Columbia; Attending Physician, Royal Jubilee Hospital, Victoria, British Columbia, Canada
Surgery for Left Ventricular Aneurysm and Remodeling

Michael P. Fischbein, MD, PhD
Assistant Professor of Cardiothoracic Surgery, Stanford University School of Medicine, Stanford, California
Type B Aortic Dissections

O. H. Frazier, MD, FACS, FACC
Clinical Professor, University of Texas M.D. Anderson Cancer Center; Professor, University of Texas Medical School Houston, Baylor College of Medicine; Director of Cardiovascular Surgical Research; Chief of Cardiopulmonary Transplantation, The Texas Heart Institute at St. Luke's Episcopal Hospital; Chief of Transplant Services, St. Luke's Episcopal Hospital, Houston, Texas
Pulsatile and Axial Ventricular Support

A. Marc Gillinov, MD
Attending Surgeon, Department of Thoracic and Cardiovascular Surgery, Cleveland Clinic; Judith Dion Pyle Chair in Heart Valve Research; Surgical Director, Center for Atrial Fibrillation, Cleveland, Ohio
Minimally Invasive Mitral Valve Replacement: Partial Sternotomy Approach
Surgery for Atrial Fibrillation

Thomas G. Gleason, MD
Associate Professor of Surgery, University of Pittsburgh Medical Center, Pittsburgh, Pennsylvania
Type A Aortic Dissections

Igor D. Gregoric, MD
Clinical Assistant Professor, University of Texas Medical School Houston; Director of Center for Cardiac Support, The Texas Heart Institute at St. Luke's Episcopal Hospital, Houston, Texas
Pulsatile and Axial Ventricular Support

John S. Ikonomidis, MD, PhD
Professor, Department of Cardiothoracic Surgery, Medical University of South Carolina; Chief of Division of Cardiothoracic Surgery, Ralph H. Johnson Veterans Administration Medical Center, Charleston, South Carolina
Aortic Arch Aneurysms

Stephan Jacobs, MD
Associate Professor, University of Leipzig; Heart Surgeon, Heart Center of Leipzig, Leipzig, Germany
Robotic Coronary Artery Bypass Grafting

Tanveer A. Khan, MD
Clinical Instructor, David Geffen School of Medicine at University of California, Los Angeles, Los Angeles, California
Heart-Lung Transplantation

Anastasios K. Konstantakos, MD
Cardiothoracic Surgeon, Billings Clinic, Billings, Montana
On-Pump Coronary Artery Bypass Grafting

Irving L. Kron, MD
Professor and Chairman, Department of Surgery, University of Virginia Health System, Charlottesville, Virginia
Surgery for Left Ventricular Aneurysm and Remodeling

Alexander Kulik, MD, MPH, FRCSC
Cardiovascular Surgery Fellow, Missouri Baptist Medical Center, St. Louis, Missouri
Tricuspid Valve Operations

Hillel Laks, MD
Professor, David Geffen School of Medicine at University of California, Los Angeles, Los Angeles, California
Heart-Lung Transplantation

Harry Lapierre, MD, FRCSC
Clinical Associate, University of Montreal Faculty of Medicine, Montreal, Quebec; University of Ottawa Heart Institute, Ottawa, Ontario, Canada
Minimally Invasive Cardiac Surgical Coronary Artery Bypass Grafting

Scott A. LeMaire, MD
Associate Professor and Director of Research, Division of Cardiothoracic Surgery, Baylor College of Medicine; Cardiovascular Surgery Staff, The Texas Heart Institute at St. Luke's Episcopal Hospital, Houston, Texas
Thoracoabdominal Aneurysms

Daniel Marelli, MD
Clinical Associate, University of Pennsylvania School of Medicine, Philadelphia, Pennsylvania; Bay Health Medical Center, Dover, Delaware
Heart Transplantation

Joseph T. McGinn, Jr., MD
Clinical Assistant Professor, State University of New
    York Downstate, Brookhaven, New York; Clinical
    Associate Professor of Surgery, New York Medical
    College, Valhalla, New York; Director of
    Cardiothoracic Surgery, Staten Island University
    Hospital; Medical Director, The Heart Institute of
    Staten Island, Staten Island, New York
    Minimally Invasive Cardiac Surgical Coronary Artery Bypass Grafting

Thierry G. Mesana, MD, PhD, FECTS, FRCSC
University of Ottawa Faculty of Medicine, Michael
    Pitfield Research Chair in Cardiac Surgery, Chief of
    Cardiac Surgery, University of Ottawa Heart
    Institute, Ottawa, Ontario, Canada
    Tricuspid Valve Operations

Tomislav Mihaljevic, MD
Attending Surgeon, Department of Thoracic and
    Cardiovascular Surgery, Cleveland Clinic
    Foundation, Cleveland, Ohio
    *Minimally Invasive Mitral Valve Replacement: Partial Sternotomy
        Approach*
    Surgery for Atrial Fibrillation

R. Scott Mitchell, MD
Professor of Cardiothoracic Surgery, Stanford
    University School of Medicine, Stanford, California
    Type B Aortic Dissections

Friedrich W. Mohr, PhD
Professor, University of Leipzig; Heart Surgeon, Heart
    Center of Leipzig, Leipzig, Germany
    Robotic Coronary Artery Bypass Grafting

Nahush A. Mokadam, MD
Assistant Professor of Cardiothoracic Surgery,
    University of Washington Medical Center, Seattle,
    Washington
    Aortic Homografts

Sorin V. Pusca, MD
Instructor in Cardiothoracic Surgery, Emory
    University School of Medicine, Atlanta, Georgia
    Off-Pump Coronary Artery Bypass Grafting

John D. Puskas, MD
Professor of Surgery, Emory University School of
    Medicine; Chief of Division of Cardiothoracic
    Surgery, Emory Crawford Long Hospital, Atlanta,
    Georgia
    Off-Pump Coronary Artery Bypass Grafting

Ladislaus Ressler, MD
Assistant Professor, Clinical Associate in Cardiac
    Surgery, University of Ottawa Heart Institute,
    Ottawa, Ontario, Canada
    Cannulation Techniques for Cardiopulmonary Bypass

Jason O. Robertson, MD
General Surgery Resident, Washington University in
    St. Louis School of Medicine; Barnes-Jewish
    Hospital, St. Louis, Missouri
    *Minimally Invasive Mitral Valve Replacement: Partial Sternotomy
        Approach*

Roberto Rodriguez, MD
Assistant Professor of Surgery, Tufts University School
    of Medicine; Cardiothoracic Surgeon, St. Elizabeth's
    Medical Center, Boston, Massachusetts
    Aortic Valve Replacement

Fraser D. Rubens, MD, MSc, FRCSC
Professor of Surgery; Director of Cardiac Surgery
    Residency and Fellowship Program, University of
    Ottawa Heart Institute, Ottawa, Ontario, Canada
    Cannulation Techniques for Cardiopulmonary Bypass

Marc Ruel, MD, MPH, FRCSC
Associate Professor of Surgery, Cellular and Molecular
    Medicine, and Epidemiology; Cardiac Surgery
    Research Chair, University of Ottawa Heart
    Institute, Ottawa, Ontario, Canada
    Incisions for Cardiac Surgery
    Minimally Invasive Cardiac Surgical Coronary Artery Bypass Grafting

Frank W. Sellke, MD
Chief of Cardiothoracic Surgery and Karl E. Karlson
    and Gloria A. Karlson Professor of Cardiothoracic
    Surgery, Alpert School of Medicine of Brown
    University, Rhode Island Hospital, and The Miriam
    Hospital; Co-Director of the Lifespan Heart Center,
    Providence, Rhode Island; Visiting Professor of
    Surgery, Harvard Medical School, Boston,
    Massachusetts
    On-Pump Coronary Artery Bypass Grafting
    Aortic Valve Replacement

Kapil Sharma, MD, FRCSC
Cardiac Surgery West Medical Corporation
    Sacramento, California
    Type B Aortic Dissections

Richard J. Shemin, MD
Robert and Kelly Day Chair of Cardiothoracic Surgery, David Geffen School of Medicine at University of California, Los Angeles; Professor and Chief of Cardiothoracic Surgery; Co-director of University of California, Los Angeles, Cardiovascular Center; Executive Vice Chair of Department of Surgery, UCLA Ronald Reagan Medical Center, Los Angeles, California
Bentall Procedure

Scott Silvestry, MD
Associate Professor of Surgery, Jefferson Medical College of Thomas Jefferson University; Surgical Director of Heart Transplant Program, Thomas Jefferson University Hospital, Philadelphia, Pennsylvania
Heart Transplantation

Vaughn A. Starnes, MD
H. Russell Smith Foundation Chair, Distinguished Professor of Surgery, Cardiovascular Thoracic Institute, University of Southern California Keck School of Medicine, Los Angeles, California
Ross Procedure

Wilson Y. Szeto, MD
Assistant Professor of Surgery, University of Pennsylvania School of Medicine, Hospital of the University of Pennsylvania, Division of Cardiovascular Surgery, Philadelphia, Pennsylvania
Thoracic Endovascular Aortic Repair for Descending Thoracic Aortic and Aortic Arch Aneurysms

Peter I. Tsai, MD
Assistant Professor of Cardiothoracic Surgery, Baylor College of Medicine; Surgical Staff, Ben Taub General Hospital, Houston, Texas
Thoracoabdominal Aneurysms

Thomas A. Vassiliades, Jr., MD, MBA
Associate Professor of Surgery, Division of Cardiothoracic Surgery, Emory University School of Medicine, Atlanta, Georgia
Endoscopic and Traditional Minimally Invasive Direct Coronary Artery Bypass

Edward D. Verrier, MD
Professor and Chief of Division of Cardiothoracic Surgery, K. Alvin and Shirley Merendino Endowed Chair of Cardiothoracic Surgery, University of Washington Medical Center, Seattle, Washington
Aortic Homografts

FOREWORD

"A picture is worth a thousand words."

Anonymous

This atlas is for practicing surgeons, surgical residents, and medical students for their review and preparation for surgical procedures. New procedures are developed and old ones are replaced as technologic and pharmacologic advances occur. The topics presented are contemporaneous surgical procedures with step-by-step illustrations, preoperative and postoperative considerations, and pearls and pitfalls, taken from the personal experience and surgical practices of the authors. Their results have been validated in their surgical practices involving many patients. Operative surgery remains a manual art in which the knowledge, judgment, and technical skill of the surgeon come together for the benefit of the patient. A technically perfect operation is the key to this success. Speed in operation comes from having a plan and devoting sufficient time to completion of each step, in order, one time. The surgeon must be dedicated to spending the time to do it right the first time; if not, there will never be enough time to do it right at any other time. Use this atlas; study it for your patients.

"An amateur practices until he gets it right; a professional practices until she can't get it wrong."

Anonymous

Courtney M. Townsend, Jr., MD
B. Mark Evers, MD

PREFACE

The heart, primary organ of life, is a complex structure. Hence, heart surgery is an inexorably technical and dramatic field, a profession that, in contrast to most other surgical specialties, involves tissue reconstruction rather than ablation. The tissues that cardiac surgeons have to fix are vascular, microvascular, fibrous, valvular, muscular, conductive, and connective, and they are often essential to every minute of human life, with little margin for error. For instance, a single-millimeter deviation in a coronary bypass, mitral valve repair, or pulmonary autograft operation can result in intraoperative death as opposed to decades of life.

Rather than teaching the interpretation of blood tests or the performance of physical examination, teachers of cardiac surgical operations must teach novices how to perform, for instance, aortic valve replacement, which can be nerve-wracking for both teacher and trainee. The level of technical and clinical mastery required of the cardiac surgeon is enormous, and atlases such as this one are important in disseminating this knowledge. We authors of this book have much benefited from our teachers, and our goal is not only to provide a state-of-the-art update on all main cardiac surgical techniques performed today, but also to pass on their legacy.

This book is meant to honor and complement the work of past, present, and future technical teachers of cardiac surgery, whose role is sometimes underestimated but who enable this specialty to be safe and therapeutically effective for our patients. We heart surgeons are collectively indebted to every one of them.

Frank W. Sellke, MD
Marc Ruel, MD, MPH, FRCSC

CONTENTS

Section IV   Operations for Aortic Disease

Section V   Miscellaneous Operations

Basic Techniques

CHAPTER 1

INCISIONS FOR CARDIAC SURGERY

Munir Boodhwani and Marc Ruel

Step 1. Surgical Anatomy

- Median sternotomy remains the most common incision used for cardiac surgical procedures because it offers easy access to all cardiac chambers and to the origins and proximal portions of the great vessels. This incision can also be used to repair aortic arch lesions and descending thoracic aortic lesions.
- A right anterolateral thoracotomy incision may be used for mitral and tricuspid valve repair or replacement, aortic valve replacement, and atrial septal defect repairs, as well as for right-sided pulmonary vein isolation procedures for atrial fibrillation.
- A left anterolateral thoracotomy incision can be used for single-vessel or multivessel (see Chapter 6) coronary artery bypass surgery, pericardial window, and left-sided pulmonary vein isolation procedures. A left posterolateral thoracotomy is the incision of choice for descending thoracic aortic procedures.

Step 2. Preoperative Considerations

- The choice of incision is influenced by a number of factors, including the urgency of the operation, the nature and extent of the surgical intervention, a history of previous cardiac surgery, patient comorbidities, and patient preferences and cosmetic reasons.
- Diabetes, obesity, chronic obstructive pulmonary disease, and use of bilateral internal thoracic arteries for coronary surgery are known risk factors for postoperative sternal wound infection. The presence of these factors may influence the choice of incision and methods of closure.
- Patients who have undergone previous sternotomy can be at high risk of damage to vital structures during sternal reentry, especially in the setting of multiple previous sternotomies, patent internal thoracic artery grafts, right ventricular dilatation, and large ascending aortic aneurysms. In these patients, preoperative computed tomography of the chest is a valuable tool to guide surgical planning and safe sternal reentry.

Step 3. Operative Steps

1. **Median Sternotomy**

- The most important consideration in performing a sternotomy is that it is done in the midline because paramedian sternotomy is a significant risk factor for sternal instability.[1]
- The patient is placed supine on the operating table. After using the suprasternal notch and xiphoid process as landmarks, a linear incision is made from just above the sternal angle to the level of the xiphoid process (Fig. 1-1). Subcutaneous fat and presternal fascia are divided using electrocautery. The linea alba is divided inferiorly for approximately 1 to 3 cm. The midline is marked by electrocautery, with close attention paid to the insertion of the pectoralis muscle, and is verified by examining the sternal width at the intercostal spaces.
- In patients without previous cardiac surgery, blunt dissection may be performed below the xiphoid process to free the pericardial and pleural attachments to the posterior table of the sternum (Fig. 1-2A). A reciprocating saw is then used to divide the sternum along the previously created midline marker, taking care to lift gently to avoid catching substernal structures with the blade (Fig. 1-2B). The sternum may be divided in a craniocaudal or a caudocranial fashion.
- After sternal division, hemostasis is obtained by cauterizing the periosteal surface of the sternum, and bone wax may be used selectively to control bleeding from the bone marrow.
- The sternotomy incision gives excellent access to all chambers of the heart as well as the great vessels and is the most commonly used incision for the majority of coronary revascularization, valvular, and ascending aortic procedures.

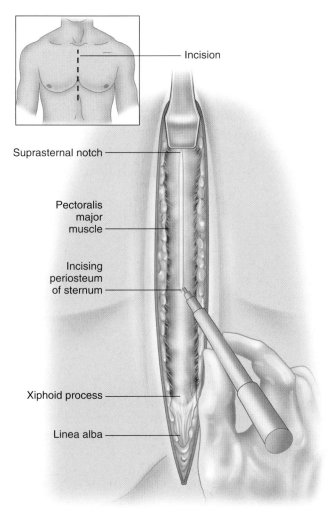

Figure 1-1

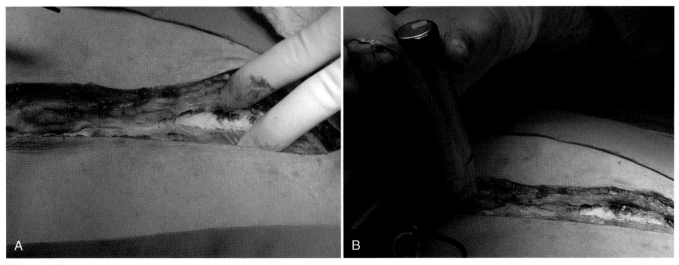

Figure 1-2

◆ This incision may be extended superiorly to provide exposure to the aortic arch, after retraction or division of the brachiocephalic vein (Fig. 1-3). Inferior extension of a median sternotomy allows entry into the peritoneal cavity for harvesting of the gastroepiploic artery.

◆ An upper or lower partial sternotomy incision may be used for certain procedures such as isolated aortic or mitral valve repair or replacement and atrial septal defect closure. This incision has the advantage of improved sternal stability and smaller incision size.

Sternotomy Closure

◆ After hemostasis and placement of chest drains, the sternum is closed using six to eight stainless steel wires. Two or three of the wires may be placed through the manubrium, and the remaining wires are placed around the body of the sternum through the intercostal spaces. It is important to stay close to the sternum and just above the superior aspect of the ribs to minimize injury to the internal thoracic artery and the intercostal neurovascular bundle.

◆ Next, the entry and exit sites of the wires are examined for bleeding, and the sternum is reapproximated. The wires are then twisted, cut, and tightened, with care taken to avoid breaking them through aggressive tightening. Wire tips are then buried into the presternal fascia.

◆ The linea alba is closed using running or interrupted fascial closure sutures, and the subcutaneous tissue is closed using an absorbable suture. Skin closure may be performed using subcuticular sutures or skin staples.

2. Thoracotomy

Anterolateral Thoracotomy

◆ The patient is placed supine on the operating table and the ipsilateral side is elevated 30 to 45 degrees with the arm placed at the side. A submammary incision is made and the pectoralis major muscle is divided using electrocautery (Fig. 1-4). The desired intercostal space (fourth or fifth) is entered after dividing the intercostal muscles on top of the rib. A partial rib resection may be performed to facilitate exposure.

◆ A small left anterior thoracotomy incision can be used for single-vessel coronary artery bypass to the anterior coronary circulation as well as for multivessel coronary revascularization in select cases (see Chapter 6). In addition, it is a common approach for a pericardial window procedure.

◆ A right anterolateral thoracotomy can be an alternative approach for mitral valve procedures and may be the desirable approach in the setting of a high-risk sternal reentry. A small right thoracotomy can be used for minimally invasive mitral valve procedures.

◆ Submammary incisions may also be chosen in women for cosmetic reasons because they are hidden by the breast fold.

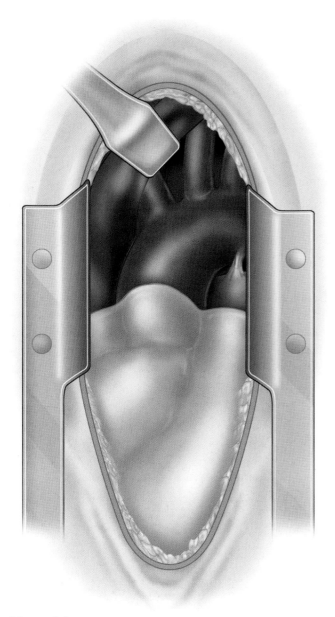

Figure 1-3

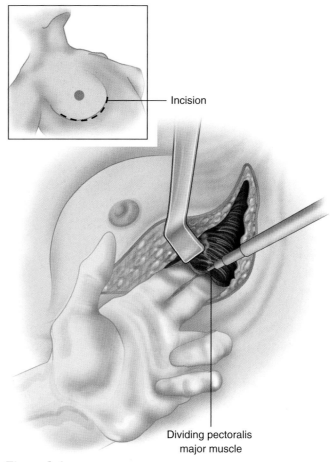

Incision

Dividing pectoralis
major muscle

Figure 1-4

Posterolateral Thoracotomy

◆ The patient is placed in the lateral decubitus position with a roll placed underneath the dependent axilla. After the patient is secured to the operating table and adequate cushioning is provided to dependent areas, the upper arm is extended anteriorly and cephalad.

◆ A curvilinear incision is started in the submammary region and extended posterolaterally, traversing 1 to 2 cm below the tip of the scapula and extending craniad midway between the spine and the scapula (Fig. 1-5).

◆ The subcutaneous tissue and the trapezius muscles are divided using electrocautery. The serratus anterior muscle is divided but may be preserved and retracted. The latissimus dorsi muscle is similarly retracted away from the surgical field. The incision may be continued posteriorly up to the level of the paraspinous muscle.

◆ The thoracic cavity may be entered through the fourth or fifth interspace at the top of the rib to avoid the intercostal neurovascular bundle. A partial rib resection may be performed to facilitate exposure.

◆ A left posterolateral thoracotomy is the incision of choice for addressing descending thoracic aortic lesions. It provides good access to the left atrium as well as the left pulmonary veins, which may be used as inflow for left heart bypass. Occasionally, this approach may be used for grafting of isolated lesions of the circumflex coronary artery territory in situations in which sternal entry carries high risk.

Thoracotomy Closure

◆ Chest drains are placed two rib spaces below the entry site and secured in place. Pericostal sutures are placed around the ribs, avoiding the intercostal neurovascular bundle. A rib approximator may be used to reduce tension as the pericostal sutures are tied (Fig. 1-6).

◆ The divided muscle layers are then reapproximated using 1-0 Vicryl suture, and the subcutaneous tissue is closed using 2-0 Vicryl. Skin may be closed using subcuticular sutures or skin staples.

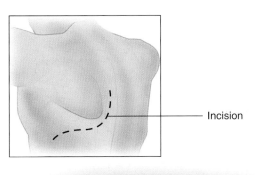

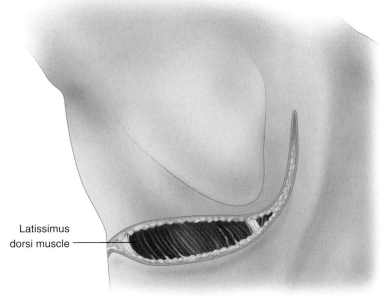

Incision

Latissimus
dorsi muscle

Figure 1-5

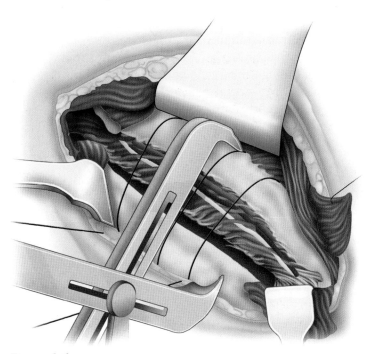

Figure 1-6

3. Other Incisions

◆ Other incisions are used occasionally for operations of the heart and great vessels. A trans-sternal bilateral anterior thoracotomy, also known as the *clamshell incision*, is typically used in the setting of trauma with suspected cardiac or great vessel injury and hemodynamic instability (i.e., when rapid access and wide exposure is desirable; Fig. 1-7). This approach has also been described for single-stage repair or aortic arch and descending thoracic aortic lesions.

◆ The midline sternotomy incision may also be extended laterally, in a "T" fashion, to facilitate better exposure of the distal aortic arch and descending thoracic aorta. Care is taken to preserve the internal thoracic artery when possible.

◆ Finally, subxiphoid access to the pericardial cavity is occasionally used for drainage of pericardial effusion and has also been described for single-vessel revascularization procedures involving the inferior circulation.

Step 4. Postoperative Care

◆ After sternotomy, patients are instructed to avoid heavy lifting with their arms as well as any movements that will exert stress on the sternal closure for a period of 4 weeks.

◆ In obese patients, particularly women, an elastic binder or other supportive garments may be used to provide comfort and reduce strain on the incision.

Step 5. Pearls and Pitfalls

◆ In cases of fragile sternal bone, inadvertent paramedian sternotomy, or sternal fractures, the sternal closure can be reinforced using the Robicsek technique.[2] With this technique, two sternal wires are placed longitudinally as a running horizontal mattress on each side and then twisted, cut, and tightened. Subsequent parasternal wires are placed around these running wires to prevent them from cutting through the fragile bone (Fig. 1-8A and B).

◆ An alternative method of placing sternal wires, the double criss-cross technique,[3] has been reported to reduce the incidence of sternal infections. Other methods or adjuncts for sternal closure have been described, including plates and screws and sternal bands. However, use of these devices may complicate and delay emergent sternal reentry in case of pericardial tamponade.

◆ In patients who are at high risk of sternal reentry, a small right or left anterior thoracotomy can aid in retrosternal dissection before sternal division.

References

1. Zeitani J, Penta de Peppo A, Moscarelli M, et al: Influence of sternal size and inadvertent paramedian sternotomy on stability of the closure site: A clinical and mechanical study. J Thorac Cardiovasc Surg 2006;132:38-42.
2. Robicsek F, Daugherty HK, Cook JW: The prevention and treatment of sternum separation following open-heart surgery. J Thorac Cardiovasc Surg 1977;73:267-268.
3. Bottio T, Rizzoli G, Vida V, et al: Double crisscross sternal wiring and chest wound infections: A prospective randomized study. J Thorac Cardiovasc Surg 2003;126:1352-1356.

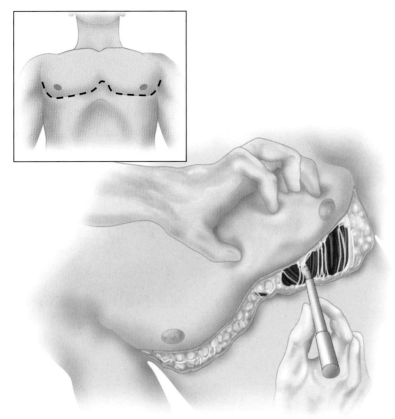

Figure 1-7

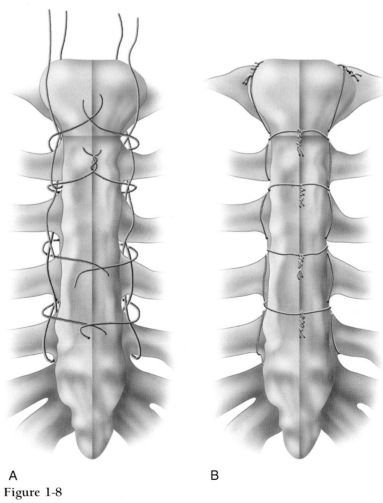

A   B

Figure 1-8

CHAPTER 2

Cannulation Techniques for Cardiopulmonary Bypass

Ladislaus Ressler and Fraser D. Rubens

Step 1. Surgical Anatomy

1. Ascending Aorta

- Cannulation sites on the ascending aorta should be as high as safely possible. Surgeons today are more frequently performing complete arterial revascularization, which in some cases may require delicate proximal anastomoses of arterial conduits (e.g., free internal thoracic arteries, radial arteries) directly to the aorta. These anastomoses are more difficult to construct if the aorta is under tension and distorted, such as may occur with a partial occluding clamp. A landmark for cannulation that is consistently successful for this approach is the pericardial reflection on the left anterolateral surface of the aorta, just below the innominate vein (Fig. 2-1). This reflection can be divided to expose an area approximately 1 cm in diameter.
- Higher sites of cannulation (arch) may be desirable in cases of demonstrated aortic disease, and this form of cannulation may be associated with fewer neurologic problems.[1]

2. Femoral/Iliac Vessels

- It is essential that all trainees be familiar with the anatomy of the common femoral artery, with emphasis on its branches and its relationship to the inguinal ligament and the common femoral vein (Fig. 2-2). We believe it is critical to identify the superficial femoral and profunda femoris arteries to ensure cannulation of the common femoral artery proper.
- In some instances part of the inguinal ligament may need to be divided to provide safe control of the proximal aspect of the vessel. However, this is not commonly required because of the availability of easier sites for cannulation (e.g., axillary artery).

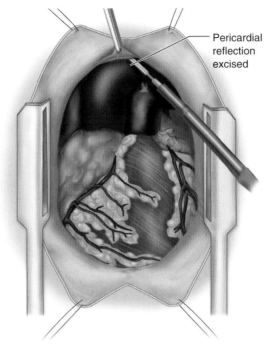

Pericardial
reflection
excised

Figure 2-1

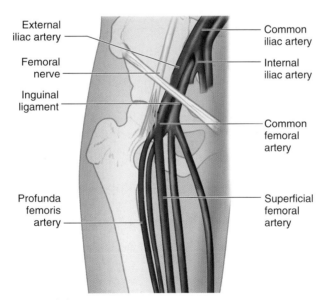

External
iliac artery

Femoral
nerve

Inguinal
ligament

Profunda
femoris
artery

Common
iliac artery

Internal
iliac artery

Common
femoral
artery

Superficial
femoral
artery

Figure 2-2

3. Axillary Artery

- Cardiac surgeons should also be familiar with the pertinent anatomy of the axillary artery. In particular, the axillary vein is anterosuperior to the artery, and the brachial plexus is posterolateral (Fig. 2-3).

Step 2. Preoperative Considerations

- It is essential to identify prospective cannulation sites, even when off-pump surgery is contemplated, and to communicate this plan with the anesthetist to allow for appropriate monitoring.
- The surgeon must anticipate vascular access problems in patients with vascular pathology and those with cerebrovascular disease. Bilateral blood pressure recording to detect subclavian stenosis is essential in every patient. The lower extremity vascular assessment should also be thorough to prepare for a potential femoral artery cannulation. A previous history of lower or upper extremity deep vein thrombosis must be elicited.
- The surgeon should assess the ascending aorta on both the chest radiograph and the angiogram. If there is any concern, echocardiography or computed tomography of the ascending aorta should be used liberally. Intraoperative epiaortic scanning, which is used by some teams routinely to guide cannulation,[2] should also be considered. Although aortic plaque may be palpated (often at the base of the innominate artery), it is the presence of mobile plaque that is most concerning, and an off-pump "no-touch aorta" approach should be considered in this situation, if possible.[3]
- High-risk patients should be appropriately draped to access alternative sites such as the axillary artery, and the surgeon should discuss all the potential approaches and strategies with the anesthetist and the perfusionist before starting to ensure readiness of cannulation and appropriate monitoring lines.
- Finally, with regard to venous cannulation, our practice has been to use two single-stage cannulae for all cases except simple coronary artery bypass. This provides the greatest flexibility if the operative strategy has to be modified in midstream (e.g., open insertion of a retrograde cannula, retrograde cerebral perfusion, control of inadvertent opening of the right atrium with left atriotomy).

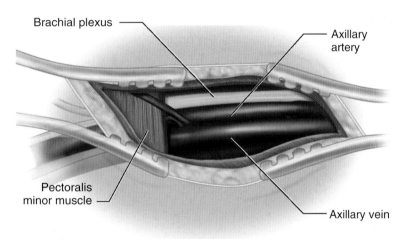

Figure 2-3

Step 3. Operative Steps

1. Arterial Cannulation

Ascending Aortic Cannulation

- The target area should be digitally palpated. The cannula should be inserted such that its flow direction and "jet" are away from the arch vessels (Fig. 2-4).
- Two sets of pursestring sutures (braided nonabsorbable 2-0) are placed around the target (8- to 10-mm diameter) with the free ends controlled with tourniquets on each side.
- There are several options for the actual cannulation, using either a no. 15 or no. 11 blade. Some surgeons prefer to incise transmurally and control the opening with their finger, passing the tip of the cannula under their digit into the aortic opening (Fig. 2-5). Some cut in an oblique manner but control the resulting flap with their pickup, directing the cannula under control into the opening. Another elegant method involves incising only the adventitia and the media, leaving the paper-thin intima to be punctured by the cannula (Fig. 2-6).

Femoral Artery Cannulation

- The safest skin incision for femoral cannulation is a vertical incision overlying and just slightly medial to the femoral pulse (Fig. 2-7). An alternative incision is a slightly oblique incision aligned with the inguinal ligament to facilitate healing.
- Lymphatic vessels should be carefully cauterized or ligated to prevent formation of a lymphocele and persistent drainage.

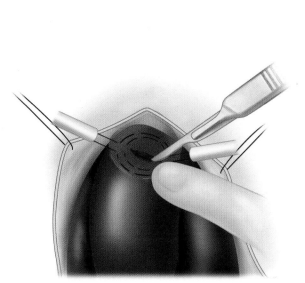

Figure 2-4

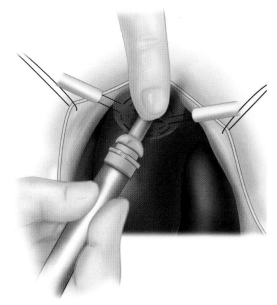

Figure 2-5

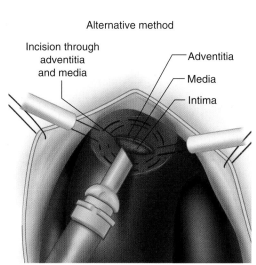

Alternative method

Incision through
adventitia
and media

Adventitia

Media

Intima

Figure 2-6

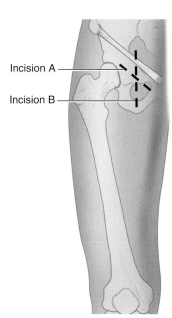

Incision A

Incision B

Figure 2-7

◆ Proximal and distal control of the femoral artery should be obtained. A target site for the arteriotomy should be chosen after considering where the proximal clamp may be safely placed and how the repair will be accomplished when the cannula is removed (Fig. 2-8A). The distal vessels may be occluded with separate clamps or tapes (Fig. 2-8B).

◆ The arteriotomy should be made in a transverse fashion and the femoral cannula gently introduced while an assistant releases the proximal clamp. The cannula is then secured by tying it to the proximal snare, with a second suture securing the tubing to the surface of the thigh.

Axillary Artery Cannulation

◆ An 8-cm transverse incision is made about 2 cm below the clavicle overlying the deltopectoral groove (Fig. 2-9). The dissection is continued between the fibers of the pectoralis major. There is often soft fat in this space, and the area should be dissected gently to avoid tearing of vessels and blood staining. The exposure is further aided by two self-retaining retractors. In an emergency, it is often necessary to sacrifice small nerves to the pectoralis major.

◆ The cephalic vein is identified in this space where it penetrates the fascia to join the axillary vein. The clavipectoral fascia is incised and the pectoralis minor muscle is retracted laterally. The axillary vein should be encircled with loops and gently retracted cephalad.

◆ The artery, which lies superior and deep to the vein, can be identified by palpation and then exposed and controlled proximally and distally with tapes. Arterial branches of the thoracoacromial trunk may be encountered and should be controlled with silk snares. Care must be taken to avoid touching the medial and lateral brachial plexus cords.

◆ After heparin is administered, the artery can be controlled with clamps, but we prefer to use a partial occluding clamp at the arteriotomy site. An 8-mm tube graft should be anastomosed to this site (Fig. 2-10A and B), and the arterial cannula inserted into the tube graft. The cannula is not advanced into the axillary artery proper, but rather perfuses from within the graft.[4]

◆ At the end of the case, the stump can be controlled with several very large hemoclips applied transversely, then oversewn with 4-0 polypropylene.

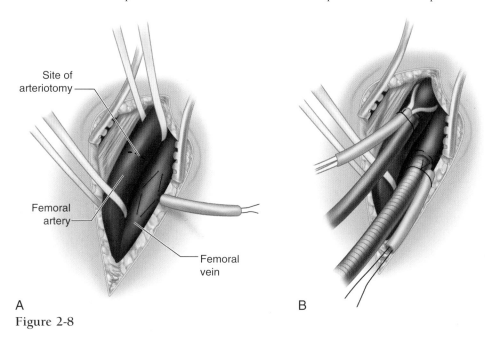

Figure 2-8

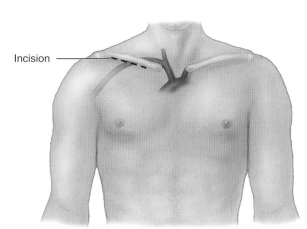

Figure 2-9

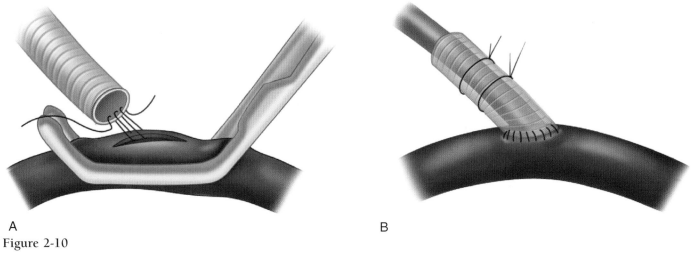

Figure 2-10

Transapical Cannulation (Fig. 2-11)

- This technique is extremely useful in situations of severe atherosclerotic disease of the aorta (porcelain aorta) or for a type A dissection in an emergency.
- Venous (right atrial) cannulation should be obtained first to allow for rapid institution of bypass after cannulating the apex. Similarly, if possible, the right superior pulmonary vein should be cannulated first for venting because it is difficult to mobilize the heart after the cannula is in place for fear of left ventricular tearing. An easy alternative is to vent the pulmonary artery.
- Manipulation of the apex may cause instability, so the equipment should be ready before proceeding.
- A 14F needle is inserted in the apex and a guidewire is passed across the aortic valve with transesophageal echocardiographic (TEE) guidance. A laparotomy pad is placed under the left ventricular apex to stabilize the heart.
- There is no need to predilate the opening. A wire-reinforced cannula with the inner dilator is passed over the guidewire and positioned across the aortic valve. The cannula is then connected to the circuit and de-aired, and bypass is commenced. Position can be verified by TEE (Fig. 2-12).
- It is not recommended to place pursestring sutures in the epicardium until after bypass has started because beating of the heart may cause tearing. Once the heart is on bypass, however, with the heart decompressed, we place two large braided pledgeted pursestrings, controlled with a tourniquet. The cannula is tied to these tourniquets and is also fixed to the skin to prevent motion.
- The strategy to deal with the relevant aortic pathology (e.g., dissection) should include provision of an alternative cannulation site (e.g., side graft to ascending aortic tube graft) to allow the apical cannula to be removed and the pursestrings tied while the heart is flaccid. We further buttress this repair with biologic glue.

2. Venous Cannulation

Femoral Vein Cannulation (see Fig. 2-2)

- We prefer to use a long double-stage cannula because it may be used for definitive perfusion. We do not routinely place tapes proximally and distally, thus avoiding posterior dissection. Two pursestring sutures (4-0 polypropylene) are placed around the target, and a 14F needle is inserted approximately 3 mm from the caudal apex of the diamond. A guidewire is inserted cephalad up to the superior vena cava (SVC). The cannula is inserted over the wire, with further minor opening of the vein wall with a scalpel superiorly up to 3 mm from the apex of the diamond. Further advancement of the cannula is guided by the TEE to ensure that the tip is just inside the SVC.
- At the completion of the procedure, the pursestrings can be gently snared as the cannula is removed and then tied with little compromise of the femoral vein lumen.

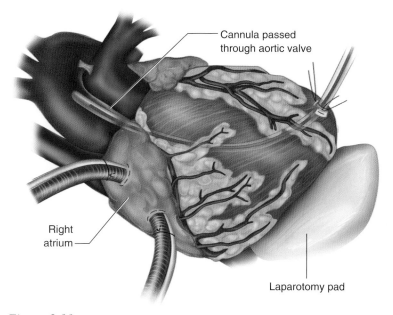

Figure 2-11

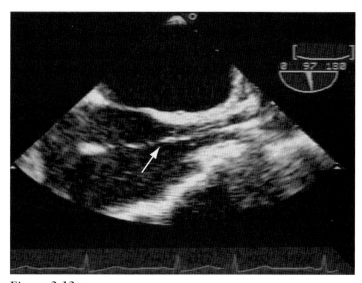

Figure 2-12

Right Atrial Cannulation

- Most commonly, a double-stage venous cannula is inserted through the right atrial appendage. The edges of the atrium can be gently grasped on each side, with an incision made using a scalpel or the scissors. The cannula is introduced with the tip directed posteriorly so that it is gently guided into the inferior vena cava (IVC). Occasionally, digital manipulation at the level of the IVC below the heart is necessary to guide the cannula into the correct position.
- If two single-stage cannulae are required, we generally place one cannula (IVC) through the atrial appendage. The second pursestring is placed approximately 1.5 cm posterior and caudal to this point so that the second cannula (SVC) crosses the IVC cannula. This orientation facilitates exposure of the tricuspid valve and the coronary sinus and provides good retraction of a left atriotomy when the caval cannulae are pulled to the left side of the incision. During preparation for orthotopic transplantation, both pursestrings should be placed as posterior in the atrial wall as comfortably possible (without a crossover orientation) to allow for the preparation of an appropriate cuff of native right atrium to facilitate the atrial anastomosis.
- If necessary, snares can be placed around the SVC and IVC after gentle circumferential dissection. We do not routinely snare for mitral valve surgery.
- Direct cannulation of the SVC may be necessary, particularly with high atrial septal defects (e.g., sinus venosus). The pursestring should be placed in a diamond fashion on the anterior surface of the SVC, well above the sinoatrial node, but in a location such that the snare will include flow through the azygos vein. The two sides of pursestring are held with forceps by the surgeon and assistant, and a vertical venotomy is completed. A right-angled cannula is inserted directly and twisted cephalad, and the pursestrings are tightened.

3. Special Cannulation Techniques

Retrograde Coronary Sinus Cannulation (Fig. 2-13A and B)

- A pursestring suture (4-0 polypropylene) is placed on the right atrial wall, caudal to the IVC cannulation site and about 1 cm from the atrioventricular junction, at the level of the acute margin of the right ventricle.
- The cannula is passed through a stab in the pursestring and is rotated such that the tip abuts on the atrial septum at a point just medial to the IVC and curls toward the left shoulder as the cannula is advanced. Proper placement is indicated by easy passage of the cannula tip and external palpation of the cannula in the coronary sinus medial to the IVC. The pressure tracing from the tip of the cannula will also be characteristic, and the position can be confirmed using TEE.
- If the cannula cannot be easily inserted, after snaring down the two single-stage cannulae, a small transverse atriotomy (1.5 cm) may be made and a pursestring suture placed around the coronary sinus ostium to secure the retrograde cannula after insertion under direct vision.

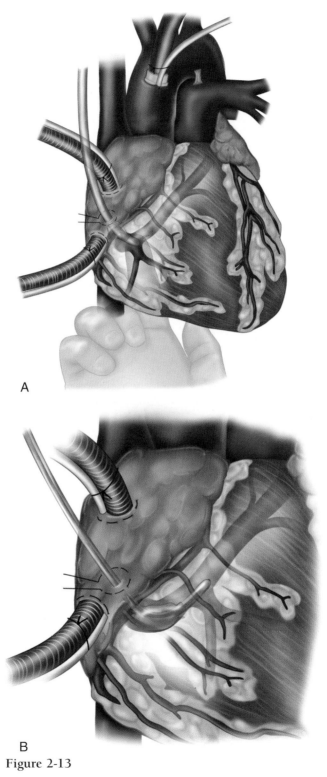

A

B

Figure 2-13

Step 4. Postoperative Care

- Surgeons should understand the pathophysiology of cardiopulmonary bypass to recognize the broad impact of this technology on virtually every organ system.
- Effective bypass should be married to proactive blood conservation strategies, including cell salvage and the use of appropriate antifibrinolytics. Surgeons may also be expected to supervise novel related techniques such as ultrafiltration[5] and retrograde autologous priming[6] and must understand the importance of well-executed cannulation to the success of these technologies.

Step 5. Pearls and Pitfalls

- Sites of arterial cannulation should be chosen with consideration to how the site of vascular entrance can be repaired should complications such as bleeding or tearing occur. For example, in the ascending aorta, the surgeon should consider whether the site chosen would be amenable to a partial occluding clamp to repair this area.
- Communication between the surgeon and the perfusionist and anesthetist is essential, particularly in complex cases. Potential strategies should be well prepared, with the appropriate equipment in the room, should cannulation sites change or emergency bypass be initiated.
- Atrial cannulation sites should be chosen carefully, particularly in fragile tissues, anticipating inadvertent tearing that can extend to the atrioventricular junction, into the second cannulation site, or, if too far inferiorly, into the IVC. On the insertion of the IVC cannula, always err on directing the cannula posteriorly, "marching" the cannula slowly forward, because initial anterior forced misplacement may lead to coronary sinus perforation, which can be lethal.
- Care must be taken in encircling the SVC and IVC to prevent posterior damage of these vessels. With the SVC, the tissue overlying the right pulmonary artery between the aorta and the SVC can be divided with cautery, and a right-angled instrument used to create the plane. Damage to the azygos vein may be extremely difficult to repair. The SVC cannula tip should be inserted only so far that, when encircled, complete drainage will occur. Similarly, care must be taken with encircling the IVC that damage to the posterior wall does not ensue. If the seal with the snare is inadequate, often a second snare will accomplish the task.
- Placement of the retrograde cannula can be facilitated by restricting the venous return somewhat to fill the right atrium.

References

1. Borger MA, Taylor RL, Weisel RD, et al: Decreased cerebral emboli during distal aortic arch cannulation: A randomized clinical trial. J Thorac Cardiovasc Surg 1999;118:740-745.
2. Zingone B, Rauber E, Gatti G, et al: The impact of epiaortic ultrasonographic scanning on the risk of perioperative stroke. Eur J Cardiothorac Surg 2006;29:720-728.
3. Gaudino M, Glieca F, Alessandrini F, et al: The unclampable ascending aorta in coronary artery bypass patients: A surgical challenge of increasing frequency. Circulation 2000;102:1497-1502.
4. Sinclair MC, Singer RL, Manley NJ, Montesano RM: Cannulation of the axillary artery for cardiopulmonary bypass: Safeguards and pitfalls. Ann Thorac Surg 2003;75:931-934.
5. Boodhwani M, Williams K, Babaev A, et al: Ultrafiltration reduces blood transfusions following cardiac surgery: A meta-analysis. Eur J Cardiothorac Surg 2006;30:892-897.
6. Rosengart TK, DeBois W, O'Hara M, et al: Retrograde autologous priming for cardiopulmonary bypass: A safe and effective means of decreasing hemodilution and transfusion requirements. J Thorac Cardiovasc Surg 1998;115:426-439.

Operations for Coronary Artery Disease

CHAPTER 3

On-Pump Coronary Artery Bypass Grafting

Anastasios K. Konstantakos and Frank W. Sellke

Step 1. Surgical Anatomy

- The coronary arteries can be found in the superficial layer of the myocardium just underneath the thin epicardial layer; occasionally, segments of the arteries may run completely intramyocardially, especially the left anterior descending artery (LAD) and, not infrequently, the lateral circumflex and ramus branches.
- The LAD can be found coursing anterior to the interventricular groove.
- The left circumflex coronary artery arises from the left main coronary artery roughly at a right angle to the LAD. It courses along the left atrioventricular groove and, in the majority of patients, terminates near the lateral margin of the left ventricle, giving off the obtuse marginal branches.
- The right coronary artery (RCA) courses from the aorta anteriorly and laterally before descending in the right atrioventricular groove and curving posteriorly at the acute margin of the right ventricle. Distal to the acute margin of the heart, the RCA turns into the posterior descending artery in right-dominant hearts.
- The posterior descending artery runs along the posterior interventricular groove, extending for a variable distance toward the apex of the heart.
- The aorta ascends to the right of the pulmonary artery at the base of the heart. It courses cephalad, where it curves leftward while giving off the arch vessels. It is at this juncture that atherosclerotic disease is commonly found and must be avoided when cannulating. The highest anterior midpoint of the aorta may be used for vent placement and proximal graft anastomoses.
- The conduits most commonly used for grafting include the internal mammary artery (IMA), the greater saphenous vein, and the radial artery.
- The IMA is located approximately 1.5 cm lateral to the sternocostal junction just inside the endothoracic fascia, running a vertical course roughly parallel to the sternum. After widely incising the pleura, it may be visualized or palpated on the anterior chest wall as a 2- to 4-mm-wide pulsatile structure running along with the internal mammary vein (IMV) and its medial and lateral venous counterparts (venae comitantes). Incision into the subfascial plane anterior to the transverse thoracic muscle permits its dissection down from the chest wall. Individual intercostal branches originate anteromedially and anterolaterally from the IMA. Medial and lateral to the artery, the parallel venae comitantes are found entering the superior intercostal space. When harvesting the IMA, both of the IMVs are taken together with the central IMA, incorporating the associated connective tissue, fat, and a portion of intercostal muscle in a single

pedicle. Proximally, the IMA emanates from the proximal subclavian artery; the subclavian vein is often encountered just anterior and medial to this junction. In addition, the phrenic nerve is located just lateral to the IMA pedicle at this level. Thus, care must be used when dissecting the proximal IMA to avoid injury to these associated structures.

- The greater saphenous vein is located on the medial side of the lower extremity just deep to the subcutaneous tissue in the thigh and just lateral to the medial malleolus in the lower leg. When harvesting with the open technique it may be initially located by making a vertical incision just lateral to the medial malleolus in the lower leg; its superficial course just underneath the skin and superficial fascia allows prompt identification. Proximally, at the upper thigh, it is found just medial to the femoral artery at its entrance into the femoral vein just underneath the deep anteromedial fascia.

- The radial artery is found laterally in the distal forearm just underneath the distal deep fascia. It courses proximally toward the antecubital fossa, taking a slightly medial course. The radial artery may be harvested as a pedicle along with the adjacent radial venae comitantes and intervening subcutaneous tissue. Care must be exerted when dissecting the artery in the lower forearm because the superficial radial nerve and lateral antebrachial cutaneous nerve may be injured.

Step 2. Preoperative Considerations

1. Preoperative Preparation

- The purpose of the preoperative evaluation is not only to prepare the patient for surgery but also to assess the risks and benefits of the anticipated procedure. A detailed evaluation of the patient's comorbid diseases should be performed. Common diseases include diabetes, hypertension, hypercholesterolemia, chronic obstructive pulmonary disease, and renal failure. Especially important is screening for a history of heparin-induced thrombocytopenia. Particular attention should be paid to blood-thinning medications that have been administered in the recent preoperative period. Glycoprotein IIb/IIIa inhibitors such as eptifibatide and abciximab should be withheld before surgery for 8 and 72 hours, respectively. Clopidogrel should be withheld for several days if possible. The use of preoperative angiotensin-converting enzyme (ACE) inhibitors may contribute to the postoperative "vasoplegia" syndrome, requiring increased use of vasopressors in the intensive care unit; some surgeons prefer to withhold ACE inhibitors for several days before surgery.

- In addition to a general assessment, the physical examination should focus on items specific to the planned operation. The chest wall should be examined for any deformities, scarring, previous surgery, and administration of radiation therapy. Patients with previous mastectomies should be carefully examined not only to plan the incision but to evaluate usage of the ipsilateral IMA. All options available for graft conduit should be thoroughly investigated. The presence of lower extremity varicosities, an abnormal Allen's test result, and unequal bilateral blood pressures predict unusable saphenous vein, radial artery, and IMA conduits. The carotid arteries should be auscultated for the presence of bruits, which may signify significant obstructive disease.

♦ Preoperative tests include serum chemistries, hematologic studies, clotting studies, and electro-cardiography (ECG). Echocardiography is done to assess regional wall motion, ejection fraction, and valvular pathology. A chest radiograph may demonstrate calcification of the aorta and show concomitant pulmonary pathology. A nuclear viability study maybe indicated to assess areas of hibernating myocardium. Obviously, the coronary angiogram should be thoroughly examined by the operating surgeon.

♦ An informed consent, including the risks and benefits of the proposed operation, should be signed by the patient after a thorough discussion with the operating surgeon. Calculation of the proposed perioperative morbidity and mortality can be obtained using the Society of Thoracic Surgeons' database (www.sts.org). In addition, the preoperative evaluation is not complete without the input of the anesthesiologist and cardiologist.

2. Intraoperative Preparation

♦ After the patient has been brought to the operating room, the appropriate monitoring devices are placed. All patients should have an arterial line inserted (in the side contralateral to the planned radial artery harvest site) before general anesthesia and intubation. For low-risk patients with normal ejection fractions, a central line is placed in the internal jugular vein. For higher risk patients, a Swan-Ganz catheter is preferred. The patient is shaved at all possible chest and extremity incisional sites with an atraumatic electric razor. ECG leads are placed away from the anterior chest wall. Defibrillator and grounding pads are placed away from the operative field, generally on the patient's posterior side. Transcranial Doppler monitoring electrodes may also be placed. A transesophageal echocardiography probe is inserted into the esophagus before preparation to avoid contamination of the anterior chest wall. When harvesting a radial artery, the arm is positioned at 45 to 60 degrees of abduction on a separate arm board. When a femoral intra-aortic balloon pump is present, the proximal portion of the line (on the thigh) is carefully resutured laterally to avoid interference with ipsilateral greater saphenous vein harvesting. Bolsters are placed underneath the knees to create a slight abduction and external rotation of the partially flexed leg; this facilitates greater saphenous vein exposure. A first-generation cephalosporin (or vancomycin in penicillin-allergic patients) is administered 30 minutes before preparation to ensure adequate circulating levels before incision. The patient is prepared anteriorly from chin to toes, with circumferential preparation of the lower extremities and selected upper extremity.

Step 3. Operative Steps

- ◆ The following discussion details the procedure of coronary artery bypass grafting using a pedicled IMA along with free greater saphenous vein or free radial artery grafts. A free IMA graft may be used when necessary. Other conduits such as the gastroepiploic artery, inferior epigastric artery, and lesser saphenous vein may also be used but are not described here.
- ◆ After the median sternotomy and before harvesting the conduits, the pericardium is entered using an inverted "T" incision (Fig. 3-1). This helps to assess the length of conduit needed, and should the patient acutely decompensate, emergent cardiopulmonary bypass can be instituted. After the pericardium is opened, the heart and aorta are grossly examined. The coronary arteries are assessed for grafting suitability by visualization and gentle palpation. The inferior and lateral coronary vessels are briefly assessed by gentle retraction and elevation of the heart; if any concern exists regarding hemodynamic stability, this step is omitted. The aorta is assessed for atherosclerotic disease by careful palpation. Epiaortic ultrasonography can be used at this point to evaluate the aorta further before cannulation. Pericardial sutures are not placed at this time.

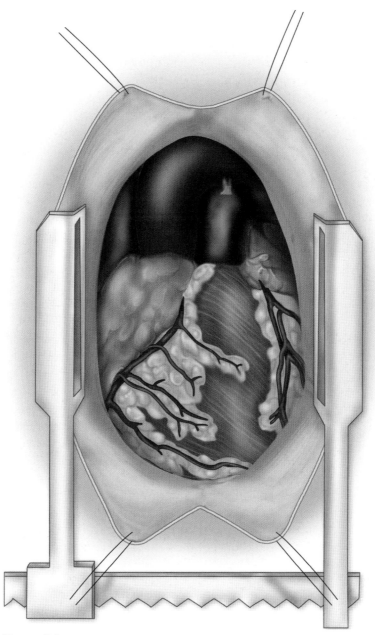

Figure 3-1

- The internal mammary retractor is placed. Wide entry into the pleural space is performed with electrocautery. The IMA is harvested along with the concomitant IMV and its venae comitantes as a 1.5-cm-wide pedicle. Alternatively, the IMA may be skeletonized when there is concern over chest wall healing (Fig. 3-2). Dissection of the IMA is performed by incising the endothoracic fascia and transverse thoracic muscle on each side of the IMA just above the bifurcation of the musculophrenic and superior epigastric arteries at the sixth intercostal space. First, a plane is developed anterior to the IMA and IMV with the spatula tip of the electrocautery. Working from distal to proximal, the pedicle is mobilized off the chest wall with selective hemoclip ligation of the IMA and IMV intercostal branches. Care is taken during branch ligation to avoid ostial avulsion of the intercostal branches and subsequent injury to the IMA proper. When approaching the subclavian vein, care is taken not to stray too far laterally and cranially in order to avoid injury to the phrenic nerve and subclavian vein, respectively. After full systemic heparinization, the distal portion of the pedicle is clamped and transected. (Alternatively, if both IMAs are to be harvested, only half the systemic heparin dose may be administered on mobilization of the first IMA.) The stump remaining on the chest wall is double ligated with 2-0 silk. After application of a distally occlusive bulldog clamp, a dilute solution of papaverine may be topically sprayed onto the pedicle to alleviate the vasospasm. The distal end is prepared by dissecting the IMA off the pedicle for a distance of approximately 1 cm, with ligation of any significant IMA side branches and terminal venae comitantes. A tapered cut is performed on the IMA tip to facilitate later anastomosis. The IMA is then carefully wrapped in a moist gauze pad and placed into the chest cavity for later use. Anterior chest wall hemostasis is thoroughly reassessed at this point to ensure no bleeding from the stumps of the intercostal vessels; any bleeding is stopped with electrocautery or ligation.
- When harvesting the right IMA, a pure skeletonized approach is preferred. This is done to obtain more length for graft use and to prevent poor chest wall healing when both IMAs are used.
- The greater saphenous vein is usually harvested simultaneously with the IMA by another member of the team. The endoscopic vein harvesting technique is preferred over the traditional open method. The endoscopic technique involves circumferential dissection of the vein using carbon dioxide insufflation to facilitate videoscopic evaluation. Once the vein is dissected along its course, the venous branches are ligated and transected, leaving at least a 5-mm stump to avoid thermal injury to the vein proper. Careful technique and operator experience are paramount to the success of this harvesting procedure. Alternatively, the vein may be harvested by the classic open technique using interrupted skip incisions, as shown in Figure 3-3. In an emergency, a single longitudinal skin incision is made along the course of the vein. It is important to stay directly anterior to the course of the vein to avoid creating extensive subcutaneous flaps that impair subsequent wound healing. Once fully exposed and mobilized, the distal end of the vein is ligated and divided, and a small catheter is inserted and secured into the distal lumen. The proximal end of the vein is double ligated with 0 silk suture and the vein is divided. After the harvested vein is free, hemostasis is checked by gentle distention using a syringe attached to the distal catheter. A solution of heparinized blood is injected into the vein while it is segmentally compressed with a small bulldog clamp to check for bleeding sites. All branches are ligated with 3-0 or 4-0 silk ties; small avulsions may be repaired using 7-0 polypropylene pursestring sutures. After the entire vein has been thoroughly prepared, it is placed in a container of heparinized blood for later use.

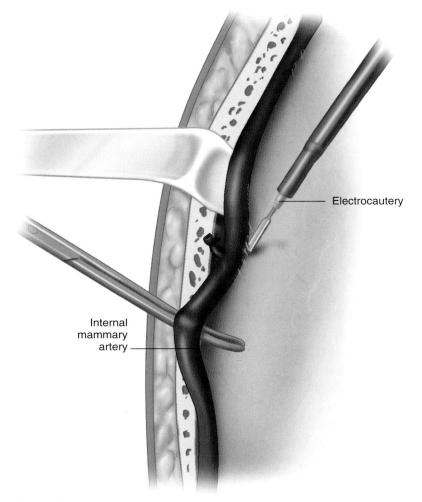

Electrocautery

Internal
mammary
artery

Figure 3-2

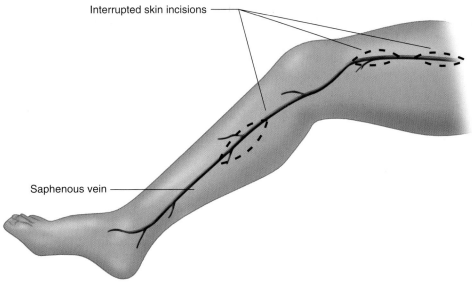

Interrupted skin incisions

Saphenous vein

Figure 3-3

♦ When indicated, the nondominant radial artery (usually the left) may be harvested. The arm, which has been prepared circumferentially, is abducted to a 45- to 60-degree angle. A longitudinal incision is made over the distal aspect of the forearm over the radial pulse (Fig. 3-4). The artery is encountered deep to the subcutaneous fascia, and a vessel loop is placed around it. The artery is temporarily occluded while the waveform produced by a sterile pulse oximeter probe on the first or second digit (modified intraoperative Allen's test) is monitored. If no significant loss of waveform is detected, exposure of the artery is continued proximally, carrying the skin incision cephalad and stopping just short of the antecubital fossa. Care is taken to avoid injury to the lateral antebrachial cutaneous nerve (which lies more superficial) and the superficial radial nerve (which is deep to the fascia) during dissection. The individual branches of the artery are double ligated with 4-0 silk or hemoclips. A harmonic scalpel may be used to facilitate the dissection of the pedicle together with the venae comitantes. After all side branches are transected, the distal end of the artery is double ligated with 3-0 silk and transected. A small olive-tip cannulation catheter is inserted into the distal radial artery lumen, and the artery is flushed retrograde with heparinized saline, with care taken not to introduce any air bubbles into the vessel. The proximal end of the artery is double ligated (1 cm distal to the brachial artery) with 2-0 silk and transected, yielding the free pedicle. The artery is once again flushed with heparinized saline, this time with dilute papaverine (40 mg/100 mL) solution, and reassessed for hemostasis under gentle syringe distention. Individual bleeding sites are repaired with 7-0 polypropylene. The artery is placed in a small cup containing the heparinized papaverine solution until ready for grafting.

♦ After the IMA retractor is replaced by a sternal retractor, a pericardial well is created by the placement of circumferential pericardial sutures around the pericardium (see Fig. 3-1); these may be fixed onto the chest wall or placed on snaps to facilitate their repositioning later. A transverse incision with electrocautery is made into the left mid-pericardium to facilitate future placement of the IMA pedicle; care is taken not to venture too far laterally to avoid injury of the phrenic nerve.

♦ If not already done, systemic heparin is administered while the cannulation sutures are placed. In the distal ascending aorta, two pursestring sutures of 2-0 Ethibond are placed in the aortic wall, without entering the lumen. The spacing of the sutures should be such that their diameter is slightly larger than that of the cannula. When adequate heparinization has been achieved (by either activated clotting time or systemic heparin concentration) and the aortic systolic pressure is less than 110 mm Hg, the aorta is cannulated (Fig. 3-5). This is done by incising the overlying adventitia inside the pursestring sutures and entering the aortic lumen with a no. 11 blade. The tip of the cannula is gently inserted into the aortic lumen. Entry into the lumen proper is corroborated by the appearance of pulsatile blood flow into the cannula under systemic pressure. The catheter is briefly bled to eliminate any entrapped air bubbles and connected to the arterial line. When no air bubbles are seen in the cannula and tubing, the surgeon asks the perfusionist to check the line pressure and flow.

♦ Using a single circumferentially placed pursestring suture of 2-0 Ethibond at the tip of the right atrial appendage, the right atrium is cannulated in a similar fashion, with care taken to advance the tip of the double-stage cannula into the inferior vena cava and ensure that the side holes remain inside the atrium (see Fig. 3-5). The cannula is then connected to the venous line.

♦ A small circumferential suture of 3-0 polypropylene or Ethibond is placed in the lateral right atrial wall or atrial appendage. Inside this area, a stab incision is made into the right atrial lumen. The retrograde cardioplegia catheter may be inserted into the coronary sinus either before or after the venous catheter has been placed into the inferior vena cava (see Fig. 3-5). This should be considered if ventricular function is poor or if there is more than trace aortic insufficiency. Advancement of the tip of the catheter into the coronary sinus is aided by palpation; the surgeon's right hand is placed gently underneath the heart while feeling the balloon pass into the sinus. Proper placement of the retrograde catheter is corroborated by an appropriately "ventricularized" venous pressure tracing on the monitor. Subsequent confirmation of appropriate catheter positioning (with the apex of the heart elevated after antegrade arrest) involves the administration of retrograde cardioplegia, which often visibly distends the posterior interventricular vein.

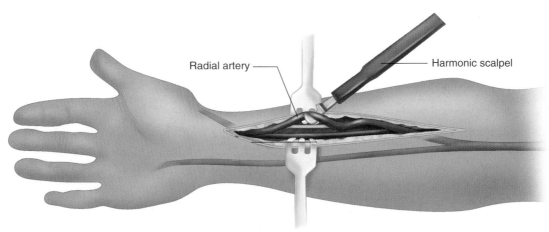

Radial artery — Harmonic scalpel

Figure 3-4

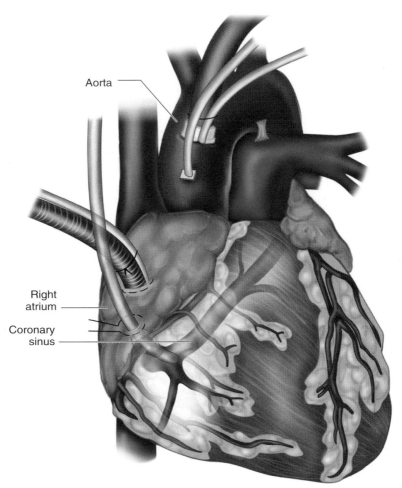

Aorta

Right atrium

Coronary sinus

Figure 3-5

◆ Cardiopulmonary bypass under mild hypothermia (32°C to 34°C) is commenced. Continuous verification of appropriate hemodynamic parameters as full flow is achieved allows ventilation to be stopped. A small pursestring suture of 4-0 polypropylene is placed on the anterior mid-ascending aorta to facilitate placement of the antegrade cardioplegia/root vent catheter (see Fig. 3-5). Once this catheter is inserted and secured, antegrade cardioplegia is begun; the distal ascending aorta is clamped proximal to the systemic arterial perfusion cannula. Retrograde cardioplegia follows. In cases of aortic valve insufficiency, larger doses of retrograde cardioplegia may be required. Cold saline (but not ice, to avoid injury to the phrenic nerve) is poured into the pericardial well to facilitate topical cooling.

◆ The general principle of distal target selection is to graft the most proximal disease-free section of the coronary artery available as long as there is no significant distal lesion. Although the order of coronary artery grafting is not as critical in on-pump (compared with off-pump) cases, the inferior circulation is usually grafted first, followed by the lateral, diagonal, and LAD circulations. Thus, in multivessel coronary artery disease, early protection of the right heart may be achieved by administration of antegrade cardioplegia down the graft. Positioning the heart to achieve optimal exposure of the distal right coronary or posterior descending artery is facilitated by placing a rolled wet laparotomy pad underneath the heart and by manual retraction of the cardiac apex by the assistant. A no. 15 blade is used to incise the epicardium over the selected region of the artery, and a no. 11 blade or smaller sharp blade is used to make a puncture into the artery itself; care should be taken not to injure the back wall of the artery. The length of the arteriotomy is chosen to match the end of the graft but is generally about 4 to 6 mm. The graft is then anastomosed onto the coronary artery using a running 7-0 polypropylene suture (Fig. 3-6). The anastomosis is checked for hemostasis by gently distending the graft with cardioplegia solution, and any needed repairs are performed at this time. The laparotomy pad is then removed from behind the heart, and the heart is filled by restricting venous return. The proximal portion of the graft is brought around the lateral side of the heart toward the aorta and sized for length before returning the venous line volume to the pump. The proximal portion of the graft is marked and transected with sharp scissors. A slight bevel is made on the proximal graft site.

◆ Antegrade cardioplegia is administered down the aortic root after complete (distal and proximal) anastomosis of each graft. This is followed by a dose of retrograde cardioplegia. A benefit of this approach is that both the native circulation and newly bypassed circulation receive myocardial protection (approximately every 10 minutes) using a single cross-clamp technique.

◆ Next, the obtuse marginal (OM), ramus, and diagonal branches are bypassed as necessary. The heart is repositioned with a wet laparotomy pad with the apex lifted cephalad and rightward by the assistant. The appropriately selected distalmost OM branch is anastomosed first with the beveled graft. Alternatively, multiple distal anastomoses may be performed using a sequential anastomotic technique, whereby the distalmost OM coronary vessel is anastomosed first in an end-to-side fashion, followed by side-to-side anastomoses of more proximally located OM, ramus, or diagonal vessels. The proximal anastomosis follows on the left anterior portion of the mid-ascending aorta.

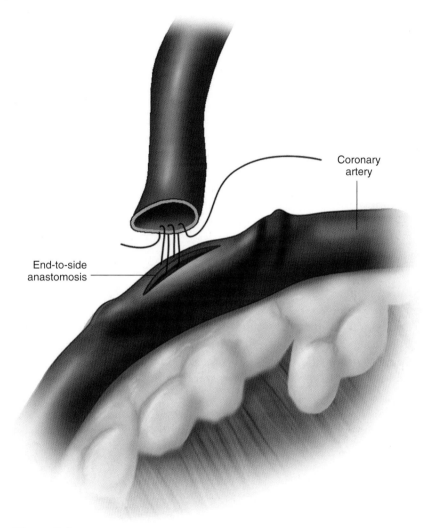

Coronary
artery

End-to-side
anastomosis

Figure 3-6

- Attention is then turned to the LAD artery. The appropriate location of the artery is chosen, and a no. 15 blade is used to incise the overlying epicardium to expose the vessel. A small spreader may be used to help retract the epicardial fat. The LAD is entered and a 4- to 6-mm arteriotomy is made. On rare occasions it may be necessary to perform an endarterectomy on the LAD or other coronary artery before performing the anastomosis (Fig. 3-7). The left IMA (LIMA) is anastomosed to the LAD in an end-to-side fashion with a 7-0 or 8-0 polypropylene running suture (Fig. 3-8). The bulldog clamp on the proximal LIMA is temporarily removed to check for anastomotic hemostasis and distal LAD blood flow (which may be seen in some transparent LAD vessels). A 5-0 polypropylene suture is passed through the lateral and medial portions of the pedicle and affixed to the epicardium to serve as a protecting mechanism against possible LIMA avulsion. This "tacking" suture should be carefully placed to avoid kinking of the anastomosis.
- For the proximal aorta–to-graft anastomoses, sites are chosen on the anterior mid-ascending aorta; a small portion of adventitia is removed at this site. This can be performed with a single-clamp technique or with a side-biting clamp placed on the aorta. A stab incision made with a no. 11 blade is followed by application of an automated punch device (usually 4.0 or 4.5 mm in diameter, according to the diameter of the graft). The anastomosis is performed with a running 5-0 or 6-0 polypropylene suture in an end-to-side fashion (Fig. 3-9). In case of a heavily calcified aorta, the proximal segment of the vein or radial artery may be anastomosed directly to the IMA or to another vein.

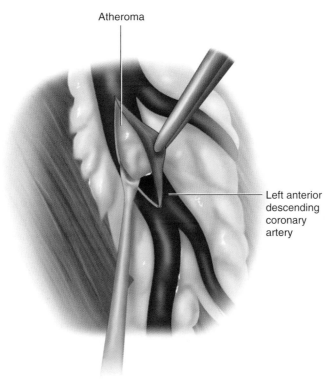

Atheroma

Left anterior
descending
coronary
artery

Figure 3-7

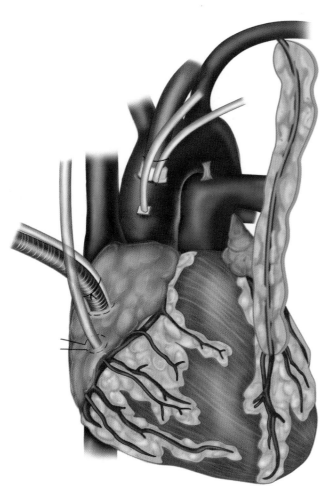

Figure 3-8

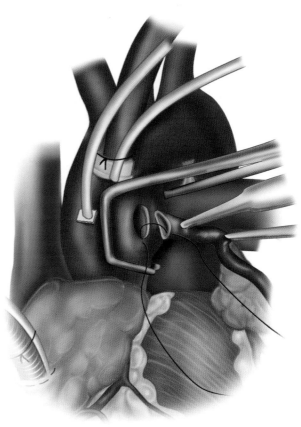

Figure 3-9

- When all anastomoses are completed (Fig. 3-10), the patient is placed in the Trendelenburg position (to prevent cerebral air embolism) and the cross-clamp is removed. Suction is applied on the aortic root vent while de-airing maneuvers are carried out; transesophageal guidance facilitates detection of air in the cardiac chambers and aorta. Alternatively, one of the proximal anastomoses may be used for venting if the suture has not been previously tied. Although some prefer to de-air the grafts directly by inserting a 25-gauge needle into the highest portion of the graft, this is not always necessary and may be harmful.
- While the patient is being rewarmed, chest tubes are placed, one in each entered pleural space and two in the mediastinum. Care is taken to prevent interference with graft positioning by the chest tubes. Although some prefer using traditional rigid chest tubes, softer Blake drains may be equally efficacious. Pacing wires are placed in the ventricular (and atrial, if needed) myocardium and brought out through the chest wall.
- Once the patient is adequately rewarmed and stable from a cardiopulmonary and metabolic perspective, he or she is weaned from cardiopulmonary bypass, and bypass is discontinued. With the patient fully decannulated, chest closure is performed. All surgical sites are once again thoroughly inspected. The bed of the IMA harvest site is thoroughly inspected, as are all grafts and anastomoses. All suture lines, pacing wire sites, and chest tube sites are also thoroughly assessed. Any suspect bleeding sites may be gently packed and reassessed if hemostasis is uncertain.
- Closure of the sternum is undertaken only when cardiopulmonary function is stable, all grafts and anastomoses are inspected, and the chest cavity is completely hemostatic. The sternum is closed according to the surgeon's preference, usually with no. 5 or 6 sternal wires, using a variety of techniques that have been described.

Step 4. Postoperative Care

- Immediate postoperative management in the intensive care unit primarily entails ensuring hemodynamic stability as the patient recovers from cardiopulmonary bypass. Intravenous fluids, blood products, inotropes, and vasopressors are used judiciously. Appropriate neurologic responsiveness is verified when the patient is hemodynamically and metabolically stable. The patient is weaned from the ventilator and extubated when ready. Transfer to the step-down unit continues the process of recovery whereby drains, catheters, and pacing wires are removed, and the patient intensifies physical activity. Judicious diuresis, beta blockade, and glycemic control are all implemented in the perioperative period. ACE inhibitors are administered to patients with low ejection fractions. Discharge either to home or to a rehabilitation/extended care facility occurs when appropriate.

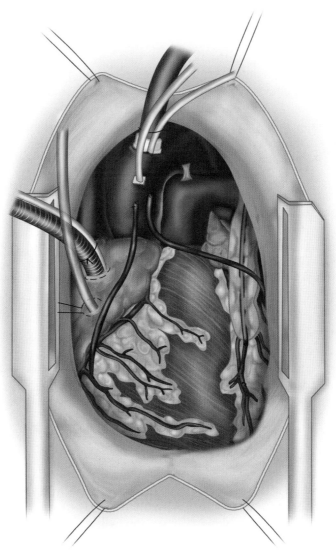

Figure 3-10

Step 5. Pearls and Pitfalls

- Careful positioning of the patient's tucked arms should include careful padding of all intravenous lines, ECG leads, and monitoring catheters to avoid excessive pressure on the skin and peripheral nerves.
- When a radial artery harvest is planned, marking should be performed before abduction of the arm because abduction can distort the skin.
- Although the use of smaller skin incisions has become popular recently, the skin incision must be long enough to allow complete exposure. Too small an incision may place excessive tension on the dermis with subsequent ischemia and impaired wound healing.
- It is important to drape widely in case exposure of the axillary or femoral vessels is required.
- Judicious use of electrocautery during sternal entry and IMA harvesting is imperative. Excessive use may promote tissue necrosis and poor healing, whereas inadequate use of electrocautery may promote excessive blood loss and hematoma formation.
- Vancomycin paste may be used as an alternative to bone wax for sternal marrow hemostasis. This paste is prepared by slowly adding 5 mL of saline to 5 g of powdered vancomycin while continuously stirring the mixture. This creates a pastelike substance that easily adheres to the marrow space and dissolves in time. This is used by surgeons who dislike leaving wax in the sternum, and there is some evidence to suggest that vancomycin paste may be helpful in preventing wound infection.
- By opening the pericardium immediately after the sternotomy, it is possible to evaluate aortic and coronary artery pathology early, thus facilitating planning for cannulation and graft use. Also, if the patient becomes hemodynamically unstable for any reason, prompt cannulation and institution of cardiopulmonary bypass may be implemented.
- Avoiding excessive retraction on the sternal spreader and the mammary retractor is of paramount importance. Adequate visualization of all pertinent structures may be obtained without excessively opening these retractors. Otherwise, brachial plexus injury, sternal fracture, rib fracture, and excessive soft tissue bleeding from overstretching may occur.
- Use of the harmonic scalpel may facilitate dissection of the radial artery pedicle. However, this should not substitute for identification and ligation of individual branches.
- In coagulopathic patients, placement of small drains in the harvested beds of the radial artery and the saphenous vein is wise.
- Placing a slight bevel on the distal graft before anastomosis to the coronary artery facilitates proper alignment and prevents kinking of the graft when the heart is placed in its normal position.
- Excessive dissection of the aortic adventitia is not advised before performance of a proximal graft anastomosis because incorporating the adventitia into the suture line may add strength to the anastomosis and enhance suture line hemostasis.
- When performing any anastomosis, it is important to avoid taking large bites at both the heel and the toe of the graft because this may lead to graft outflow obstruction.

- Excessive epicardial dissection is avoided before performance of the distal coronary anastomosis. By taking bites that incorporate a small portion of the adjacent epicardial fat, suture line hemostasis is improved.
- Sizing the proper length of the graft is facilitated by performing the proximal anastomosis immediately after the distal anastomosis. This also allows administration of antegrade cardioplegia through the aortic root and down the new graft.
- If there is any evidence of bleeding, oversewing all cannulation sites with an extra suture of pledgeted 4-0 or 3-0 polypropylene may be beneficial in preventing unexpected postoperative hemorrhage.
- Before closing the chest, it is prudent to double-check the IMA harvesting site to ensure hemostasis.
- A single-clamp technique may be associated with less chance of postoperative neurocognitive dysfunction or stroke.

Bibliography

Aranki SF, Rizzo RJ, Adams DH, et al: Single-clamp technique: An important adjunct to myocardial and cerebral protection in coronary operations. Ann Thorac Surg 1994;58:296-302; discussion 302-303.

Vander Salm TJ, Okike ON, Pasque MK, et al: Reduction of sternal infection by application of topical vancomycin. J Thorac Cardiovasc Surg 1989;98:618-622.

CHAPTER 4

OFF-PUMP CORONARY ARTERY BYPASS GRAFTING

Sorin V. Pusca and John D. Puskas

- Off-pump coronary artery bypass (OPCAB) established itself over the past 10 years as a standard technique in the armamentarium of cardiac surgeons. Over 20% of all surgical coronary revascularization in the United States is performed off-pump. The technique has superior results in experienced hands in both routine[1-6] and high-risk cases,[5-9] but it has a steep learning curve; excellent on-pump surgeons could have marginal results early in their OPCAB experience.[10]
- Cardiac positioning and stabilization are key elements for good visualization, precise anastomosis. and the success of this technique. Understanding the use of the pericardium as the key element of positioning and retraction is critical to successful OPCAB.

Step 1. Surgical Anatomy

- The pericardium has a parietal part and a visceral part, contiguous with each other. Traction on the parietal component is transmitted to the visceral component. Furthermore, the pericardium is attached to the diaphragm and restricts the lateral movement of the heart. Transecting these attachments gives mobility to the heart.
- The right and left phrenic nerves travel on the corresponding lateral aspects of the pericardium. Any incision on the pericardium has to avoid injuring them.

Step 2. Preoperative Considerations

- OPCAB can be used in any instance when coronary artery bypass is indicated. Patients who benefit most from OPCAB are those with pre-existing renal insufficiency, cerebrovascular disease, diseased ascending aorta, and low ventricular ejection fraction, as well as female patients in general.
- OPCAB can be a taxing procedure for the anesthesiologist. Frequent changes in the position of the table and of the heart create variable hemodynamics, requiring rapid response and constant monitoring of the surgical field by the anesthesiologist to understand the causes of the altered hemodynamics.

- ◆ Anesthesia setup includes readily available alligator clips for temporary atrial or atrioventricular sequential pacing and internal defibrillation paddles for prompt cardioversion–defibrillation should sustained arrhythmias occur. The goal is a steady, regular rate of 80 to 90 beats/min. This makes the heart smaller and improves lateral wall visualization. Bradycardia increases diastolic filling time, distends the heart chambers, impairs visualization, and ultimately results in hypotension.
- ◆ The ability to avoid the cardiopulmonary bypass machine in off-pump cases, combined with the desire to decrease postoperative bleeding, prompted many OPCAB surgeons to decrease the heparin dose from the standard 400 units/kg to 180 to 200 units/kg (half-dose protocol). The advantage of this method is decreased postoperative bleeding. The disadvantage is that if rapid conversion to a pump case needs to be performed, additional heparin must be rapidly administered.

Step 3. Operative Steps

1. Incision

- ◆ We routinely perform OPCAB using a standard median sternotomy.
- ◆ Alternatively, OPCAB can be performed using a left anterior or anterolateral thoracotomy or a left anterior 3-cm minithoracotomy (endoscopic atraumatic coronary artery bypass [Endo-ACAB]). Such techniques require prior mastery of standard OPCAB strategies.

2. Exposure, Cardiac Positioning, and Stabilization

- ◆ Displacing or rotating the heart without compressing it means creating enough space inside the chest so that the heart is not squeezed against the pericardium, sternal border, or retractor. Space is created by the following techniques:
  - ▲ Widely opening the anterior pericardium at the diaphragm (reverse "T" incision) from the right heart margin to slightly *past* the apex of the heart (Fig. 4-1), including transection of the left pericardial fat pad, while visualizing and preserving the left phrenic nerve (Fig. 4-2).
  - ▲ Elevating the right side of the sternal retractor with rolled towels, thus elevating the right sternal margin 2.5 to 4 cm.
  - ▲ Releasing all pericardial stay sutures on the right side when lifting or rotating the heart toward the right.
  - ▲ Transecting the right pericardium at its reflection on the diaphragm (ensuring careful hemostasis and avoiding right phrenic nerve injury).
  - ▲ Excising the right pericardial fat pad, particularly when it is excessive.
  - ▲ Opening the entire right pleura if needed (usually for large hearts and hearts with poor ejection fraction), thus allowing right-sided cardiac structures and sometimes even the apex of the heart to "roll" in the right pleural cavity, underneath the sternal border.

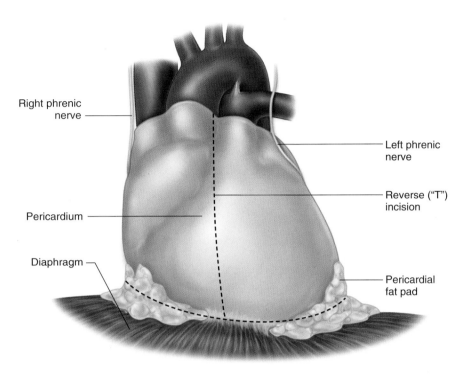

Right phrenic nerve

Left phrenic nerve

Reverse ("T") incision

Pericardium

Diaphragm

Pericardial fat pad

Figure 4-1

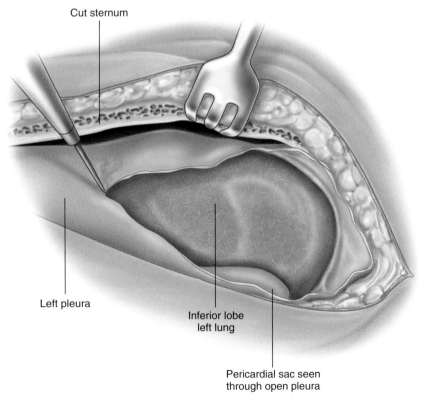

Cut sternum

Left pleura

Inferior lobe left lung

Pericardial sac seen through open pleura

Figure 4-2

- Epiaortic ultrasonography of the ascending aorta is performed in all cases after opening the pericardium to define the strategy for the proximal anastomosis (side-biting clamp, HeartString device (Guidant Corporation, St. Paul, Minn) or inflow from sources other than the ascending aorta [Table 4-1]). If the aorta is grade I or II, we separate it from the pulmonary artery in anticipation of using a side-biting clamp. Such a separation in the loose areolar plane between the two vessels is helpful to prevent the side-biting clamp from slipping during completion of the anastomosis.
- Methods used for cardiac displacement include apical suction devices, traction sutures, and operating table tilt (both side-to-side and craniocaudal). It is of paramount importance that cardiac displacement be done slowly, gently, and incrementally, giving the cardiac muscle time to adjust to the new loading conditions.
- Deep traction sutures allow the use of the pericardium as a "cradle" and position the heart to expose various coronary arteries. Pulling toward the left shoulder on a single deep traction suture, positioned two thirds of the way between the inferior vena cava and the left inferior pulmonary vein at the posterior reflection of the pericardium on the left atrium (Fig. 4-3A), helps expose the left anterior descending artery (LAD) and ramus intermedius territories. Pulling it laterally to the left exposes the circumflex territory; caudad traction on this suture toward the patient's feet exposes the posterior descending territory. Alternatively, four deep pericardial sutures—immediately anterior to the left superior and left inferior pulmonary veins, midway between the inferior pulmonary vein and inferior vena cava close to the left atrium, and immediately anterior to the inferior vena cava—can be used in concert to expose various cardiac regions by alternating placing tension on one or two sutures and releasing the others (Fig. 4-3B).
- Apical suction devices (cardiac positioners) help surgeons rotate the heart to expose various territories without compressing the heart. In spite of their name, "apical" suction devices may be used on any surface of the heart and can be used in multiple configurations. It is advantageous to place them relatively close to the artery to be exposed. However, because their profile is relatively high, they may interfere with the surgeon's view or with the placement of coronary stabilizers if placed too close. It is important to place them on smooth regions of the epicardium, without epicardial fat crevices that can disrupt the vacuum created by the positioner.
- The average suction required ranges from 100 to 250 mm Hg. Suctions in excess of 350 mm Hg can create serious subepicardial hematomas, particularly in the elderly or in patients with frail tissues.
- Small subepicardial hematomas can be ignored. Large or freely bleeding subepicardial hematomas should be repaired with local manual pressure and with fibrin sealants after heparin reversal. It should not be assumed that a bleeding epicardial hematoma will stop bleeding after chest closure. If an epicardial tear occurs, the suction on the cardiac positioner should be disconnected (opening the stopcock to air toward the suction cup) and the tear repaired with pledgeted sutures.

TABLE 4-1. **Strategies for Providing Arterial Inflow to the Coronary Bypasses in OPCAB**

ASCENDING AORTIC GRADE*	SIDE-BITING CLAMP	HEARTSTRING	EXTRA-AORTIC INFLOW	OBSERVATIONS
I (wall < 2 mm)	Yes	Yes	Yes	All strategies adequate
II (wall ≥ 2 mm but < 3 mm)	Yes	Yes	Yes	All strategies adequate
III (wall ≥ 3 mm but < 4 mm)	No	Yes[a]	Yes	[a]Should be inserted *only* in a region where aorta is grade I or II by epiaortic ultrasonography
IV (wall ≥ 4 mm)	No	No[b]	Yes	[b]*Could be* inserted *only* in a region where aorta is grade I or II by epiaortic ultrasonography, if no other strategy is appropriate
V (mobile atheroma with free-floating tip)	No	No[c]	Yes	[c]*Could be* inserted *only* in a region where aorta is grade I or II by epiaortic ultrasonography, at least 2 cm away from the mobile atheroma, if no other strategy is appropriate after extensive search

*By epiaortic ultrasound.

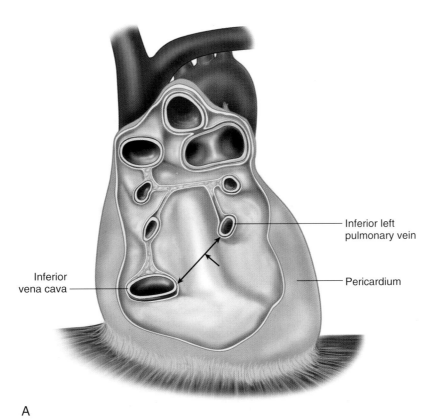

Inferior left
pulmonary vein

Inferior
vena cava

Pericardium

A

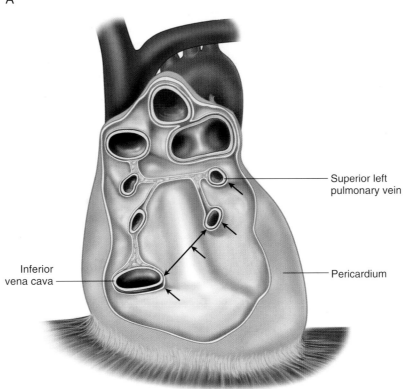

Superior left
pulmonary vein

Inferior
vena cava

Pericardium

B

Figure 4-3

◆ Coronary artery suction-based stabilization devices (stabilizers) currently in use immobilize a small portion of the surface of the heart by using suction, not compression (like the old stabilizers). This allows OPCAB to be performed with significantly less aggressive administration of intravenous fluid, which decreases volume overload and makes opening the right pleural cavity less often necessary.

◆ The malleability of the stabilizer pods is useful on curved surfaces of the heart or on irregular epicardial fat. It is important to mold the malleable pods to the surface of the territory to be exposed in such a way that all the suction cups can make uniform contact with the epicardium. The two pods should be as close together as possible for best stabilization. The suction on the stabilizers should initially be set around 150 mm Hg (one half to two thirds that of the positioner) and may be increased as needed.

◆ The suction pods should be applied on the heart before the mechanical arm of the stabilizer is tightened. The motion of the pods attached to the epicardium should be studied carefully in systole and diastole. The mechanical arm should be tightened with the pods in the median position of the oscillation between systole and diastole (the "mechanical median"). This detail and the notion of the mechanical median (Fig. 4-4) are crucial for optimal immobilization without compression of the heart. Furthermore, it is important to understand that more compression can result paradoxically in more—not less—movement of the stabilized anastomotic site as well as deterioration of hemodynamic stability.

◆ The following are examples of commonly used configurations for traction sutures, positioners, and stabilizers by territories (assuming that the retractor is positioned with the transverse bar at the caudal end of the sternotomy):
  ▲ LAD/diagonal territory: Single deep stitch (Fig. 4-5) pulled to the left and/or cephalad, lap pad sometimes placed under the apex of the heart, stabilizer on the transverse bar of the sternal retractor. The positioner is usually not needed but can be placed on the right side of the sternal retractor.
  ▲ Circumflex territory (Fig. 4-6): Single deep stitch pulled laterally to the left, positioner (always needed) on the cranial end of the right side of the sternal retractor, with the apical cup on the obtuse margin of the heart (the apex of the heart can be placed under the right sternal margin, with the right pericardial diaphragmatic reflection and right pleura widely open if needed), stabilizer on the transverse bar of the sternal retractor toward the right.

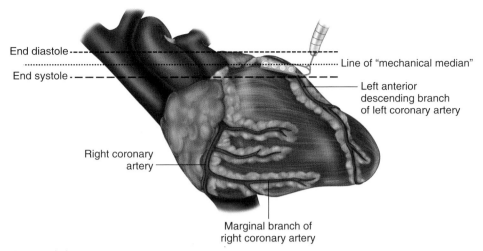

End diastole ----------------------------------

.... Line of "mechanical median"

End systole -------------------------------

Left anterior descending branch of left coronary artery

Right coronary artery

Marginal branch of right coronary artery

Figure 4-4

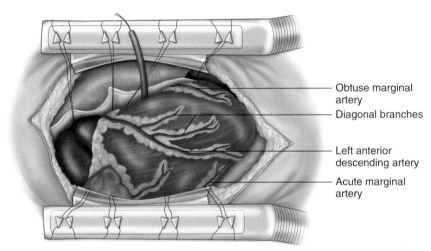

Obtuse marginal artery

Diagonal branches

Left anterior descending artery

Acute marginal artery

Figure 4-5

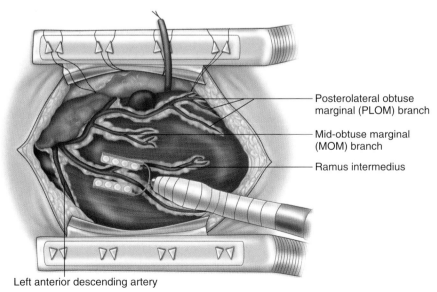

Posterolateral obtuse marginal (PLOM) branch

Mid-obtuse marginal (MOM) branch

Ramus intermedius

Left anterior descending artery

Figure 4-6

▲ Posterior descending artery territory (Figs. 4-7A and B and 4-8): Inferior right pericardial stay suture taut, left-sided pericardial sutures relaxed, single deep stitch pulled inferiorly (caudad) and to the left, positioner (always needed) on the cranial end of the right side of the sternal retractor, with the apical cup on the apex lifting it straight up, stabilizer on the upper half of either the right or the left bar of the sternal retractor.

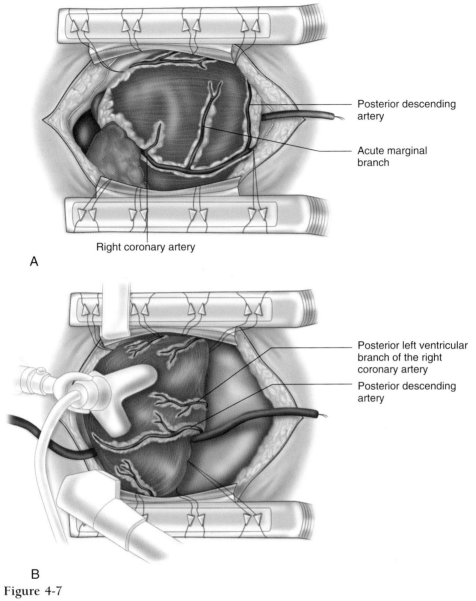

Posterior descending
artery

Acute marginal
branch

Right coronary artery

A

Posterior left ventricular
branch of the right
coronary artery

Posterior descending
artery

B

Figure 4-7

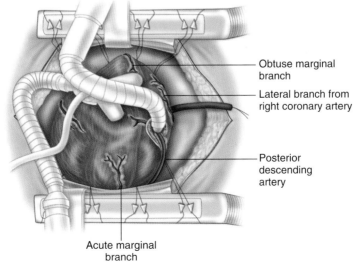

Obtuse marginal
branch

Lateral branch from
right coronary artery

Posterior
descending
artery

Acute marginal
branch

Figure 4-8

▲ Distal right coronary territory (Fig. 4-9): Single deep stitch pulled inferiorly (caudad) and to the left, positioner (always needed) on the cranial end of the right side of the sternal retractor, with the apical cup on the acute margin of the right ventricle lifting it up and slightly cephalad, stabilizer on the lower half of either the right or the left bar of the sternal retractor.

3. Control of Coronary Blood Flow and Visualization of Arteriotomy

- In most cases, there is significant blood flow through a stenotic coronary artery. Even an incision in an artery with complete proximal occlusion can result in significant blood loss because of collateral flow.
- Elastic (Silastic) tapes can be looped one or more times around the target artery immediately proximal to the planned arteriotomy (i.e., Retract-o-tape; Quest Medical, Inc., Allen, Tex); such tapes are effective at limiting the blood loss and improve stabilization and exposure. The principal disadvantage of using Silastic tapes is their potential for causing injury to the coronary artery—intimal disruption and even dissection. Such tapes should not be applied distal to the anastomosis.
- Temporary arterial clips, like the MyOcclude device (Vascular Therapies, US Surgical Corporation, Norwalk, Conn), can be inserted vertically in the myocardium, and when the spring is released, they compress the coronary artery between their jaws. Their depth of penetration is at minimum 5 mm and therefore they should be avoided on thin ventricles in general and on the right ventricle in particular for fear of ventricular perforation.
- A temporary shunt can be inserted through the arteriotomy, maintaining perfusion of the territory distal to it (or proximal to it if the artery has a complete proximal occlusion and is fed by collaterals). The shunts range in diameter from 1.5 to 3 mm. They are deformable and have an attached tether that facilitates removal after the anastomosis is completed (but before the sutures are tightened). Some surgeons believe that off-pump coronary anastomosis is safer with a shunt in place because it limits the ischemia associated with temporary occlusion of the coronary artery and also prevents inadvertent suture bites through the back wall of the target coronary artery. However, insertion of the shunt necessarily causes some degree of endothelial damage to the target coronary artery. Furthermore, it is sometimes more difficult to complete the anastomosis because of confined space through which to pass the needle between the shunt and the wall of the artery.
- The blower-mister (Clear View Misted Blower; Medtronic, Inc., Minneapolis, Minn) is a device that delivers a jet of CO_2 under pressure in the middle of a jet of pH-balanced saline solution, resulting in atomization of the liquid. The resulting stream of mist and CO_2, when directed over the arteriotomy, clears the blood from the anastomosis without resulting in air embolism because the CO_2 is rapidly resorbed. The device does not prevent blood loss, but it is essential for completion of a good anastomosis under direct vision.

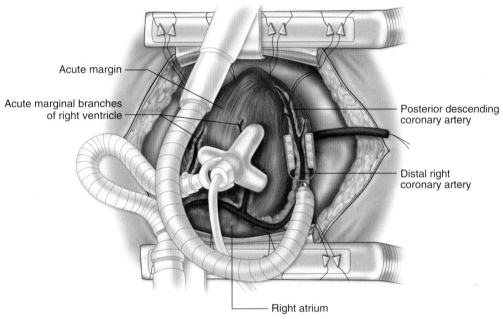

Acute margin

Acute marginal branches
of right ventricle

Posterior descending
coronary artery

Distal right
coronary artery

Right atrium

Figure 4-9

4. Conduct of Routine OPCAB

- The anastomosis of the left internal mammary artery (LIMA) to the LAD usually should be constructed first, particularly when the LAD stenosis is very severe and very proximal. This ensures immediately available new blood flow to the anterior wall and septum and allows the heart to better tolerate further manipulation.
- The left lateral pericardial traction sutures are pulled taut and the right ones released. A folded wet, warm laparotomy pad can be placed underneath the apex of the heart to displace it to the right and out of the chest. It is important that the laparotomy pad not compress the left inferior pulmonary vein, the left atrium, or the lateral wall of the heart and that it not result in significant torque on the heart.
- The stabilizer is positioned over the chosen anterior wall target. A positioner is usually not needed for the LIMA-to-LAD anastomosis.
- The epicardium is opened over the LAD with a no. 15 blade, and two small stab incisions are made on each side of the LAD proximal to the planned arteriotomy.
- The blunt needle of the Silastic vessel tape is passed through one of these incisions, then underneath the artery and exiting through the other incision; the needle is passed a second time through the same openings to create a double loop around the artery.
- A small arteriotomy is performed in the LAD with a diamond-shaped ophthalmic blade, then the Silastic tape previously looped around the artery is gently pulled taut to occlude the inflow. The arteriotomy is enlarged in standard fashion with forward- and back-biting coronary scissors. Retrograde flow from collateral circulation is *not* occluded by the proximal tape, and use of the blower-mister is essential to provide a clear field.
- We perform all of our distal anastomoses with running 8-0 Surgi-Pro II sutures. The anastomoses are performed in exactly the same fashion as those completed using cardiopulmonary bypass; each bite, through both the graft and the target artery, should be taken under direct vision.
- At completion of the anastomosis and before tying the suture, the Silastic tape is released and the anastomosis is allowed to expand. The suture is then tied, and the temporary soft clip applied on the LIMA is removed to establish perfusion through the newly created anastomosis.
- Vein grafts may be difficult to de-air after the distal suture has been tied; they should be allowed to back-bleed before that knot is tied. Inadvertent flushing of air down the distal coronary artery can result in air embolism and cause significant hemodynamic instability. A small atraumatic vascular bulldog clamp should be applied to each vein graft as close to the aortic (proximal) end as possible when the graft has been de-aired by back-bleeding (this distance is determined by the location of venous valves). These small clamps will be removed after final de-airing of conduits after the proximal anastomoses are completed.
- To perform the proximal anastomosis, we release the caudal pericardial traction sutures on both sides and place under tension the cranial ones to expose the ascending aorta. The operating table is placed in the reverse Trendelenburg position (i.e., head up and feet down) to produce a systolic blood pressure of 90 to 100 mm Hg and to improve aortic visualization. Adjustments in table position are preferred over use of vasodilators for this purpose because wide pressure swings may result with the latter.
- The proximal anastomosis using a side-biting clamp is completed in standard fashion. It may be prudent to make only one aortotomy at a time, in case the clamp slips. It is also important to realize that multiple attempts to reposition the clamp, particularly if the clamp is closed or released suddenly, can result in damage of the aortic wall and increased risk of stroke.
- If the aorta is grade I or II, use of a side-biting clamp carries little risk of serious atheroembolism. However, for higher grades, alternative strategies should be used (see Table 4-1).

♦ The aorta can be left undisturbed and only a small portion of the anterior wall cleaned of epiaortic fat in order to use a HeartString device. The automatic aortotomy cutter of the Heart-String kit should be used to perform the aortotomy, taking care to inspect the device for the presence of a full aortic wall "doughnut" in its cutting cylinder, proof of an adequate and safe aortotomy. The appropriately folded HeartString should then be inserted through the aortotomy. It is important to use a needle with small radius (i.e., very curved) to perform the anastomosis because the suture bite cannot extend beyond the diameter of the HeartString umbrella. It is critical to remain within the area of this umbrella while performing the anastomosis. The device is removed after completion of the anastomosis by pulling on the string that unravels the umbrella and cutting the monofilament suture that secures its strut.

♦ Alternative proximal inflow becomes mandatory in high-grade aortic disease. One or both internal mammary arteries as well as the gastroepiploic artery can be used as pedicled (or skeletonized) sources of inflow. In addition, the left subclavian or right innominate artery or the descending aorta can be used as a site for proximal anastomosis in unusual circumstances.

Step 4. Postoperative Care

♦ Patients who underwent uncomplicated OPCAB can be extubated in the operating room or shortly thereafter in the recovery room. Early extubation allows for faster recovery and a shorter intensive care unit stay.

♦ Overall, patients who underwent OPCAB tend to have a smoother postoperative course than patients who required cardiopulmonary bypass. Their capillary permeability is maintained, and they will mobilize fluids more easily. Routine transfer to the cardiothoracic step-down unit the morning after surgery can be expected.

Step 5. Pearls and Pitfalls

♦ Impaired right ventricular filling is the root cause of poor hemodynamics during lateral wall exposure in many cases[11,12] and must be scrupulously avoided. Lateral wall exposure, which is required in approximately 80% of coronary bypass cases, is a fundamental hurdle that the novice OPCAB surgeon must master.

♦ Common mistakes during heart positioning for OPCAB include the following:
  ▲ Not opening the pericardium past the apex of the heart.
  ▲ Retracting the apex of the heart to the right without releasing the right-sided superficial pericardial traction sutures. A common mistake of the novice is to manipulate the heart with an apical suction device while the right pericardial stay sutures are taut.
  ▲ Trying to place the apex of the heart under the right sternal margin without opening the right diaphragmatic pericardial reflection and the right pleura.
  ▲ Compressing the heart with the stabilizer to achieve immobility of the desired arterial segment (compression below the mechanical median).

- It is critical for the anesthesia and surgical teams to constantly monitor the heart rate, systemic and pulmonary blood pressures, and ST segment on the continuous electrocardiogram tracing. Abnormalities in each of those values require prompt correction; accepting delays in correction can lead to emergency conversion to cardiopulmonary bypass with increased mortality and morbidity.
- An audible sucking sound is a clear indication that there is loss of contact between the cups on the pods of the suction devices and the epicardium. Visually identify which cup has lost contact and mold the pods accordingly. It is helpful to use a dry gauze to blot the region where the stabilizer will be applied; a wet, bloody, or slippery surface can result in loss of suction in the stabilizer.
- When using the stabilizers, it is helpful to first apply one pod and then gently compress the two pods toward each other, laying down the second pod on the heart in such a way that the pods recoil slightly away from each other and the epicardium between the two pods is stretched. This allows easier exposure of the underlying coronary artery.
- At Emory, we use coronary shunting selectively:
  - ▲ If there is evidence of myocardial ischemia on temporary occlusion of the coronary artery (i.e., ST segment elevations >2 mm; pulmonary artery pressure elevation, particularly if associated with systemic hypotension; ventricular arrhythmias; atrial bradyarrhythmia on occlusion of the right coronary artery).
  - ▲ If there is low-grade (60% to 70%) stenosis of a large coronary artery (occlusion of such an artery would result in significant ischemia in its territory because collateral circulation has not developed yet).
  - ▲ If the artery to be occluded supplies a large territory (either directly or through collaterals).
  - ▲ If the target coronary artery is very calcified, thus preventing effective occlusion by the elastic tape.

References

1. Puskas J, Cheng D, Knight J, et al: Off-pump versus conventional coronary artery bypass grafting: A meta-analysis and consensus statement from the 2004 ISMICS Consensus Conference. Innovat Cardiothorac Surg 2005;1:3-27.
2. Hart JC, Puskas JD, Sabik JF III: Off-pump coronary revascularization: Current state of the art. Semin Thorac Cardiovasc Surg 2002;14:70-81.
3. Puskas JD, Williams WH, Duke PG, et al: Off-pump coronary artery bypass grafting provides complete revascularization with reduced myocardial injury, transfusion requirements, and length of stay: A prospective randomized comparison of two hundred unselected patients undergoing off-pump versus conventional coronary artery bypass grafting. J Thorac Cardiovasc Surg 2003;125:797-808.
4. Puskas JD, Thourani VH, Marshall JJ, et al: Clinical outcomes, angiographic patency and resource utilization in 200 consecutive coronary bypass patients. Ann Thorac Surg 2001;71:1477-1483.
5. Mack MJ, Brown P, Houser F, et al: On-pump versus off-pump coronary artery bypass surgery in a matched sample of women. Circulation 2004;110(Suppl 2):II1-II6.
6. Brucerius J, Gummert JF, Walther T, et al: Impact of off-pump coronary bypass grafting on the prevalence of adverse perioperative outcome in women undergoing coronary artery bypass surgery. Ann Thorac Surg 2005;79:807-812.
7. Morris CD, Puskas JD, Pusca SV, et al: Outcomes after off-pump reoperative coronary artery bypass grafting. Innovat Cardiothorac Surg 2006;1:181-182.
8. Vohra HA, Kanwar R, Khan T, et al: Early and late outcome after off-pump coronary artery bypass graft surgery with coronary endarterectomy: A single-center 10-year experience. Ann Thorac Surg 2006;81:1691-1696.
9. Rastan AJ, Eckenstein JI, Hentschel B, et al: Emergency coronary artery bypass graft surgery for acute coronary syndrome: Beating heart versus conventional cardioplegic cardiac arrest strategies. Circulation 2006;114(Suppl I):I477-I485.
10. Khan NE, De Souza A, Mister R, et al: A randomized comparison of off-pump and on-pump multivessel coronary-artery bypass surgery. N Engl J Med 2004;350:21-28.
11. Grundeman PF, Borst C, Verlaan CW, et al: Exposure of circumflex branches in the tilted, beating porcine heart: Echocardiographic evidence of right ventricular deformation and the effect of right or left heart bypass. J Thorac Cardiovasc Surg 1999;118:316-323.
12. Grundeman PF, Borst C, van Herwaarden JA, et al: Vertical displacement of the beating heart by the octopus tissue stabilizer: Influence on coronary flow. Ann Thorac Surg 1998;65:1348-1352.

ENDOSCOPIC AND TRADITIONAL MINIMALLY INVASIVE DIRECT CORONARY ARTERY BYPASS

Thomas A. Vassiliades, Jr.

Step 1. Surgical Anatomy

- Because the vast majority of cardiac operations are performed through a median sternotomy, small variations in chest wall anatomy from patient to patient are largely irrelevant to the conduct of the procedure. In contrast, the technical success of minimally invasive approaches to the heart often hinges on the recognition of unique chest wall anatomy and the consequential procedural adjustments. The minimally invasive cardiac surgeon should have an in-depth understanding of "normal" anatomic variation and its surgical relevance.

1. Chest Wall

- Surgically relevant variations of chest wall anatomy include (1) the cross-sectional geometry of the thorax, (2) the widths of the ribs and interspaces and their three-dimensional relationships about the bony surface of the thoracic cage, (3) the quantity (thickness) of the soft tissue on both sides of the bony thorax, and (4) the three-dimensional spatial relationship of the chest wall, the intended target area (such as the internal mammary artery or mitral valve), and other nearby structures (e.g., the lung or diaphragm).
- The minimally invasive cardiac surgeon needs to have a radiologist's perspective of the thorax, with a clear mental "computed tomography scan" image of the patient's anatomy, before making the skin incision. Much of the success of thoracoscopically proficient surgeons stems from their ability to understand not only what is on the video monitor but what lies beyond the edges.

◆ I have found it helpful to perform a thorough physical examination of the patient's thorax at the time of consultation and before committing to any particular minimally invasive approach. In general, patients have either a circular/oval cross-sectional thoracic geometry (Fig. 5-1A) or one that more closely resembles a rectangle (Fig. 5-1B). Recognition of the differences in thoracic shapes has important surgical implications for port placement and the subsequent conduct of the operation. In patients with a rectangular thorax, the front and back of the chest are relatively flat—that is, the ribs and interspaces lie nearly in the space plane anterior to posterior. Reaching the internal mammary artery (IMA) in this situation requires placing the ports more posteriorly in interspaces that have more effacement with the intended target area: specifically, placing the ports along the mid-axillary line rather than along the anterior axillary line. The adjustment provides a more favorable angle of approach.

2. Internal Mammary Artery

◆ With experience, the surgeon performing thoracoscopic harvesting gains a deeper understanding of the subtle anatomy of the IMA. The left IMA (LIMA) lies within 2 cm of the left sternal edge in 95% of patients. Variations in the course of the IMA away from the sternum tend to occur primarily along its distal half, with lateral deviation creating a potentially challenging situation for thoracoscopic harvesting.

◆ The LIMA arises from the left subclavian artery, which can be seen in a thin patient without significant amounts of adipose tissue (Fig. 5-2). The LIMA then travels laterally and anterior to the subclavian vein and left phrenic nerve before crossing under the first rib. It is at the first rib, and often slightly more superior to the left subclavian vein, that most surgeons typically harvest the LIMA when using an open sternotomy incision.

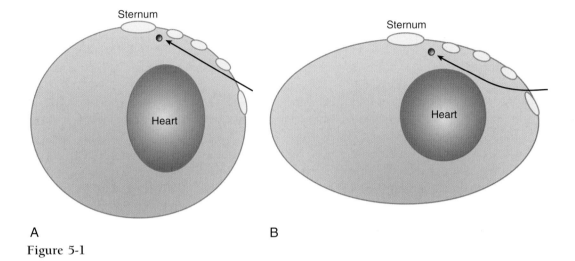

Figure 5-1

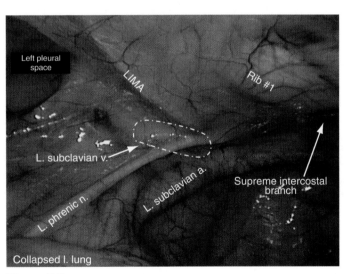

Figure 5-2

- As discussed later, the LIMA can be thoracoscopically harvested more superiorly than in the open technique by virtue of the lateral view's providing clear identification of the subclavian vein and artery, phrenic nerve, and supreme intercostal branch of the IMA. For the most part, the IMA courses beneath a layer of endothoracic fascia. However, in the first intercostal space, it is not uncommon to see a loss of endothoracic fascia development and the IMA "freely floating" in adipose tissue. It is in this region that one occasionally encounters acute turns or loops in the course of the IMA (Fig. 5-3).
- As the LIMA courses into the second and third intercostal spaces, it becomes less visible, traveling anterior (deep) to the transversus thoracis muscle, but posterior (superficial) to the intercostal muscles. Many times, it is easier to see one or both of the accompanying veins of the IMA or see the area of pulsation of the IMA beneath the muscle. At the level of the sixth rib, the IMA then divides into the superior epigastric and musculophrenic arteries, which marks the extent of the IMA harvest. During its course, the IMA gives off numerous anterior intercostal branches that vary in size, number, and location. However, these branches arise only within the intercostal spaces themselves, usually close to the rib edges, both superiorly and inferiorly. The arterial branches are almost always accompanied by at least one venous branch. The portions of the IMA that course directly over the ribs are sometimes densely adherent to the periosteum, but no branches arise in these areas.

3. Surface Anatomy of the Heart (Thoracoscopic)

- A thoracoscopic, lateral view of the surface of the beating heart can be disorienting to the novice minimally invasive cardiac surgeon. Even in the open sternotomy scenario, correctly correlating the anatomy as depicted in the coronary angiograms with the intraoperative findings may not always be straightforward, particularly for the trainee.
- Coronary arteries are often partially or completely intramyocardial as well as hidden by epicardial fat. For example, the proximal one third to one half of the left anterior descending coronary artery (LAD) and its diagonal branches are often intramyocardial or covered by a layer of epicardial fat. Viewed through a thoracoscope positioned in the fifth intercostal space along the left mid-axillary line, the diagonal coronary artery will be in direct view and the LAD will be in the background coursing away from the camera, with the distal portion not completely visible unless the anterior surface of the heart is depressed with an instrument or an angled scope is used. When there is a large, prominent diagonal coronary artery coursing parallel to the LAD, the surgeon must be careful not to mistake the diagonal for the LAD.

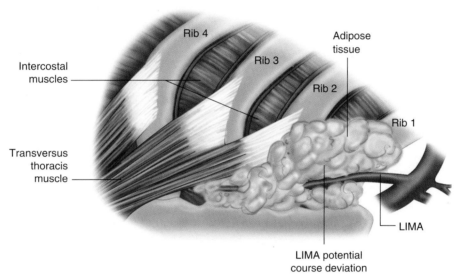

Figure 5-3

4. Procedural Definitions

- *Minimally invasive direct coronary artery bypass* (MIDCAB) is one of the original terms denoting the use of a nonsternotomy and off-pump approach to coronary artery bypass grafting. In light of several more contemporary variations of this original operation, we will use MIDCAB to refer to harvesting the LIMA under direct vision through a small anterior thoracotomy and then using that incision to perform the LIMA-to-LAD anastomoses off-pump.
- *Endoscopic atraumatic coronary artery bypass* (EndoACAB) denotes a thoracoscopic LIMA harvest followed by off-pump LIMA-to-LAD anastomoses under direct vision, using a non–rib-spreading thoracotomy.
- *Totally endoscopic coronary artery bypass* (TECAB) denotes a ports-only, thoracoscopic approach to the entire procedure, including harvesting of the LIMA and performance of the anastomosis between the LIMA and LAD. TECAB can be performed on-pump with an arrested heart, or off-pump.

Step 2. Preoperative Considerations

1. Patient Selection

- Patients with single-vessel disease involving the LAD or its diagonal branches comprise the largest group in which one of the minimally invasive coronary artery bypass procedures (MIDCAB, EndoACAB, TECAB) is performed. With growing interest in hybrid coronary revascularization, we may see these procedures performed more commonly in patients with multivessel disease, in which the LAD is grafted with the LIMA and the non-LAD stenoses are stented.
- In general, there are a few clinical situations in which a minimally invasive approach is less appealing or even a contraindication. Previous surgery in which the left pleural space has been entered can present challenges, particularly if a thoracoscopic approach is planned. However, patients with previous bypass surgery in which the LIMA remains intact can still undergo a minimally invasive bypass operation. Women with large breasts are another subgroup of patients that can be challenging for a nonsternotomy approach in that either a larger submammary incision is required, or an incision or ports need to pass through the breast itself.
- It remains unclear whether patients with severe chronic lung disease would tolerate single-lung ventilation, and whether a thoracotomy would be superior to a sternotomy. In general, the EndoACAB operation, which requires single-lung ventilation, can be well tolerated by patients with chronic obstructive pulmonary disease with a forced expiratory volume in 1 second (FEV_1) as low as 1 L. Overall, patient selection is partially dictated by the surgeon's level of experience. In general, thinner patients (body mass index <30) with normal heart size and function are the easiest and safest patient population to operate on early in the learning curve. Patients with mild to moderate chronic obstructive pulmonary disease tend to have a more barrel-shaped chest and wider interspaces, making thoracoscopic LIMA harvesting easier.

2. Specialized Equipment

- The list of specialized equipment required for a minimally invasive bypass operation largely depends on the particular approach. For the MIDCAB operation, a chest wall elevator device can be used to retract the ribs sufficiently to expose the LIMA for harvesting. Although this technique was popular when it was first introduced, most centers have abandoned it. The degree of force and displacement of ribs required to harvest the LIMA is often so excessive that the resultant pain and chest wall disruption nullify any potential advantage of avoiding a sternotomy or hemisternotomy.
- Most centers that perform a significant volume of nonsternotomy coronary bypass procedures use a thoracoscopic harvest technique, either robotically assisted, in which a robotic arm controls the movement of the scope and the surgeon operates manually, or completely robotic, using the da Vinci telemanipulator (Intuitive Surgical, Mountain View, Calif).
- An off-pump stabilization system designed for use in a small thoracotomy or under complete thoracoscopic control is another important piece of equipment required for these procedures. Table 5-1 provides a short list of the instruments required for minimally invasive coronary bypass operations.

TABLE 5-1.	**Specialized Equipment for Minimally Invasive Coronary Artery Bypass Procedures**

Double-lumen endotracheal tube

Patient temperature management system

External (R2) defibrillator pads

Video tower equipment: monitor, carbon dioxide insufflator, light source, video camera control (EndoACAB and TECAB)

Three chip surgical telescopes (EndoACAB and TECAB)

Endoscopic positioner, optional (EndoACAB)

Robotic telemanipulator, optional (TECAB)

Trocars (EndoACAB and TECAB)

Cutting and sealing technology: electrosurgery, harmonic scalpel, clip applier

Suction/smoke evacuator (EndoACAB and TECAB)

Extra-long surgical instruments (MIDCAB)

Thoracoscopic instruments (EndoACAB and TECAB)

Chest wall retractor for left internal mammary artery exposure (MIDCAB)

Off-pump stabilization system

Graft assessment technology, optional

EndoACAB, endoscopic atraumatic coronary artery bypass; MIDCAB, minimally invasive direct coronary artery bypass; TECAB, totally endoscopic coronary artery bypass.

3. Anesthetic Considerations

- There are two important primary differences between minimally invasive coronary artery bypass operations and off-pump coronary artery bypass (OPCAB) grafting through a sternotomy that have important ramifications for intraoperative patient management: (1) minimally invasive approaches using thoracoscopy rely on one-lung ventilation (OLV) and carbon dioxide insufflation; and (2) the heart is not significantly repositioned or anatomically distorted during the performance of a minimally invasive approach, unlike multivessel OPCAB surgery. In the case of the former, OLV and carbon dioxide insufflation make the anesthesiologist's job more challenging, particularly in the presence of chronic lung disease. Usually hypoxemia can be mitigated by increasing the percentage of oxygen delivered, verifying proper tube placement, optimizing ventilation, and suctioning the ventilated lung. For recalcitrant cases, positive end-expiratory pressure to the ventilated lung or continuous positive airway pressure to the non-ventilated lung rectifies the hypoxemia.
- Although minimal to no manipulation of the heart usually translates into stable hemodynamics, occlusion of the proximal LAD alone can cause ischemia and left ventricular dysfunction, leading to hemodynamic collapse. For these reasons, transesophageal echocardiography is an invaluable adjunct in assessing contractility throughout the procedure. The surgeon should be prepared immediately to insert a shunt, or to insert one prophylactically in cases in which the LAD supports circulation to more than one territory.

Step 3. Operative Steps

1. Minimally Invasive Direct Coronary Artery Bypass

- For the purposes of comparing operative techniques, the MIDCAB approach is defined as a thoracotomy with a direct-vision harvest of the LIMA and an off-pump LIMA-to-LAD anastomosis. Technically speaking, the left anterior small thoracotomy (LAST) approach, described by Calafiore and colleagues in 1996, is the original and perhaps most common MIDCAB technique used today. However, modifications of this theme have also been described, such as a lower hemisternotomy or a subxiphoid (transabdominal) approach. Each of these procedures begins by positioning the patient either supine, as for a median sternotomy, or in a slight right lateral decubitus position to elevate the left chest.

- In the case of the LAST approach, a 6- to 10-cm incision is made within the left fourth intercostal space starting from the left sternal border and extending laterally and parallel to the ribs. A chest wall retractor designed for LIMA harvesting (e.g., Thoralift; US Surgical Corp., Norwalk, Conn) is then inserted to lift the fourth rib anteriorly and deflect the second and third ribs posteriorly, thereby exposing the LIMA for harvesting under direct vision. In my experience, the fourth rib often requires disarticulation with the sternum for adequate exposure and complete harvesting superiorly, or the rib eventually becomes disarticulated during the course of the LIMA harvest. Adequate exposure of the LIMA can be challenging, and the potential for serious chest wall injury exists unless the surgeon carefully monitors the force of retraction. The history of this procedure reveals that many surgeons abandoned this technique as a result of wound complications ultimately caused by this part of the procedure. The amount of chest wall disruption often led to prolonged periods of postoperative pain exceeding that seen after a median sternotomy. Further, a small but not insignificant number of patients developed chronic pain syndrome, chronic rib dislocations, or lung hernias. On the other hand, the attraction to harvesting the LIMA with this direct-vision approach is that it does not require one-lung ventilation, thoracoscopic instrumentation, or any endoscopic experience.
- Once the LIMA is harvested during a MIDCAB procedure, the patient is systemically heparinized, the end of the LIMA is prepared for anastomosis, and the LAD is exposed much as in an OPCAB performed by a full median sternotomy. The LIMA-to-LAD anastomosis is then performed on the beating heart with the assistance of one of the many commercially available stabilizer systems. The details of performing an off-pump coronary anastomosis are described in Chapter 4. With experience and the assistance of cardiac positioner devices, additional coronary targets can be accessed through the same incision. However, the advantages to the patient of performing multivessel OPCAB grafting through a thoracotomy compared with a sternotomy appear limited. Another potential drawback of the original LAST approach is that if conversion to an on-pump procedure is necessary, the patient may require a sternotomy in addition to the anterior thoracotomy.

2. Endoscopic Coronary Artery Bypass

- The EndoACAB operation consists of a thoracoscopic LIMA harvest followed by a direct-vision, off-pump coronary anastomosis performed through a 3- to 4-cm, non–rib-spreading thoracotomy. The goals of this operation are to harvest the entire LIMA, use the thoracoscopic view of the LAD to pinpoint the incision for the eventual anastomosis, and then perform the anastomosis using the hand-sewn, direct-vision technique, but through an incision as atraumatic to the patient as a ports-only approach. Hence, the idea is to achieve the benefits of a totally endoscopic operation, but with fewer technical hurdles and in a more cost-effective manner.

Preparation and Patient Positioning

- As previously mentioned, a left-sided, double-lumen endotracheal tube is placed for OLV. Although the size of the tube is based on the patient's size and sex, the goal is to place the largest tube that will fit in the mainstem bronchus with only a small air leak when the cuff is deflated. Typically, the sizes used are 35F to 39F for women and 39F to 41F for men. In my experience, a double-lumen tube provides more reliable lung collapse than either an Arndt bronchial blocker or a Univent tube, although these are the preferred alternatives in cases in which a double-lumen tube cannot be inserted.

- Once the endotracheal tube is secured in place, the defibrillator (R2) pads are placed—one pad on the right anterior chest (leaving room for a sternotomy if necessary) and the other pad on the left posterolateral chest, posterior to the left mid-axillary line, the usual sites of the ports (Fig. 5-4). *It is imperative that the heart lie between the pads.* Verify with the anesthesiologist that the pads are connected to the defibrillator box. In addition, if it becomes necessary to defibrillate during the operation, *the left lung must be reinflated first* because the electrical current will not pass through a gas-filled chest, and defibrillation will be unsuccessful.

- We also place energy transfer pads (The Arctic Sun; Medivance, Inc., Louisville, Colo) on the back or the posterior thigh for patient temperature management. Electrocardiogram electrodes and defibrillator pads can be placed under these pads. Alternatively, a sterile forced-air patient warming system (Bair Hugger; Augustine Medical, Inc., Eden Prairie, Minn) can be placed over the legs once the patient is completely draped.

- The patient is placed in the supine position with the left chest elevated 15 to 20 degrees by a folded blanket or roll. The roll must come up to the level of the shoulder so that it supports the scapula and protects the brachial plexus. The right arm is tucked alongside the patient (except in morbidly obese patients), and the left arm, bent at the elbow, is supported above the head using a standard operating room arm support (Fig. 5-5). When the patient is positioned in this manner, the left chest area is exposed to provide space for maximal instrument range of motion through the ports. Using this configuration, postoperative brachial plexus palsy is extremely rare. If a robotic arm is being used to control the thoracoscope (AESOP; Intuitive Surgical), it is attached to the bed rail to the right of the patient at the level of the xiphoid. The patient should be positioned close to the AESOP (toward the right side of the bed) to maximize robotic arm length because this can be a concern in obese patients.

- To optimize surgical ergonomics during the thoracoscopic IMA harvest, a chair is draped and the surgeon is seated facing the patient's left side (Fig. 5-6A). The monitor, chest, and surgeon are then configured in a straight line (Fig. 5-6B). When applying the sterile drapes, the sternum is left exposed as a point of reference and for easy access in the event of an emergency. The legs are prepared as usual for possible vein harvesting. A specialized drape is supplied with the AESOP arm. At the time of draping, ventilation to the left lung is discontinued to allow time for the egress of residual air in the lung.

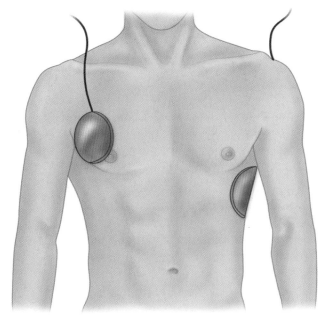

Figure 5-4

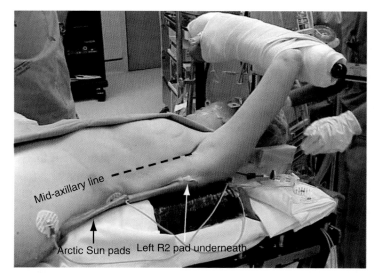

Figure 5-5

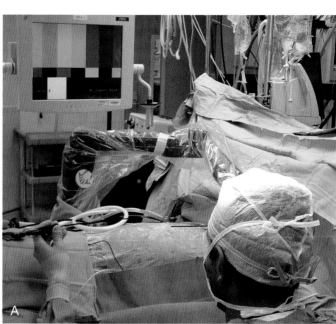

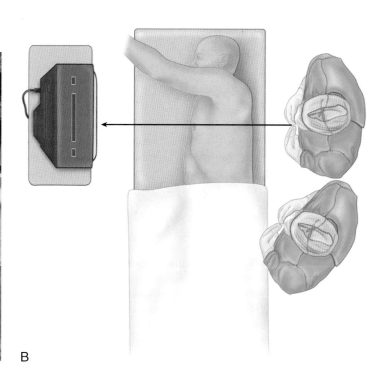

Figure 5-6

Port Placement

- A 5.5-mm port is inserted in the fifth intercostal space along the left mid-axillary line. Carbon dioxide insufflation is set at 8 to 10 mm Hg, which is tolerated by nearly all patients as long as the preinsufflation central venous pressure is a minimum of 8 mm Hg. A 5-mm, zero-degree scope is inserted and the anatomy of the left pleural cavity is assessed. Two additional 5.5-mm ports are then placed for the left and right instruments. A port is placed over the fourth rib along the mid-axillary line to allow the use of the third and fourth intercostal spaces (ICS) (Fig. 5-7)
- Occasionally, patients have narrow rib spaces requiring that the uppermost port be moved (using the same skin incision) back and forth between intercostal spaces three and four. The right-hand instrument can be either a long monopolar cautery with an attached smoke evacuator chamber (Opti4 Handset and Electrodes; Valleylab, Boulder, Colo) or a harmonic scalpel (Ethicon, Inc., Somerville, NJ).
- The lowermost port for the left-hand instrument is placed in the seventh intercostal space. This provides sufficient space for the robotic arm to hold the scope and camera without colliding with the left-hand port. The left-hand instrument is either a grasper or endoscopic Kitner dissector used for simple tissue manipulation.

Left Internal Mammary Artery Harvest

- The LIMA is harvested superiorly above the level of the first rib, stopping medially at the left phrenic nerve, but continuing the dissection laterally up to the subclavian artery if desired. All branches can and should be divided, including the highest (supreme) intercostal branch. The dissection of the LIMA should extend inferiorly to the bifurcation at the level of the sixth rib.
- My technique of harvesting the LIMA thoracoscopically differs somewhat from my open technique. I prefer to remove the layer of adipose tissue superficial to the endothoracic fascia before harvesting the LIMA. This provides better visualization of the entire course of the LIMA and decreases the chances of inadvertent injury to it. I then dissect superiorly and inferiorly along the entire length of the LIMA, separating the pedicle a small distance at a time to avoid excessive retraction of the LIMA. An endoscopic view of the completed LIMA harvest is shown in Figure 5-8.

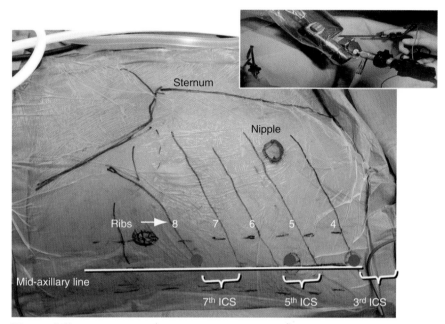

Figure 5-7

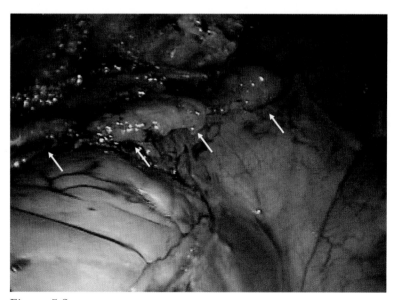

Figure 5-8

Pericardiotomy and Coronary Target Identification

- Opening the pericardium longitudinally approximately 3 to 4 cm from the midline puts the opening very close to the LAD. Because of the port placement and the lateral vantage point of the endoscope, the coronary vessel most readily visible is usually the diagonal. The LAD lies in the background and courses away from the camera, as previously discussed and illustrated in Figure 5-9.
- The pericardium is opened widely from the great vessel down close to the apex. To prevent inadvertent herniation of the heart out of the pericardium, the apex is not exposed. Once the LAD has been clearly identified, the next task is to pinpoint the location of the small thoracotomy such that it will be directly over the LAD.
- The surgeon must be aware that with insufflation turned on, the heart is displaced from its normal location. In most cases, chest insufflation tends to push the heart medially (to the right) and downward toward the diaphragm. Therefore, the best way to estimate the location of the LAD with respect to the chest wall is to disconnect the insufflation temporarily before passing a finder needle (long spinal needle) through the chest wall. Usually the middle LAD lies in the third or fourth intercostal space near the left nipple, but this can vary considerably from one patient to the next.
- Once the site of the anticipated working port (small thoracotomy) has been selected and marked on the skin, the patient is systemically heparinized (150 units/kg), and the distal LIMA is clipped (Hemolock clips; Weck Systems, Triangle Park, NC) and divided thoracoscopically just proximal to the bifurcation. A grasper or long vascular clamp passed through the highest port holds the harvested and divided LIMA, preventing twisting and maintaining the proper orientation until the small thoracotomy has been created.

Small Thoracotomy

- With the anticipated site of the LAD now identified on the skin, a 5-cm incision is created in the center of the interspace, parallel to the ribs. The pectoralis major muscle is separated in the direction of its fibers in order to preserve the muscle. In older women, this muscle is usually thin. However, in younger men, the pectoralis major muscle is often thick: preserving it avoids atrophy and added postoperative disability. The intercostal muscles are divided and the thoracic cavity is entered.
- At this point, the options for exposure include using a non–rib-spreading opening, spreading the ribs using a small rib retractor, or resecting a short segment of rib. If the incision has been placed close to the LAD and the rib space is at least 18 mm wide (the width of an average index finger), I perform the anastomoses without spreading the ribs. A small soft tissue retractor (CardioVations, Somerville, NJ) is placed through the interspace and attached to the skin using the adhesive backing. This retracts the subcutaneous tissue and muscle without moving the ribs and provides a clear path to the epicardial surface of the heart (Fig. 5-10). A Weitlaner retractor (Codman, Raynham, Mass) can be inserted within the soft tissue retractor, outside the rib spaces, to keep the leaves of cloth taught against the tissue.

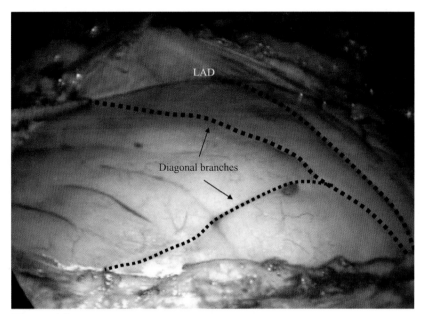

Figure 5-9

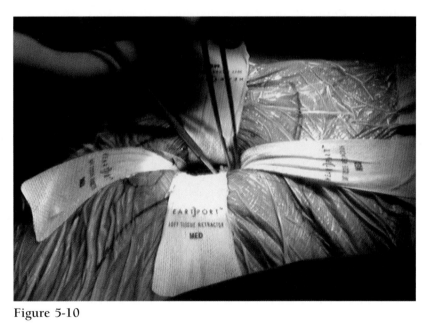

Figure 5-10

♦ The general approach is to place the stabilizer, the LIMA holder, and sometimes the carbon dioxide blower through the previous port sites so that the small thoracotomy remains unobstructed. As demonstrated in Figures 5-11 and 5-12, the previous camera port becomes the port for the stabilizer arm, and the highest port provides access to the clamp holding the harvested LIMA.

Coronary Stabilization and Anastomosis

♦ The stabilization system consists of two parts: the epicardial foot plate and the arm. Several systems are commercially available, and all work in a similar fashion. The stabilizer plate (either compression or suction based) is introduced through the small thoracotomy while the arm is brought through one of the previous port sites (usually the middle or upper port works best). The plate and arm are connected inside the chest, and the entire system is attached to a clamp attached to the bed rail. This approach moves the stabilization system out of the view of the surgeon, allowing more space for hand suturing the anastomosis.

♦ From this point onward, the conduct of the operation is similar to an open-sternotomy, off-pump anastomosis. Vessel occlusion can be accomplished however the surgeon prefers, and a shunt may be used if necessary. To keep the LIMA occluded during the anastomosis, one can use the long clamp holding the LIMA through the port or remove this clamp and place a bulldog clamp further distally along the LIMA. With either technique, the clamp needs to be sufficiently distant (≥3 cm) from the end of the LIMA to keep it from obstructing the surgeon's view once the LIMA is brought down to the epicardial surface. The anastomosis begins by placing five sutures around the LIMA and LAD heals and then bringing the LIMA down to the LAD. The remainder of the anastomosis is completed using a running suture technique.

Closing and End-Procedure Checklist

♦ Once the LIMA-to-LAD anastomosis is completed, flow is assessed using a transit-time flow probe (MediStim AS; Medtronic, Inc., Minneapolis, Minn). I first assess the flow with the native flow occluded and then assess both the proximal and distal limbs of the LAD, as clinically relevant. The stabilization system is carefully withdrawn. The LIMA pedicle is secured to the epicardial surface on both sides using interrupted sutures. A 20F chest tube is inserted in the most inferior port and directly posteriorly.

♦ Once hemostasis of all surgical sites has been verified, the left lung is slowly reexpanded, ensuring that it slides anterior to the LIMA pedicle. If necessary, the pericardium should be incised where the pedicle enters the pericardial space to prevent kinking of the graft. The chest wall is carefully examined for bleeding. Intercostal nerve blocks are injected at this time. The pectoralis major muscle can then be reapproximated with a single suture and the remainder of the subcutaneous layers closed using standard techniques. If a segment of rib has been resected, it is advisable to place a suture around the ribs to prevent future lung herniation.

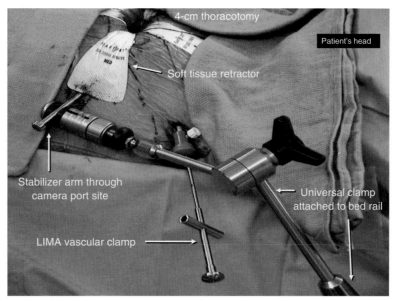

Figure 5-11

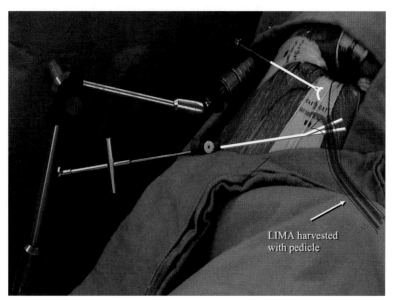

Figure 5-12

3. Totally Endoscopic Coronary Artery Bypass

- The TECAB can be performed on the arrested or beating heart, on-pump or off-pump. In general, the on-pump, arrested-heart TECAB is technically easier and is used as a transitional operation in the learning curve for the off-pump TECAB. In the on-pump, arrested-heart TECAB, the patient is positioned in a 30-degree right lateral decubitus position.
- After setup of the da Vinci system (Fig. 5-13), a camera port is introduced in the left fifth intercostal space along the anterior axillary line while the left lung is collapsed. Carbon dioxide is insufflated at target pressures of 10 to 12 mm Hg. Instrument ports are then inserted through the third and seventh intercostal spaces along the mid-clavicular line under thoracoscopic vision.
- The IMA is identified and the endothoracic fascia and transverse thoracic muscle are removed from the IMA pedicle so that the vessel can be adequately visualized. Complete harvesting is accomplished using electrocautery at 20 W and endoscopic clips for division of pedicle side branches. Heparin is administered, and after endoscopic placement of a temporarily occluding bulldog clamp, preparation of the distal graft portion is carried out and IMA flow is assessed.
- Concurrently, the left femoral artery and vein are exposed. After systemic heparinization, the right atrium is cannulated (through the femoral vein) using a 25F or 27F Medtronic venous return cannula (96370 Medtronic). A 21F Remote Access Perfusion (ESTECH, Danville, Calif) cardiopulmonary bypass system is inserted under transesophageal echocardiographic guidance. The pericardial fat pad is grasped with a long-tip endoscopic forceps and removed from the pericardium using electrocautery.
- After incision of the pericardium at the sternal border and further lateral incision of the visible pericardium, the LAD is identified. Cardiopulmonary bypass is started, and the ascending aortic occlusion balloon is inflated for induction of cardioplegia. The target vessel is then exposed and incised with a lancet endoscopic knife while giving cardioplegia.
- The LIMA is then sutured robotically to the target vessel using 7-0 Pronova (PN 8713; Johnson & Johnson, Somerville, NJ) running suture. The aortic occlusion balloon is deflated and the heart defibrillated if necessary. After rewarming and weaning from cardiopulmonary bypass, the patient is decannulated and heparin is fully reversed. A chest tube is inserted into the left pleura through the lower instrument port and the left lung is reinflated. The other two thoracic ports are closed.
- More recently, an additional 5-mm assistance port has been inserted in the fourth intercostal space parasternally through which suture material can be brought in and out, and transthoracic assisting carried out.
- The off-pump, beating-heart TECAB procedure is technically more challenging in part because the heart is not unloaded. For exposure and stabilization of the LAD, an endoscopic suction stabilizer (Octopus TE; Medtronic) is introduced through a subxiphoid port. The revascularization target is occluded locally with Silastic snares and incised.
- The anastomosis is performed using 7-0 Pronova as previously described. Another successful anastomotic technique involves the interrupted use of U-Clips (Medtronic). The recent addition of a second-generation da Vinci system with fourth robotic arm capability controlling the endoscopic stabilizer has greatly facilitated this operation.
- Despite significant technological improvements, the EndoACAB and TECAB procedures require steep learning curves in the first 10 to 20 cases. Operative times for single-vessel revascularization in these early cases can be expected to be 4 to 5 hours.

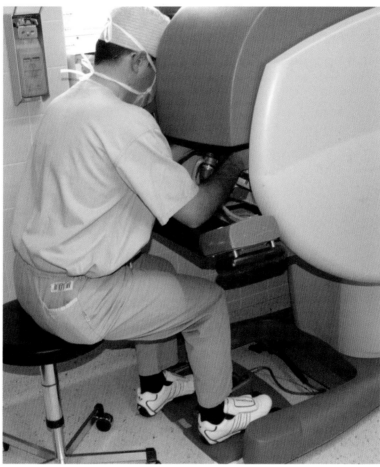

Figure 5-13
(Courtesy of Dr. J. Bonatti.)

Step 4. Postoperative Care

- After the MIDCAB, EndoACAB, or TECAB, procedure, the patient may be safely extubated in the operating room or soon thereafter in the intensive care unit (ICU). Reasons for not extubating immediately include postoperative hypothermia, a difficult intubation, or a prolonged, complicated operative course.
- Postoperative care in the ICU is similar to that for most off-pump revascularization patients. An uncomplicated patient can be safely discharged to the telemetry floor within 6 hours after surgery if he or she meets the following criteria: (1) no significant arrhythmias, (2) adequate pain control, (3) an oxygen requirement of 3 L/min or less, (4) no inotropic support, (5) an alert and cooperative mental status, and (6) minimal chest tube drainage (<100 mL/hr).

Step 5. Pearls and Pitfalls

1. Skill Sets

- Overall, there are three primary skill sets required in performing minimally invasive coronary artery bypass surgery: (1) thoracoscopy with or without robotics, (2) approaching the coronary arteries through a nonsternotomy approach, and (3) off-pump coronary anastomoses. Each of these skills should be learned individually, one at a time.
- Complications occur more often when the novice surgeon attempts to push through multiple learning curves simultaneously during the same procedure. It is critical that the surgeon new to the minimally invasive coronary bypass operation have a solid background in off-pump bypass techniques performed through a sternotomy.
- Twenty to 30 OPCAB cases should provide adequate knowledge and experience to begin the task of grafting through a limited-access approach. In the case of EndoACAB and TECAB, knowledge and experience using laparoscopy and thoracoscopy greatly facilitate the learning process. This is particularly relevant to the established, practicing cardiac surgeon who trained before the introduction of endoscopic techniques.
- Finally, familiarity and comfort with approaching the heart through a small nonsternotomy approach also come with a learning curve. My recommendation is for the novice surgeon to perform the early procedures with a more generous incision, scaling down as knowledge and experience are acquired.

2. Hemodynamic Collapse

◆ Perhaps the most feared intraoperative complication during minimally invasive coronary bypass procedures is sudden hemodynamic collapse. Although hemodynamic collapse occurs rarely, there must always be a contingency plan. With all three minimal access techniques, the sternum is exposed, prepared, and draped within the operative field to facilitate easy and rapid access. Similarly, the groin and legs must always be prepared and draped. As previously mentioned, defibrillator pads are placed on all patients as well.

◆ A LIMA-to-LAD anastomosis performed using a minimally invasive approach usually involves less mechanical manipulation than one performed through a sternotomy. However, significant ischemia can still occur. The generous use of shunts, particularly when occluding large vessels with only moderately severe stenoses, is highly recommended.

Bibliography

Bonatti J, Schachner T, Bonaros N, et al: Technical challenges in totally endoscopic robotic coronary artery bypass grafting. J Thorac Cardiovasc Surg 2006;131:146-153.

Boyd WD, Rayman R, Desai ND, et al: Closed-chest coronary artery bypass grafting on the beating heart with the use of a computer-enhanced surgical robotic system. J Thorac Cardiovasc Surg 2000;120:807-809.

Calafiore AM, Giammarco GD, Teodori G, et al: Left anterior descending coronary artery grafting via left anterior small thoracotomy without cardiopulmonary bypass. Ann Thorac Surg 1996;61:1658-1665.

Falk V, Jacobs S, Gummert J, et al: Robotic coronary artery bypass grafting (CABG): The Leipzig experience. Surg Clin North Am 2003;83:1381-1386.

Nataf P, Lima L, Regan M, et al: Thoracoscopic internal mammary artery harvesting: Technical considerations. Ann Thorac Surg 1997;63(Suppl):S104-S106.

Subramanian V, Patel NU, Patel NC, et al: Robotic assisted multivessel minimally invasive direct coronary artery bypass with port-access stabilization and cardiac positioning: Paving the way for outpatient coronary surgery? Ann Thorac Surg 2005;79:1590-1596.

Vassiliades T: Endoscopic-assisted atraumatic coronary artery bypass. Asian Cardiovasc Thorac Ann 2003;11:359-361.

Vassiliades T: Multivessel, all-arterial, off-pump surgical revascularization without disruption of the thoracic skeleton. Ann Thorac Surg 2004;78:1441-1445.

Vassiliades T: Technical aids to performing thoracoscopic internal mammary artery harvesting. Heart Surg Forum 2002;5:119-124.

CHAPTER 6

Minimally Invasive Cardiac Surgical Coronary Artery Bypass Grafting

Marc Ruel, Vincent Chan, Harry Lapierre, and Joseph T. McGinn, Jr.

Step 1. Surgical Anatomy

- A comprehensive understanding of thoracic and coronary anatomy is vital to the successful performance of minimally invasive coronary artery bypass grafting.
- The multivessel small thoracotomy (MVST) operation, recently renamed *minimally invasive cardiac surgical coronary artery bypass grafting* (MICS CABG), is based on spatial relationships between the left internal thoracic artery, the coronary arteries and their branches, the apex of the heart, and the ascending aorta. All of these structures can be accessed through the fourth or fifth left anterolateral intercostal space.
- The MICS CABG operation is different from a minimally invasive direct coronary artery bypass (MIDCAB).
  - ▲ First, it is a multivessel operation that allows complete revascularization, even in the presence of diffuse and/or triple-vessel coronary disease.
  - ▲ Second, the thoracotomy is often smaller and much more lateral, allowing for adequate rib spreading without risk of costochondral or rib injury and allowing for the use of the space normally occupied by the left lung (deflated during the procedure) when working within the closed chest.
  - ▲ Third, the left internal thoracic artery, skeletonized or not, is harvested over its entire length—that is, from the level of the subclavian vein or higher, down to the bifurcation—as in a regular CABG operation.
  - ▲ Fourth, all coronary arteries and their relationships are directly visualized and identified, because the pericardium is opened widely, as in a regular CABG operation.
  - ▲ Fifth, the operation allows for proximal anastomoses to be routinely performed on the ascending aorta, as in a regular CABG procedure.
- In essence, within a patient's closed thorax, the result of a MICS CABG operation should be equivalent to that of a regular CABG operation; however, the MICS CABG is minimally invasive, avoids cardiopulmonary bypass, and does not involve a sternotomy.

- ◆ Figure 6-1 illustrates the key anatomic structures of the thorax.
- ◆ Figure 6-2 demonstrates the coronary anatomy.
- ◆ Currently, four commercially available instruments are desirable for performance of the MICS CABG procedure:
  - ▲ Thoratrak MICS Retractor System (Medtronic, Minneapolis, Minn)

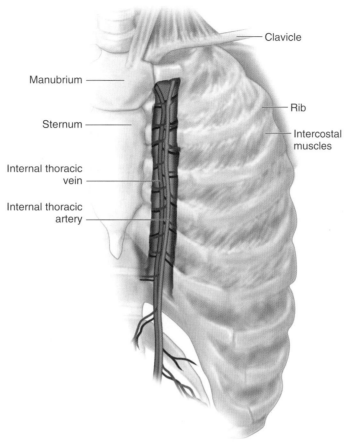

Clavicle

Manubrium

Rib

Sternum

Intercostal muscles

Internal thoracic vein

Internal thoracic artery

Figure 6-1

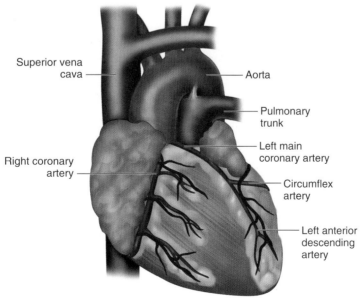

Superior vena cava

Aorta

Pulmonary trunk

Left main coronary artery

Right coronary artery

Circumflex artery

Left anterior descending artery

Figure 6-2

▲ Starfish Non-Sternotomy (NS) Heart Positioner (Medtronic) (Fig. 6-3)
▲ Octopus NS Tissue Stabilizer (Medtronic) (Fig. 6-4)
▲ Rultract Skyhook Retractor (Rultract, Cleveland, Ohio)
- Coronary arteries may be accessed by moving the apex of the heart within the closed chest in order to bring the arteries to be grafted, including the ascending aorta for proximal arteries, into the "window" created by the lateral thoracotomy. To reach the right coronary artery (RCA), it is important that its posterior descending or left ventricular branch be sufficiently developed for it to be accessible. This can readily be determined on the preoperative angiogram by the presence of at least one RCA terminal branch vessel extending beyond the crux, preferably at least halfway toward the apex of the heart.
- Cardiac apex movements include displacing the Starfish NS positioner toward the patient's left shoulder to expose the posterior descending artery, or toward the right hip to expose the marginal branches of the circumflex artery. The left anterior descending artery usually lies spontaneously within the surgeon's field of view. If not, it can easily be visualized by modifying ventilatory parameters on the isolated right lung (see below) or by gently displacing the apical positioner toward the patient's right hip.
- Notably, we have also developed a method by which the ascending aorta can be directly and routinely accessed in the MICS CABG operation. This is our favored modality if ascending aortic atherosclerosis is not present. This method allows the MICS CABG operation to be of the same configuration, completeness, and quality as a regular off-pump coronary artery bypass operation, without the invasiveness and the sternotomy. Alternatively, T- or Y-grafts can be made between the internal thoracic artery and radial artery or arteries.

Step 2. Preoperative Considerations

1. Indications and Contraindications

- The indications for and contraindications to MICS CABG are similar to those for conventional coronary artery bypass grafting with open sternotomy, with the following exceptions:
  ▲ In patients with peripheral vascular disease, special attention should be given during the history and physical examination to the detection of possible left subclavian artery stenosis. When stenosis is suspected, Doppler or angiographic examination, or both, of the left subclavian–internal thoracic artery (ITA) axis is indicated. This is important for occasional patients in whom the ITA may serve as the sole source of blood flow to all grafts, if a Y- or T-graft configuration is elected because of concomitant disease in the ascending aorta. If use of a radial artery is contemplated, the ulnar pulse and Allen's test should be compatible with its safe use.
  ▲ A good left femoral pulse is desirable, as the left side is easier to proceed with should a period of peripheral cardiopulmonary bypass assistance be contemplated during the grafting period. If a good left femoral pulse is not detected, the right femoral artery and vein are used. Extreme caution and planning should be taken with patients who have no femoral pulses. In this case, an off-pump coronary artery bypass approach may be safer, unless only one or two very accessible coronary vessels need grafting.

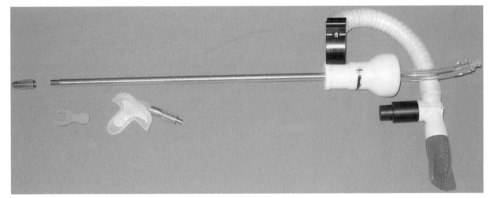

Figure 6-3

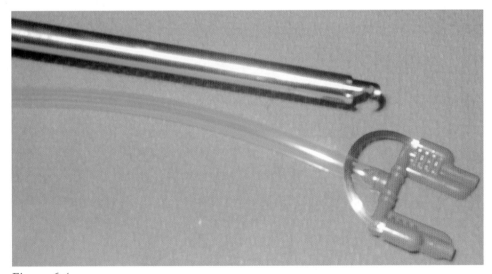

Figure 6-4

▲ Pulmonary disease, if present, should be carefully evaluated, as the tolerance of single-lung ventilation, although not absolutely necessary, is highly desirable during the operation.

▲ In patients with a large body mass index, it may be difficult to adequately visualize and harvest the left internal thoracic artery and to adequately expose lateral coronary targets. Patients with significant cardiac hypertrophy also present unique challenges when mobilizing the heart through the "closed" chest.

▲ As mentioned, if a bypass to the RCA is contemplated, the angiogram should show that the posterior descending artery or main left ventricular branch of the RCA is of sufficient length for it to be adequately visualized through the left chest.

Step 3. Operative Steps

1. Anesthetic Induction

◆ Patients may be given paravertebral thoracic (T2-T3) blockade.

◆ Intubation is performed with either a double-lumen endotracheal tube or a regular endotracheal tube plus a left bronchial blocker, to allow for selective decompression of the left lung. Endotracheal tube or blocker placement is verified by bronchoscopy.

◆ Transesophageal echocardiography is used routinely. This will help monitor cardiac function and also allow for safe and optimal placement of guidewire-guided femoral venous and arterial cannulae, should cardiopulmonary bypass assistance be contemplated.

2. Patient Positioning

◆ Patients are positioned in a 15- to 30-degree right lateral decubitus position, with the right arm extended to allow harvest of the radial artery. The patient's left arm is either elevated over the head or slightly flexed along the patient's side, according to the surgeon's preference (Fig. 6-5A and B).

◆ The patient is draped to allow access to the left groin and right thigh or leg for femoral cannulation and saphenous vein harvest, respectively.

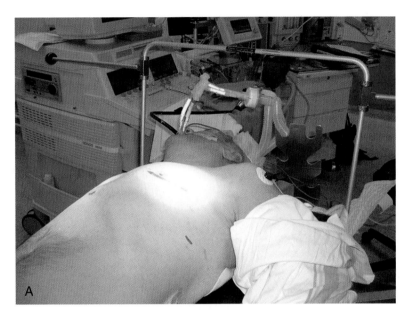

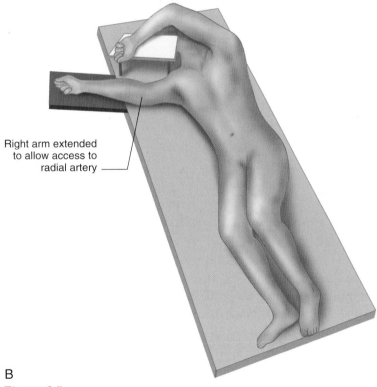

Right arm extended
to allow access to
radial artery

B
Figure 6-5

3. Incision

- A 5- to 6-cm incision is made in the fifth intercostal space in the anterior portion of the left chest, started approximately at the mid-clavicular line and extended laterally. Note that this incision is lateral to where a minimally invasive direct coronary artery bypass incision is typically performed (Fig. 6-6).
- A Finochietto or Thoratrak rib spreader is inserted, and an incision in the pericardium is made approximately 1 to 2 cm anterior to the left phrenic nerve, extending cephalad to the level of the left atrial appendage and anterocaudad to the diaphragmatic reflection (Fig. 6-7).
- The Thoratrak is progressively pulled cephalad and leftward by the Rultract Skyhook retractor (Rultract, Inc., Independence, Ohio). Using long instruments and a long electrocautery blade, the entire length of the left internal thoracic artery is taken down from a lateral approach under direct vision. Care is taken to identify and avoid the phrenic nerve.
- Heparin is given prior to left internal thoracic artery division, with activated clotting time targets based on the surgeon's preference if no pump assist is used.
- An 8-mm incision is made in the left seventh intercostal space (Fig. 6-8) to allow introduction of the Endoscopic Octopus Tissue Stabilizer. This allows for presentation of the ascending aorta and subsequently for stabilization of target epicardial coronary vessels in the chest cavity.

4. Grafts

- Once the left internal thoracic artery is harvested, proximal anastomoses can be performed by using a proximal connector or hand-sewn/tangential clamp approach, directly onto the ascending aorta. To do so, one first retracts the pericardium inferolaterally toward the thoracotomy "window" by using multiple progressive sutures and by bringing the Thoratrak retractor in a cephalomedial direction by corresponding traction on the Rultract Skyhook. Then, one of two methods can be used to bring the aorta within finger reach of the surgeon for performance of hand-sewn proximal anastomoses.
  - ▲ The Ottawa method involves gently packing an open 4 × 4 in the right lateral aspect of the aorta, anterior to the superior vena cava, and asking the anesthetist to use positive end-expiratory pressure (up to 10 to 12 cm H_2O) on the isolated right lung, as well as a 1:1 inspiratory/expiratory ratio, which together effectively bring the mediastinal structures toward the left and into the thoracotomy "window."
  - ▲ The Staten Island method involves dissecting behind the aorta and passing an open 4 × 4 in that space for left anterior retraction of the aorta.
- Either of these methods is combined with gentle pressure and left posteroinferior depression of the pulmonary artery trunk or right ventricular outflow tract with the Octopus NS, followed by tangential clamping. This way, up to three hand-sewn proximal anastomoses can be readily performed, using 6-0 polypropylene, as in a regular off-pump coronary artery bypass or CABG operation.

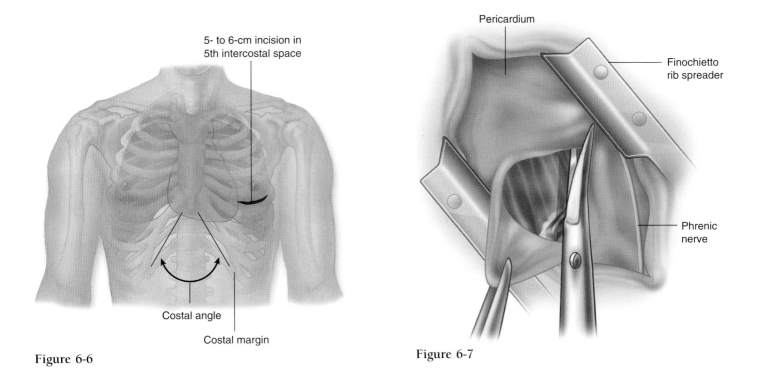

Figure 6-6

Figure 6-7

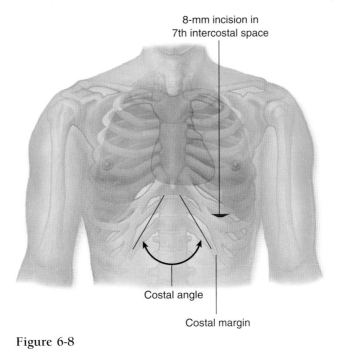

Figure 6-8

◆ If pump assistance is needed, a minimally invasive femorofemoral approach is chosen, with the use of high-performance cannulae providing full or near-full perfusion flows. No aortic cross-clamping is performed at any point.

◆ The Starfish NS is inserted just under the xiphoid process (via a 5-mm incision) and connected to the apex of the heart. Retraction of the apex toward the left shoulder allows visualization of the posterior interventricular branch of the right coronary artery. Retraction of the apex inferiorly toward the right hip allows visualization of the circumflex system.

◆ A Silastic occluder with knotted pledget is placed around the coronary artery to be bypassed, just proximal to the anastomosis, and anchored with a clip (Fig. 6-9).

◆ The coronary arteriotomy and anastomosis are performed in usual fashion. Visualization is obtained by use of an intracoronary shunt and a blower-mister (Fig. 6-10).

◆ The flow of each conduit is assessed with a flow probe.

◆ A pleural chest tube is placed through the orifice created for the Octopus NS, and a pericardial drain is left in the hole created for the Starfish NS.

◆ The left lung is reinflated, and all grafts are inspected under direct vision to rule out kinking or tension.

◆ Our preferred grafting sequence starts with the left anterior descending artery and then proceeds from collaterized to collaterizing remaining vessels. However, if pump assistance is elected from the start, the Ottawa preference is to *finish* the grafting sequence with the left internal thoracic artery/left anterior descending artery, as with the regular on-pump CABG operation, in order to "move and shake" the left internal thoracic artery–left anterior descending artery axis as little as possible.

4. Closure

◆ The thoracotomy incision is closed with a single 2 Vicryl stitch around the intercostal space.

◆ The anterior pectoralis muscle fascia is closed with 0 Vicryl.

◆ The subcutaneous tissue and skin are closed in the usual fashion.

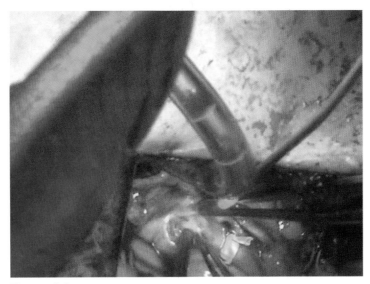

Figure 6-9

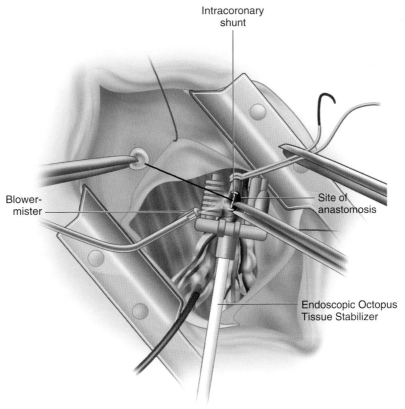

Figure 6-10

Step 4. Postoperative Care

- Local pain management with the On-Q pain relief system (I-Flow, Lake Forrest, Calif) allows for next-day discharge in many patients.
- Pain is also managed with oral administration of nonsteroidal anti-inflammatory agents. Use of paravertebral thoracic block also improves postoperative pain.
- All patients undergoing MICS CABG should be treated with medical therapy standard to conventional coronary bypass with open sternotomy, including aspirin, beta blockers, and anticholesterol agents.
- Patients undergoing MICS CABG with a radial artery graft are placed on dihydropyridine calcium channel blockers for 6 months to help prevent graft spasm.

Step 5. Pearls and Pitfalls

- Preoperative assessment is crucial to identify patients with an unsuitable anatomy or with peripheral, ascending, aortic, or subclavian artery disease, or those who cannot tolerate prolonged single-lung ventilation.
- In patients with severe cardiac hypertrophy, favorable exposure of the lateral and inferior coronary arteries may not be possible. Pump-assist MICS CABG is desirable in these patients.
- As with standard off-pump surgical revascularization, patients with significant ischemia or instability associated with manipulation of the heart should be treated with pump assistance, or if unsuitable, with conventional open sternotomy and on-pump bypass grafting.

References

1. Lapierre H, Chan V, Ruel M: Off-pump coronary surgery through mini-incisions: Is it reasonable? Curr Opin Cardiol 2006;21:578-583.
2. McGinn JT, Reddy V, Lapierre H, Ruel M. Three hundred consecutive cases of multi-vessel small thoracotomy coronary artery bypass grafting. Circulation 2008;118(18Suppl 2):2280.

CHAPTER 7

ROBOTIC CORONARY ARTERY BYPASS GRAFTING

Stephan Jacobs, Volkmar Falk, and Friedrich W. Mohr

- The rationale underlying minimally invasive robotic bypass surgery is to reproduce the excellent results of classic operations with less trauma. The goal is to avoid the three maneuvers that generate most of the "invasiveness" and, therefore, complications for the patient—sternotomy, cardiopulmonary bypass (CPB), and aortic manipulation.
- The surgical telemanipulator is designed to provide the bypass surgeon with stereoscopic vision, full dexterity, unimpaired hand–eye alignment, and tactile feedback in a confined space through ports only.[1] It enables the fine, controlled soft tissue manipulation that is needed in bypass grafting. The preserved integrity of the chest allows for quick progression to ambulation and patient discharge.

Step 1. Surgical Anatomy

- Because of the rapid development of technology and the increasing requirement for less traumatic surgery, robotic coronary artery bypass grafting provides the means and the opportunity to graft the left internal thoracic artery (ITA) to the left anterior descending coronary artery (LAD) without opening the chest.
- The telemanipulator-assisted procedure can be performed through four 1-cm port incisions.

Step 2. Preoperative Considerations

- The patient is placed in the supine position, with the left side raised 30 degrees. The camera port is placed in the fourth intercostal space 2 cm medial to the anterior axillary line for a 30-degree angled scope. Under direct vision, the right instrument port is placed in the second intercostal space medial to the anterior axillary line and thus in the center of a triangle created by the manubrium, acromion, and the camera port. The left instrument port is placed in the sixth/seventh intercostal space medial to the anterior axillary line. The port for the endostabilizer is introduced subxiphoidally 2 cm to the left under endoscopic guidance (Fig. 7-1).
- To maximize space in a closed chest environment (Fig. 7-2A), single-lung ventilation using the right lung is required, with CO_2 insufflation to increase the available space between the sternum and the heart to enhance exposure (Fig. 7-2B).
- Insufflation pressures in the range of 10 to 12 mm Hg are usually well tolerated, despite an increase in right ventricular filling pressures and a decrease of intrathoracic blood volume index and right ventricular ejection fraction.[2]
- Avoiding cardiopulmonary bypass and aortic manipulation minimizes the cardiovascular, renal, and neurologic morbidity associated with conventional bypass surgery. On the other hand, inadequate space is one of the main reasons for conversion to open bypass.[3]
- Male patients with a huge chest should anatomically be considered ideal for the totally endoscopic coronary artery bypass (TECAB) procedure.

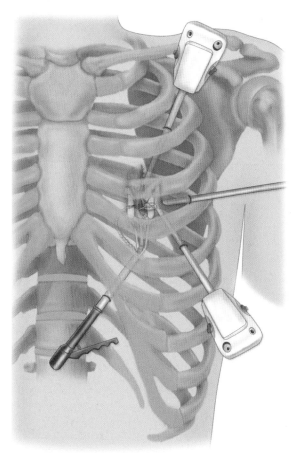

Figure 7-1

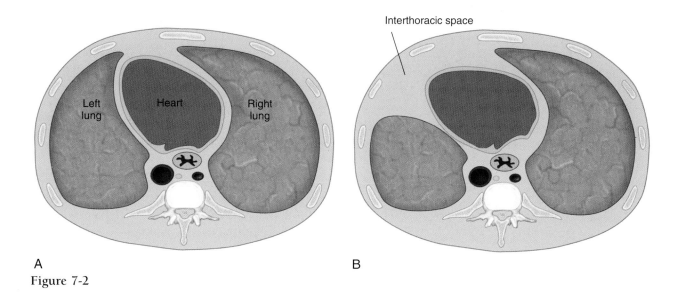

A

B

Figure 7-2

Step 3. Operative Steps

- After the system is set up and the ports placed, the anatomic structures are identified (Fig. 7-3).
- Left ITA (LITA) takedown starts by retracting and incising the fascia. Splitting the fascia frees the LITA and facilitates dissection off the anterior thoracic wall, moving from the lateral to the medial edge. A small pedicle is kept. Following the correct tissue plane, the path of the LITA is always known, and it can be safely harvested (Fig. 7-4).
- The next step is pericardial lipectomy. Epicardial fat is removed, beginning medially, by taking down the mediastinal attachments (Fig. 7-5).
- Opening the pericardium longitudinally and identifying the LAD is facilitated by identifying anatomic landmarks such as the apex of the heart and the groove between the medial aspect of the left atrial appendage and the pulmonary artery. Care must be taken to avoid injury of the phrenic nerve and not to extend the pericardiotomy too far laterally over the apex because the heart may drop out of the pericardial sac (Fig. 7-6).

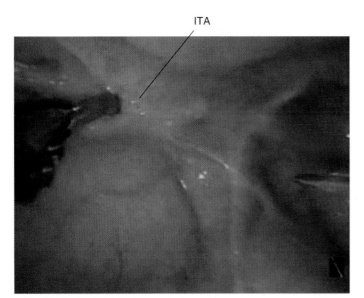

Figure 7-3

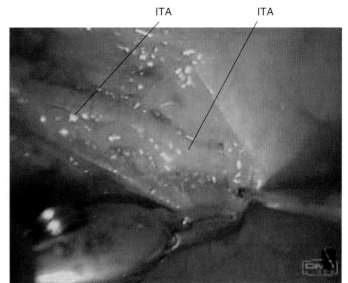

Figure 7-4

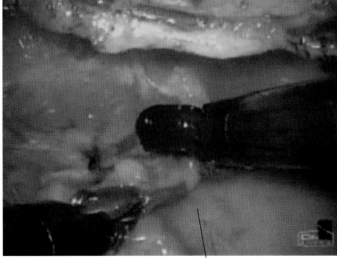

Figure 7-5

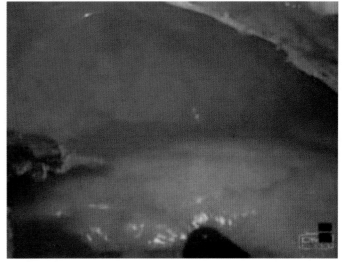

Figure 7-6

- The ideal length of the graft can be assessed after the anastomotic spot is determined. After heparinization, a vascular clamp is placed and the distal end of the ITA is prepared by skeletonizing and clipping the concomitant veins (Fig. 7-7).
- The endostabilizer, temporary Silastic occlusion tapes, and a 7-cm 7-0 double-armed polypropylene suture are inserted and stored in the mediastinum, and the endostabilizer is then introduced under endoscopic vision onto the target site. The stabilizer pads should be equidistant from and run parallel to the LAD (Fig. 7-8).
- After dissection of the anastomotic target site, the Silastic tapes are placed proximal and distal to the anastomotic site and tightened, occluding the LAD (Fig. 7-9).

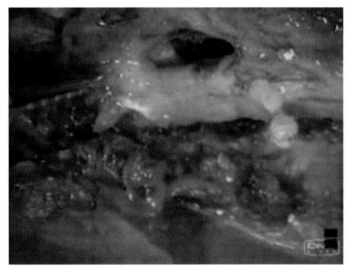

Figure 7-7

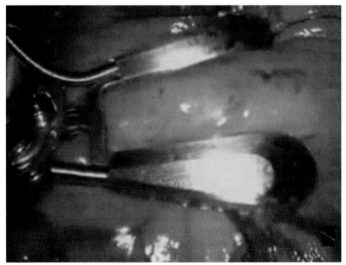
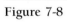

Figure 7-8

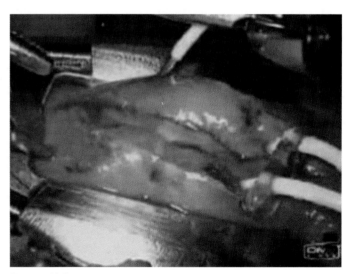

Figure 7-9

- The arteriotomy is performed, transection of the LITA is completed, and the graft is brought close to the target site to start the anastomosis (Fig. 7-10).
- The anastomosis is best performed by beginning at the middle of the medial wall (12 o'clock position; Fig. 7-11).
- Suturing inside-out on the LITA and outside-in on the LAD toward and around the heel is recommended (Fig. 7-12).
- After the circumference of the anastomosis has been sutured, the needles are broken off and an instrument knot is tied (Fig. 7-13).
- At the end of the procedure, occlusion tapes and the vascular clamp are released and evacuated, the stabilizer and instruments are withdrawn, and the left lung is ventilated. A chest tube is inserted through one of the port holes, all other holes are closed, and protamine is given.

Step 4. Postoperative Care

- The patient is transferred to the anesthetic recovery room and extubated, on average, after 70 minutes.
- Particular care regarding single-lung ventilation must be taken during the procedure to ensure that no atelectasis develops.
- Recovery time and length of hospital stay are decreased, and the average patient is discharged after 3 days.

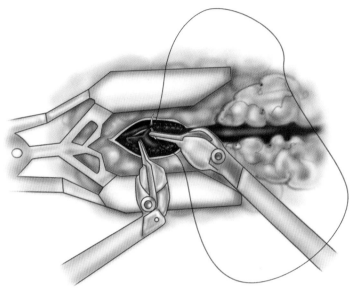

Figure 7-10

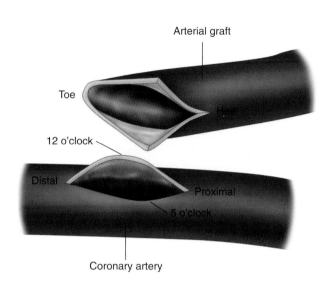

Figure 7-11

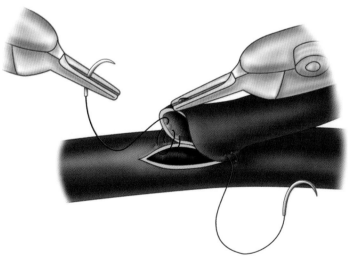

Figure 7-12

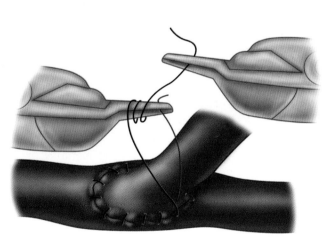

Figure 7-13

Step 5. Pearls and Pitfalls

- The da Vinci telemanipulation system is designed to provide the human operator with dexterity in a confined space. After initial successes with internal mammary artery takedown and some on-pump TECAB cases, the technique was underestimated by surgeons. Patency rates equaled the patency rates with conventional bypass surgery; however, operating times ranged from 4 to 6 hours for a single bypass graft.[4]

- Endoscopic coronary artery bypass grafting on the beating heart is technically more challenging. Based on an intention-to-treat analysis, the conversion rate (elective conversion to a minimally invasive direct coronary artery bypass [MIDCAB] procedure) is still 30%. Conversions result mostly from inability to locate or dissect the LAD owing to the presence of heavy target vessel calcification.[3]

- LITA takedown is now a routine procedure that can be performed in 30 to 40 minutes. Total operating time for a beating heart TECAB procedure ranges from 2.5 to 3.5 hours, with a patency rate of 92% to 94%.[5]

- The use of a robotic system is currently restricted to few indications (single-vessel bypass grafting of the LAD, occasionally double-vessel grafting), but it may be used for endoscopic multivessel procedures in the near future.[6]

- Lack of assistance, limited space, and the lack of fine tactile feedback render this procedure challenging. Among the difficulties are determination of the optimal site for an anastomosis, target vessel calcification, back-bleeding from septal branches, and incomplete immobilization.

- A low threshold for conversion is mandatory to avoid any risk to the patient. Elective conversion is safe and should not be considered a failure.

- To overcome the learning curve, a structured course of training is considered essential for procedural success. Takedown of the ITA should be routinely accomplished before aiming at a complete TECAB procedure.

- Continued rapid development in image-guided, computer-enhanced endoscopic bypass surgery may be expected. The application of multimodal three-dimensional imaging and surface registration will optimize preoperative planning of the procedure and may allow for intraoperative navigation.[7]

References

1. Falk V, Mintz D, Grünenfelder J, et al: Influence of 3D vision on surgical telemanipulator performance. Surg Endosc 2001;15:1282-1288.
2. Raumanns J, Diegeler A, Falk V, et al: Hemodynamic effects of CO_2 insufflation under one lung ventilation for robot-guided surgery. Anesth Analg 2000;90:SCA55.
3. De Cannière D, Wimmer-Greinecker G, Cichon R, et al: Feasibility, safety and efficacy of closed chest CABG: Early European experience. J Thorac Cardiovasc Surg 2007;134:710-716.
4. Falk V, Diegeler A, Walther T, et al: Total endoscopic coronary artery bypass grafting. Eur J Cardiothorac Surg 2000;17:38-45.
5. Kappert U, Cichon R, Schneider J, et al: Closed chest coronary artery bypass surgery on the beating heart with the use of a robotic system. J Thorac Cardiovasc Surg 2000;120:809-811.
6. Stein H, Cichon R, Wimmer-Greinecker G, et al: Totally endoscopic coronary artery bypass surgery using the da Vinci surgical system: A feasibility study on cadaveric models. Heart Surg Forum 2003;6:E183-E190.
7. Falk V, Mourgues F, Adhami L, et al: Cardio navigation: Planning, simulation and augmented reality in robotic assisted endoscopic bypass grafting. Ann Thorac Surg 2005;79:2040-2047.

CHAPTER 8

POSTINFARCTION VENTRICULAR SEPTAL DEFECT

Arvind K. Agnihotri

Step 1. Surgical Anatomy

- Postinfarction ventricular septal defects are classified as occurring in three locations: apical, anterior, and posteroinferior (Fig. 8-1). Most common is an anterior or apical defect caused by anterior/septal myocardial infarction after occlusion of the left anterior descending coronary artery. In about one third of patients, the rupture occurs in the posterior septum after an inferior septal infarction. The inferior septal infarction is usually due to occlusion of a dominant right coronary or, less frequently, of a dominant circumflex artery. An apical septal defect can be considered a variant of an anterior defect, but it presents the opportunity for a modified, and less involved, surgical technique.
- Associated with the septal defect is a variable amount of adjacent (both septal and free wall) myocardial damage. In addition, the posterior papillary muscle is often involved in a posterior postinfarction septal defect. When the free wall infarction involves the papillary muscle, special techniques must be used to anchor the repair, or a mitral valve replacement should be undertaken.

Step 2. Preoperative Considerations

- Without surgery, 50% of patients with postinfarction ventricular septal defect will die within 24 hours, and 80% will die within 4 weeks. Therefore, the presence of this defect is considered an urgent indication for operation.
- The goal of preoperative management is to reduce the left-to-right shunt by reducing both the systemic vascular resistance and the left ventricular pressure. In addition, efforts are made to maintain cardiac output and arterial pressure to aid in end-organ perfusion. Placement of an intra-aortic balloon pump is greatly beneficial and should be done as soon as the diagnosis is made.

◆ To prevent postpump coagulopathy, an antifibrinolytic is administered before commencing cardiopulmonary bypass and is continued as an infusion. The use of surgical sealants on the epicardial surface of the heart at the location of felt buttresses is also recommended.

◆ Areas of full-thickness myocardial infarction will not hold suture against pressure. Regardless of the operative technique or location of the defect, it is critical to anchor suture lines to non-infarcted tissue. In the endocardium this is done by taking stitches at least 5 mm from the zone of necrosis. When this is not possible, stitches are taken through the full thickness of the free wall and a buttress of Teflon felt is used. In this way, strength is afforded by the epicardial portion of the ventricular wall, and the stress distributed.

◆ Repairs must minimize tension at the suture lines. This often involves the use of prosthetic material.

◆ There are two general approaches to treatment of the necrotic muscle. The first approach emphasizes debridement of necrotic tissue and tension-free repair, and it usually involves a prosthetic patch to replace excised tissue. The second approach is to leave the necrotic tissue in place, but to "exclude" it by placing a bovine pericardial patch that circumscribes the infarction. Both techniques are described.

2. Standard Technique: Debridement of Necrotic Tissue

Anterior/Apical Defects
- The ventricular septal defect is approached through an incision through the anterior/apical left ventricle, passing through the area of necrosis. After debridement of necrotic tissue, smaller defects, particularly at the apex, can be closed by approximating the free walls of the right ventricle (RV) and left ventricle (LV) with the septum using interrupted 0 polypropylene sutures over Teflon felt strips (Fig. 8-2A and B). It is critical that the stitches pass through healthy muscle.
- More commonly, the size of the necrotic tissue prevents a primary tension-free repair, requiring use of prosthetic patch material. Low-porosity Dacron is used most commonly, although glutaraldehyde-treated bovine pericardium is an alternative. The patch is fashioned to be slightly larger than the defect. Pledgeted sutures of 1-0 Tevdek are passed from the right ventricle through the intraventricular septum and then through the patch material (Fig. 8-3A). In the apical portion, pledgeted sutures are taken through the free wall of the right ventricle (Fig. 8-3B). The ventriculotomy is then closed with Teflon felt strips and #1 Tevdek using first interrupted mattress sutures, then a running suture as a second layer (Fig. 8-3C).

Posteroinferior Defects
- Closure of posteroinferior septal defects poses the greatest technical challenge. Simple plication of these defects is rarely possible. With large defects, this results in unacceptable tension and reopening or catastrophic disruption. Depending on the size and location of the defect, one or two patches may be required. In addition, rupture of the posterior papillary muscle occasionally requires replacement of the mitral valve.

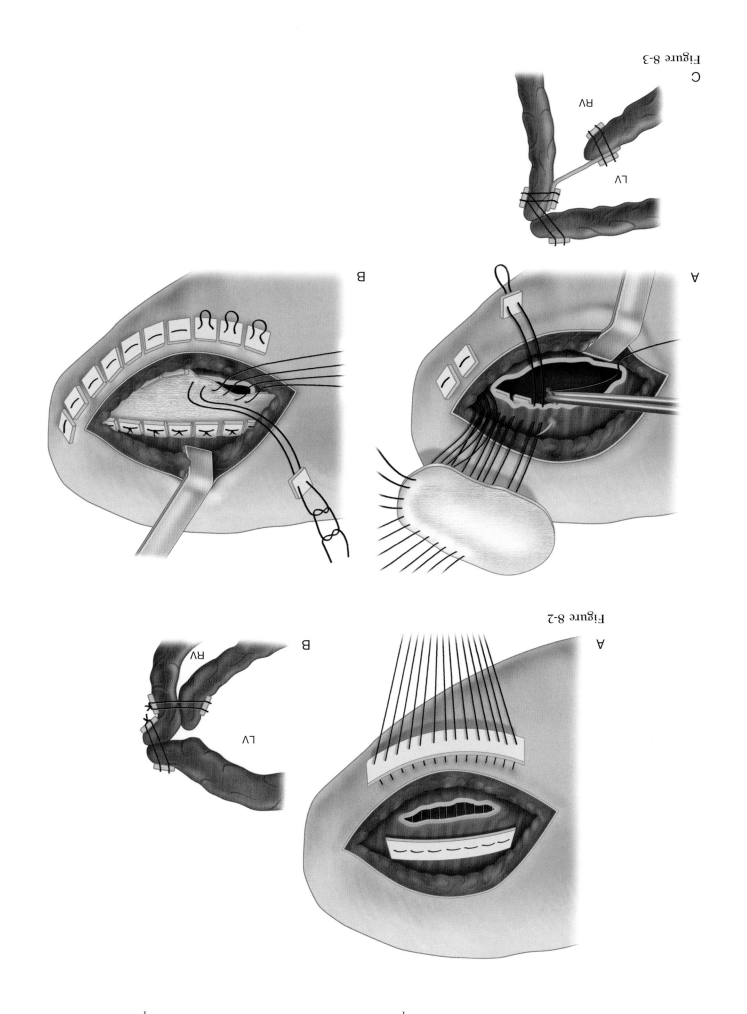

C

RV

LV

Figure 8-3

B

A

Figure 8-2

B

RV

LV

A

- A transinfarct posterior incision is made just to the left ventricular side of the posterior descending coronary artery (Fig. 8-4A). This incision is started at the mid-portion of the posterior wall and extended toward the mitral annulus and apically. Most commonly, rupture is found in the proximal half of the posterior septum (Fig. 8-4B) and involves the posteromedial papillary muscle. The necrotic portion of the ventricular septum is excised along with the involved portion of the posterior ventricular free wall (Fig. 8-5A). The free edge of the right ventricle is shaved back to expose the margins of the defect clearly.
- Rarely, repair of a small septal rupture can be undertaken primarily. An appropriate lesion would appear as an "unhinging" of the posterior attachment to the septum with little adjacent myocardial necrosis. The repair is accomplished by approximating the posterior septum to the free wall of the right ventricle with felt-buttressed mattress sutures of 1-0 Tevdek. The left ventricle can then be closed with a separate suture line, again with interrupted mattress sutures of #1 Tevdek buttressed with felt. A second running suture line is then taken to reinforce the ventriculotomy closure.
- More commonly, patches are required. A single patch can be added to aid in a tension-free closure of the LV after primary closure of the septum (Fig. 8-5B).

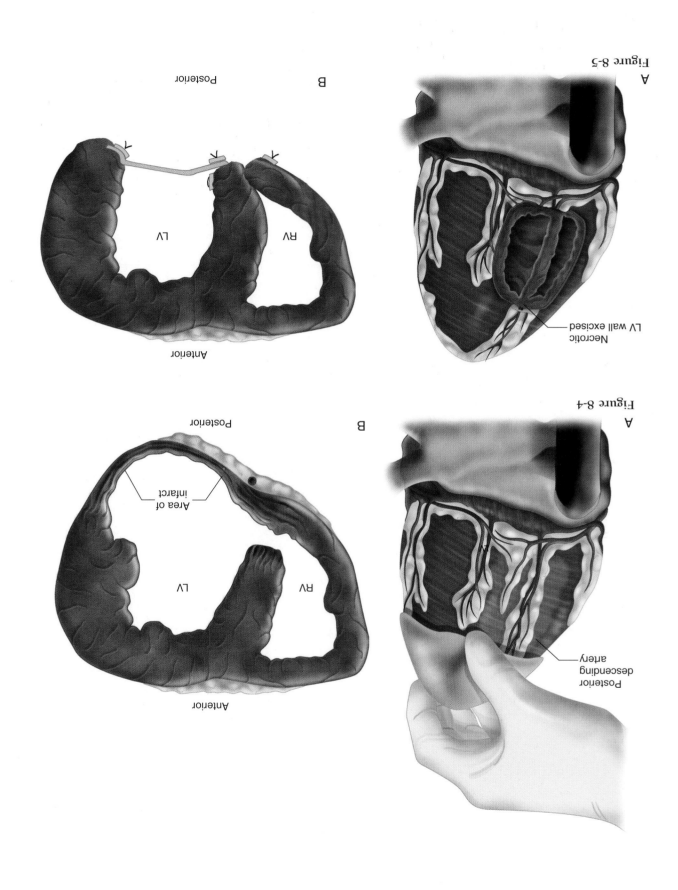

Figure 8-4

A

B

Anterior

Posterior

Area of
infarct

LV

RV

Figure 8-5

A

Necrotic
LV wall excised

B

Anterior

Posterior

LV

RV

Posterior
descending
artery

- When the defect in the septum is larger, a two-patch technique is used. Interrupted mattress sutures of buttressed 2-0 Tevdek are placed circumferentially around the defect. The sutures are placed on the right ventricular side of the septum and then transitioned to the epicardial surface of the diaphragmatic right ventricular free wall. An appropriately shaped patch of Dacron is parachuted down after passage of the stitches. Use of additional felt on the exterior of the patch cushions the sutures and aids in even distribution of forces (Fig. 8-6A).

- A second patch is now required for closure of the remaining defect into the left ventricle. Mattress sutures of buttressed 2-0 Tevdek are placed circumferentially around the margins of the posterior left ventricular free wall. The stitches are taken from the endocardial surface through the ventricular wall so that the patch will lie on the epicardial surface when the repair is complete (Figs. 8-6B and 8-7). Again, use of additional felt on the outside of the patch may be advantageous (Fig. 8-8).

- Involvement of the posterior medial papillary muscle may preclude the placement of stitches through infarcted tissue. In these cases, as in the case of papillary muscle rupture, a mitral valve replacement is performed after patch placement. The mitral valve is exposed through an incision in the dome of the left atrium. The valve is excised and replaced with a low-profile mechanical valve. Interrupted, felted 2-0 Tevdek sutures are used, with the needle passing from the left atrium through the annulus.

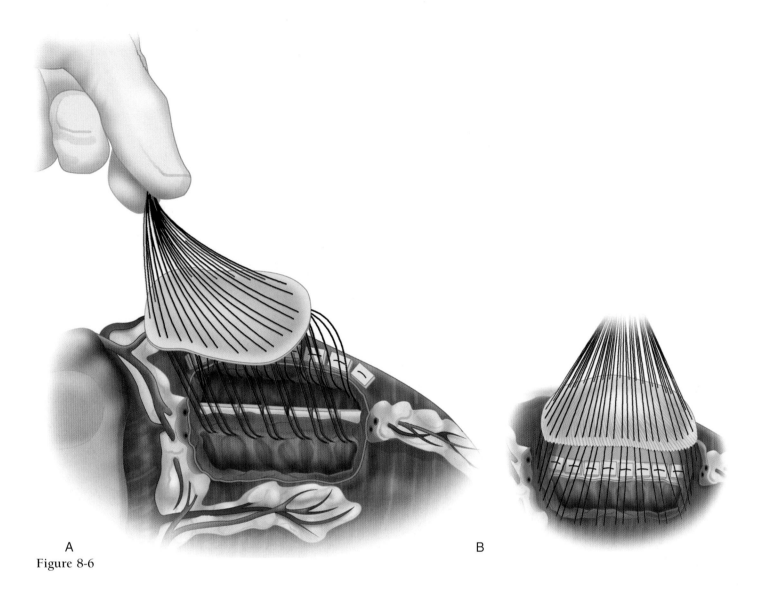

A

B

Figure 8-6

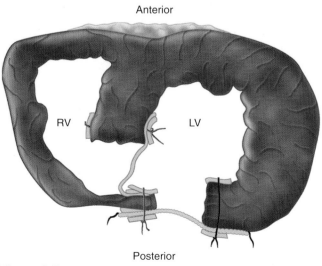

Figure 8-7

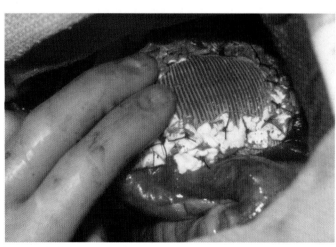

Figure 8-8

3. Modification of Technique: Infarct Exclusion

Anterior/Apical Defects

- The apical portion of the ventricle is opened through the infarction with extension onto the anterior left ventricle. A glutaraldehyde-preserved bovine pericardial patch is secured to non-infarcted areas of the left ventricular septum using a running 3-0 polypropylene stitch. The stitches should be inserted 5 to 7 mm deep in the muscle and 4 to 5 mm apart. The stitches in the patch should be 5 mm from its free margin to allow the patch to cover the area between the entrance and exit of the suture (Fig. 8-9A).
- The suture line is begun at the most proximal part of the septum, and suturing begins traveling toward the apex. The suture line continues from the septum onto the left ventricular free wall. If the infarct involves the anterior papillary muscle at its base, the suture is brought outside the heart at this point and continued as full-thickness interrupted 2-0 polypropylene stitches buttressed on the epicardial surface with a strip of bovine pericardium or Teflon felt. The left ventricle is then closed with interrupted mattress sutures of 2-0 polypropylene buttressed by Teflon felt strips, followed by a running 2-0 polypropylene stitch (Fig. 8-9B).

Posteroinferior Defects

- A transinfarct incision is made in the inferior wall of the left ventricle just lateral to the posterior descending coronary artery to expose the defect and is extended toward both the mitral valve and the apex. Care is taken to avoid damage to the posterior lateral papillary muscle.
- A bovine pericardial patch is tailored in a triangular shape. Its size will be approximately 4 × 7 cm in most patients. The base of the triangle is sutured to the mitral valve annulus with a continuous 3-0 polypropylene suture. The medial suture line then transitions from the mitral annulus to the endocardium of the ventricular septum and is continued along that structure apically. Laterally, the suture line transitions to the endocardium of the posterior left ventricle. After several stitches, the posterior papillary muscle is encountered. If the area of necrosis is small and if healthy tissue allows for continuation, the running suture is continued toward the apex.
- More commonly, on reaching the posterior papillary muscle, it is necessary to bring the running stitch through the muscle to the outside of the left ventricle. The suture line is then continued with interrupted full-thickness 2-0 polypropylene stitches and buttressed with felt on the outside (Fig. 8-10A).
- The suture line continues until the patch is completely secured, and then the ventriculotomy is closed in two layers of full-thickness sutures buttressed on strips of Teflon felt. The infarcted right ventricular wall is left undisturbed (Fig. 8-10B).

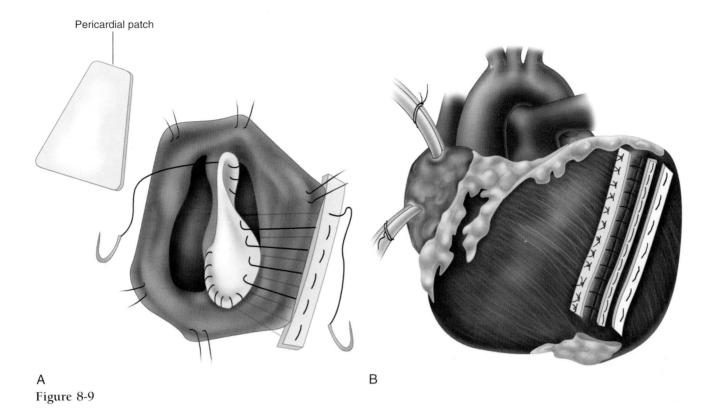

Figure 8-9

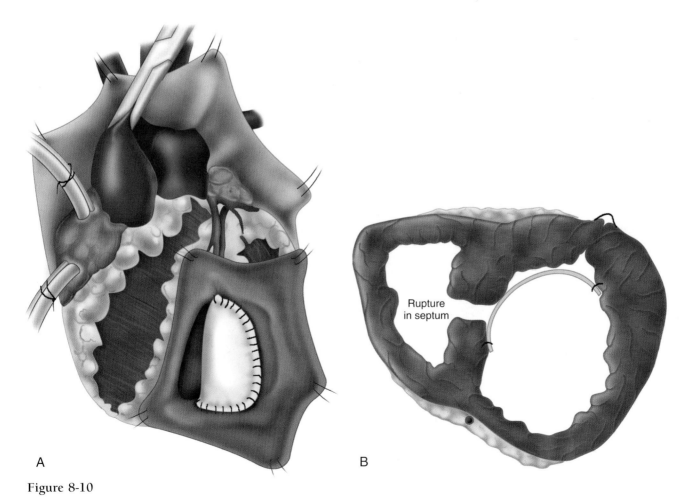

Figure 8-10

Step 4. Postoperative Care

- If an intra-aortic balloon pump was not inserted before surgery, one should be placed now.
- Inotropic support is instituted with milrinone (phosphodiesterase inhibitor). This drug is preferred because in addition to its inotropic properties, it has vasodilatory properties in the pulmonary vascular bed.
- Posterior defects are associated with a right ventricular infarction and more often result in right heart failure on separation from bypass. In such circumstances, inhaled nitric oxide (20 ppm) is instituted before attempted separation. Additional maneuvers may include right-sided infusion of prostaglandin E_1 (0.5 to 2 µg/min) and left-sided norepinephrine infusion through a left atrial line.
- Extubation usually requires aggressive early postoperative diuresis. After fully rewarming, intravenous infusion of furosemide at doses of 5 to 20 mg/hr is used to maintain urine output greater than 100 mL/hr. Continuous venovenous hemofiltration is used for nonresponders.

Step 5. Pearls and Pitfalls

- The common problems during separation from bypass are low cardiac output with or without right ventricular failure and bleeding.
- Recurrent or severe ventricular ectopy is common. Before attempted separation from cardiopulmonary bypass, amiodarone is begun with a bolus of 150 mg followed by ongoing infusion at 1 mg/min. The bolus may be repeated up to six times for malignant ectopy.
- Inadequate hemodynamics on separation from cardiopulmonary bypass may require placement of a ventricular assist device. A left ventricular assist device usually is sufficient.

Bibliography

Agnihotri AK, Madsen JC, Daggett WM Jr: Surgical treatment of complications of acute myocardial infarction: Postinfarction ventricular septal defect and free wall rupture. In Cohn LH (ed): Cardiac Surgery in the Adult, 3rd ed. New York, McGraw-Hill, 2008, pp 753-784.

Cooley DA: Postinfarction ventricular septal rupture. Semin Thorac Cardiovasc Surg 1998;10:100-104.

Daggett WM: Postinfarction ventricular septal defect repair: Retrospective thoughts and historical perspectives. Ann Thorac Surg 1990;50:1006-1009.

David TE, Armstrong S: Surgical repair of postinfarction ventricular septal defect by infarct exclusion. Semin Thorac Cardiovasc Surg 1998;10:105-110.

Kouchoukos NT, Blackstone EH, Doty D, et al: Postinfarction ventricular septal defect. In Kirklin/Barratt-Boyes Cardiac Surgery, 3rd ed. Philadelphia, Churchill Livingstone, 2003, pp 456-471.

Michel-Behnke I, Trong-Phi L, Waldecker B, et al: Percutaneous closure of congenital and acquired ventricular septal defects: Considerations on selection of the occlusion device. J Intervent Cardiol 2005;18:89-99.

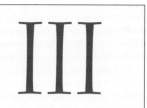

Operations for Valvular Heart Disease

CHAPTER 9

AORTIC VALVE REPLACEMENT

Roberto Rodriguez and Frank W. Sellke

Step 1. Surgical Anatomy

- The aortic valve is the last valve in the heart through which the blood is pumped before it goes to the body. The purpose of the aortic valve is to prevent backflow of blood from the aorta to the left ventricle.
- The normal aortic valve is tricuspid, with left coronary, right coronary, and noncoronary leaflets each attached just beneath one of three sinuses of Valsalva. The sinuses of Valsalva are slight dilations of the aorta above the valve associated with each of the leaflets. These dilations create the vortex of blood flow required for valve closure.
- The sinuses end at the sinotubular junction, which is the narrowest portion of the ascending aorta.
- The aortic valve is supported by a fibrous skeleton with a shallow "U"-shaped configuration at each leaflet, and this skeleton is continuous with the anterior leaflet of the mitral valve.
- The atrioventricular conduction system passes through the interventricular septum below the noncoronary cusp near the right noncoronary commissure.
- The left main coronary artery arises from the left sinus of Valsalva. Its ostium lies directly posterior near the level of the sinotubular junction. The left main coronary artery runs to the left beneath the pulmonary artery. The left main coronary artery should be avoided because it runs for short distance along the posterior aspect of the aorta and comes very close to the commissure between the left and right coronary cusps. Deep sutures must be avoided in this area. The right coronary ostium is an anterior structure located above the right coronary cusp. Its location tends to be more variable than that of the left main coronary artery.

◆ The ventricular septum is located beneath the right coronary cusp and contains the conduction system. Deep sutures in the muscle below the right coronary leaflet may damage the conduction system, in particular the left bundle and the bundle of His (Fig. 9-1).

Step 2. Preoperative Considerations

1. Indications for Aortic Valve Replacement for Aortic Stenosis

◆ In the vast majority of adults, aortic valve replacement (AVR) is the only effective treatment for severe aortic stenosis (AS). Although there is some lack of agreement about the optimal timing of surgery, particularly in asymptomatic patients, it is possible to develop rational guidelines for most patients.

◆ In the absence of serious comorbid conditions, AVR is indicated in virtually all symptomatic patients with severe AS. There are many ways in which AVR benefits these patients. These benefits depend partly on the state of left ventricular (LV) function. The outcome is similar in patients with normal LV function and in those with moderate depression of contractile function. The depressed ejection fraction in many of these patients is caused by excessive afterload, and LV function improves after AVR in such patients. If LV dysfunction is not caused by afterload mismatch, improvement in LV function and resolution of symptoms may not be complete after valve replacement,[1] but survival is still improved in this setting.[2]

◆ Symptomatic patients with angina, dyspnea, or syncope exhibit symptomatic improvement and an increase in survival after AVR.[1-6]

◆ In patients who have severe AS, even those with a low transvalvular pressure gradient, AVR results in hemodynamic improvement and better overall patient functional status.

◆ In summary, symptomatic patients with severe AS should undergo AVR. These patients will have improved LV function, improved symptoms, and improved survival after AVR.

◆ Many clinicians are reluctant to proceed with AVR in an asymptomatic patient, whereas others are concerned about conservative treatment of a patient with severe AS. Insertion of a prosthetic aortic valve is associated with low perioperative morbidity and mortality. Despite this, some difference of opinion persists among clinicians regarding the indications for corrective surgery in asymptomatic patients. Irreversible myocardial depression or fibrosis may develop during a prolonged asymptomatic stage, and this may preclude an optimal outcome.[5,7] Still others attempt to identify patients who may be at especially high risk of sudden death without surgery, although data supporting this approach are limited. Patients in this subgroup include those who have an abnormal response to exercise (e.g., hypotension), those with LV systolic dysfunction or marked/excessive LV hypertrophy, or those with evidence of very severe AS.

◆ We recommend that asymptomatic patients with an aortic valve area of less than 0.8 cm^2 should undergo replacement. Similarly, any evidence of impaired LV function (e.g., decreased ejection fraction, LV dilation, or significantly elevated LV diastolic pressure at rest or with exercise) is an indication for AVR. In the absence of symptoms, a peak aortic gradient of 70 mm Hg may be an indication for surgery, but this is controversial.

◆ Patients with mild to moderate AS (a peak gradient >10-20 mm Hg), with or without symptoms, who are undergoing coronary artery bypass surgery should undergo AVR at the time of the revascularization procedure.

◆ Similarly, patients with moderate AS or AI (aortic insufficiency) undergoing surgery on other valves (e.g., mitral valve repair) or the aortic root should also undergo AVR as part of the surgical procedure, and it is generally accepted practice to perform AVR in patients with moderate AS (e.g., mean gradient 25-40 mm Hg or an AVA <1.3 cm^2) who are undergoing mitral valve or aortic root surgery. Such patients with moderate AS may also warrant AVR at the time of coronary artery bypass surgery, but there are limited data to support this policy.

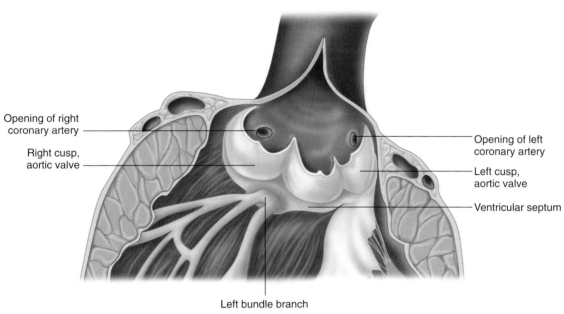

Opening of right
coronary artery

Right cusp,
aortic valve

Opening of left
coronary artery

Left cusp,
aortic valve

Ventricular septum

Left bundle branch

Figure 9-1

2. Indications for Aortic Valve Replacement in Aortic Regurgitation

- The indications for AVR for aortic regurgitation in the range of +3 to +4 include the presence of symptoms or any impairment of LV function, LV dilation, or significant elevation of LV end-diastolic pressure.
- Symptomatic patients with advanced LV dysfunction (ejection fraction <0.25 or end-systolic dimension >60 mm) present difficult management issues. Some patients manifest meaningful recovery of LV function after operation, but many will have developed irreversible myocardial changes. The mortality rate associated with valve replacement approaches 10% in these patients, and the postoperative mortality rate over the subsequent few years is high.
- AVR should be considered more strongly in patients with New York Heart Association (NYHA) functional class II and III symptoms, especially if symptoms and evidence of LV dysfunction are of recent onset and intensive short-term therapy with vasodilators, diuretics, or intravenous positive inotropic agents results in substantial improvement in hemodynamics or systolic function. However, even in patients with NYHA functional class IV symptoms and ejection fraction less than 0.25, the high risks associated with AVR and subsequent medical management of LV dysfunction are usually a better alternative than the higher risks of long-term medical management alone.[8]
- AVR in asymptomatic patients remains a controversial topic, but it is generally agreed that valve replacement is indicated in patients with LV systolic dysfunction.[8-14] As noted previously, for the purposes of these guidelines, LV systolic dysfunction is defined as an ejection fraction below normal at rest.
- Valve replacement is also recommended in patients with severe LV dilation (end-diastolic dimension >75 mm or end-systolic dimension >55 mm), even if ejection fraction is normal. The majority of patients with this degree of dilation have already developed systolic dysfunction because of afterload mismatch and thus are candidates for valve replacement on the basis of the depressed ejection fraction. The elevated end-systolic dimension in this regard is often a surrogate for systolic dysfunction. The relatively small number of asymptomatic patients with preserved systolic function despite severe increases in end-systolic and end-diastolic chamber size should be considered for surgery because they appear to represent a high-risk group with an increased incidence of sudden death,[15,16] and the results of valve replacement in such patients have thus far been excellent. In contrast, postoperative mortality is considerable once patients with severe LV dilation develop symptoms or LV systolic dysfunction.[17]

Step 3. Operative Steps

- Once exposure of the cardiac structures has been achieved, the patient is heparinized and cannulated through the distal ascending aorta and right atrial appendage. If the aorta is heavily calcified, the surgeon must consider femoral or axillary cannulation, deep hypothermia, and circulatory arrest without cross-clamping to avoid stroke. Transesophageal or epiaortic echocardiography can be useful in this case[18] or if there is some uncertainty about the state of the aorta. A retrograde cardioplegia cannula is placed into the coronary sinus. Cardiopulmonary bypass is instituted and an LV vent is placed through the right superior pulmonary vein. An aortic cannula is placed for the delivery of cardioplegia and de-airing. The aorta is cross-clamped, and the heart is arrested with antegrade and retrograde cardioplegia. Intermittent doses of cardioplegia are given throughout the case. In patients with significant aortic insufficiency, antegrade cardioplegia is often not effective, and arrest can be initiated with retrograde cardioplegia, followed by direct injection of cardioplegia down the coronary ostia, if needed.
- Access to the aortic valve can be through either an oblique or a transverse aortotomy. The aortotomy is placed at least 1 cm (above the sinotubular junction) above the right coronary ostium. This circumvents compromise on closure and injury to the right coronary artery. The aortotomy can be extended to the noncoronary sinus of Valsalva (Fig. 9-2).

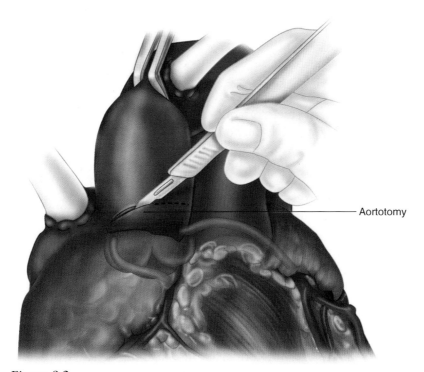

Aortotomy

Figure 9-2

- With the aortic valve exposed, the leaflets are resected and the annulus is debrided of calcium. The surgeon must leave a thin rim of valve tissue and not excise the annulus completely. Resection of the valve is initiated at the commissure between the right and the noncoronary sinuses. The commissure is excised from the aortic wall, and the right coronary cusp is excised (Fig. 9-3). The commissure between the left and right coronary cusps is excised, and the left coronary cusp is removed. Resection is completed with excision of the noncoronary cusp, performed toward the commissure between the left and noncoronary cusps (Fig. 9-4). When calcification is encountered, careful debridement is required to avoid detaching the aorta from the ventricle. A rongeur can be used to crush the calcium into smaller pieces to facilitate removal. All debris must be accounted for; this will minimize the possibility of stroke or coronary ostial occlusion. Extensive and vigorous irrigation must be performed after valve excision. A small gauze cloth may be placed into the left ventricle to prevent calcified particulate matter from entering the cavity, especially if the valve is severely calcified. Retrograde cardioplegia is given during irrigation to prevent debris from entering the coronary ostia.
- Several suturing techniques have been used, but the most common uses horizontal pledgeted sutures with pledgets on the aortic or ventricular aspect of the annulus, depending on the type of valve being inserted.
- Traction sutures can be placed at the sinotubular junction above the commissures. This provides maximum exposure of the annulus. The annulus is measured and the appropriate-sized valve is selected for the replacement. If the annulus is too small, various aortic root enlargement techniques can be used (see Chapter 10).
- We use an interrupted suture technique that affords maximum strength of prosthetic attachment and has a low incidence of perivalvular leak. We place sutures from below the annulus, exiting slightly above it into the aorta. Double-needle, pledgeted 2-0 Dacron sutures are used, with little space between them. The sutures are alternating green and white to simplify identification of the suture pairs. The pledgets are placed below the annulus in the LV outflow tract. This secures the prosthesis by compressing the annulus between the sutures and the prosthesis (Fig. 9-5).

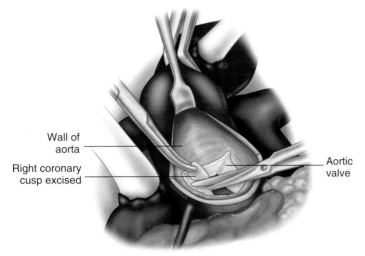

Figure 9-3

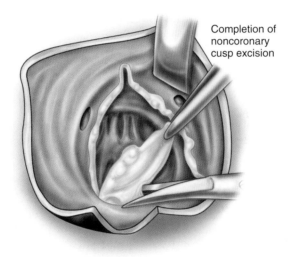

Figure 9-4

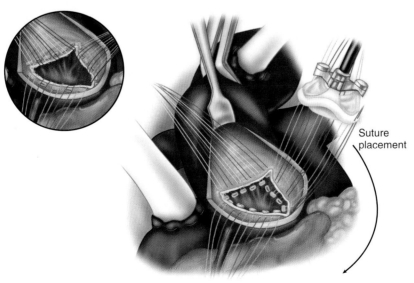

Figure 9-5

- Sutures are placed in the right coronary annulus toward the commissure between the right and noncoronary sinuses. In a similar fashion, the left coronary annulus is sutured toward the non-coronary sinus. Finally, the noncoronary sutures are placed (Fig. 9-6). The left main coronary artery should be avoided because it runs for short distance along the posterior aspect of the aorta and comes very close to the commissure between the left and right coronary cusps. Deep sutures must be avoided in this area. Also, deep sutures in the muscle below the right coronary leaflet may damage the conduction system (see Fig. 9-1).
- The sutures are then passed through the sewing ring of the prosthesis, which is tied down in the supra-annular position (Fig. 9-7). Supra-annular valves allow for a larger orifice area and tend to seat well in the annulus. We prefer to tie down the commissure sutures first, followed by the left, right, and noncoronary sinuses.
- Once the prosthesis has been tied down into place, the aortotomy is closed. We use two running polypropylene sutures. Pledgeted, double-needle polypropylene sutures are placed at the lateral aspects of the aortotomy and tied down. A horizontal mattress stitch is used from the lateral aortotomy toward the middle. A second continuous stitch is placed as a second layer for the closure (Fig. 9-8). When a friable or thin aorta is encountered, consideration should be given to using felt strips for closure.
- After release of the cross-clamp, transesophageal echocardiography is used to assess the position of the prosthesis and evaluate for the possibility of perivalvular leak. Intraventricular air volume can also be assessed. If a significant quantity of air remains in the ventricle, this can be aspirated using a needle in the ventricular apex. Atrial and right ventricular pacing wires are placed. After recovery of a suitable heart rhythm, the patient is weaned from cardiopulmonary bypass, and transesophageal echocardiography is used to monitor for ventricular function. Cannulae are removed, heparin is reversed with protamine, and the incision is closed.

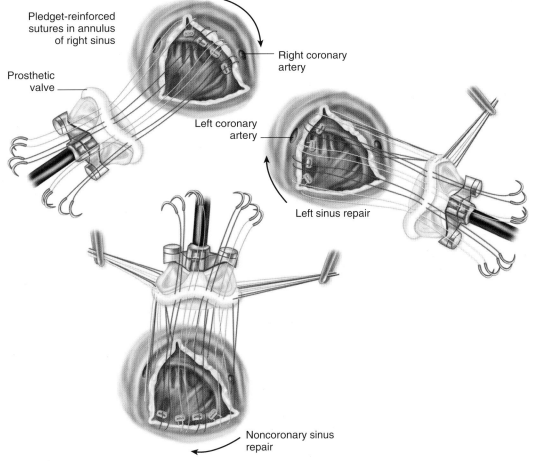

Pledget-reinforced
sutures in annulus
of right sinus

Right coronary
artery

Prosthetic
valve

Left coronary
artery

Left sinus repair

Noncoronary sinus
repair

Figure 9-6

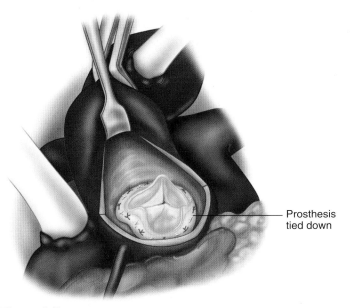

Prosthesis
tied down

Figure 9-7

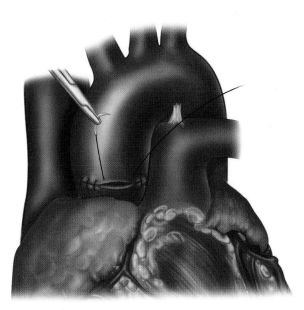

Figure 9-8

Step 4. Postoperative Care

- The postoperative management for a patient having undergone AVR is routine and standard for most postcardiac surgical patients.
- However, several points should be addressed. A patient with AS has a hypertrophied left ventricle and thus will likely be very sensitive to the state of volume load. In addition, atrial fibrillation is often not well tolerated in such patients with a stiff, hypertrophic left ventricle. Although a Swan-Ganz catheter may not always be required, it may help to assess the degree of volume loading in such a patient and should be considered in complex cases.
- Wide fluctuations in blood pressure are not uncommon, and any sudden increase in bleeding from the chest tubes or mediastinal tubes should alert the surgeon to the possibility of aortotomy suture line bleeding.
- In cases in which a mechanical valve has been placed, warfarin is begun on the first or second postoperative day. If the international normalized ratio (INR) has not increased by the fourth day, we usually begin intravenous heparin until the patient is anticoagulated with warfarin. The pacing wires are removed on or about the third postoperative day, while the INR is generally still less than 2.

Step 5. Pearls and Pitfalls

- Solitary AVR is usually a straightforward procedure. However, attention to several points can improve the outcome. Because the aortic valve is often calcified, the surgeon should take care not to lose calcified debris in the ventricle or down the coronary arteries. A gauze pad can be placed in the ventricle during debridement to prevent embolization, and the ventricle should be copiously irrigated with cold saline after debridement. In addition, retrograde cardioplegia should be administered during irrigation.
- When using one of the high-profile valves currently on the market, the surgeon needs to ensure that the coronary arteries are not occluded by the sewing ring, the pledgets, or the sutures. In the event of a regional wall motion abnormality after bypass, it may be necessary to rearrest the heart and inspect the coronary ostia or to bypass the vessel supplying the dysfunctional region.
- In the presence of a small aortic root, it is not advised to force a valve into the root. This may result in a perivalvular leak or, worse, aortic or ventricular disruption. This is especially true in elderly, frail patients with a calcified annulus. If the surgeon is concerned with the possibility of patient-prosthesis mismatch (predicted aortic valve area index <0.8 cm^2/m^2), he or she should consider enlarging the aortic root annulus (see Chapter 10).
- Transesophageal echocardiography has become a standard part of the procedure. It allows the surgeon and anesthesiologist to assess the adequacy of replacement in terms of possible perivalvular leak, abnormal leaflet motion, or regional or global myocardial dysfunction. In our opinion, it should be used in every case of valve replacement or repair unless contraindicated.

References

1. Connolly HM, Oh JK, Orszulak TA, et al: Aortic valve replacement for aortic stenosis with severe left ventricular dysfunction: Prognostic indicators. Circulation 1997;95:2395-2400.
2. Smith N, McAnulty JH, Rahimtoola SH: Severe aortic stenosis with impaired left ventricular function and clinical heart failure: Results of valve replacement. Circulation 1978;58:255-264.
3. Schwartz F, Baumann P, Manthey J, et al: The effect of aortic valve replacement on survival. Circulation 1982;66:1105-1110.
4. Murphy ES, Lawson RM, Starr A, Rahimtoola SH: Severe aortic stenosis in patients 60 years of age or older: Left ventricular function and 10-year survival after valve replacement. Circulation 1981;64:II-184-II-188.
5. Lund O: Preoperative risk evaluation and stratification of long-term survival after valve replacement for aortic stenosis: Reasons for earlier operative intervention. Circulation 1990;82:124-139.
6. Kouchoukos NT, Davila-Roman VG, Spray TL, et al: Replacement or the aortic root with a pulmonary autograft in children and young adults with aortic-valve disease. N Engl J Med 1994;330:1-6.
7. Lund O, Larsen KE: Cardiac pathology after isolated valve replacement for aortic stenosis in relation to preoperative patient status: Early and late autopsy findings. Scand J Thorac Cardiovasc Surg 1989;23:263-270.
8. Bonow RO, Nikas D, Elefteriades JA: Valve replacement for regurgitant lesions of the aortic or mitral valve in advanced left ventricular dysfunction. Cardiol Clin 1995;13:73-83.
9. Ross J Jr: Afterload mismatch in aortic and mitral valve disease: Implications for surgical therapy. J Am Coll Cardiol 1985;5:811-826.
10. Nishimura RA, McGoon MD, Schaff HV, Giuliani ER: Chronic aortic regurgitation: Indications for operation—1988. Mayo Clin Proc 1988;63:270-280.
11. Bonow RO: Asymptomatic aortic regurgitation: Indications for operation. J Card Surg 1994;9:170-173.
12. Rahimtoola SH: Valve replacement should not be performed in all asymptomatic patients with severe aortic incompetence. J Thorac Cardiovasc Surg 1980;79:163-172.
13. Carabello BA: The changing unnatural history of valvular regurgitation. Ann Thorac Surg 1992;53:191-199.
14. Gaasch WH, Sundaram M, Meyer TE: Managing asymptomatic patients with chronic aortic regurgitation. Chest 1997;111:1702-1709.
15. Turina J, Turina M, Rothlin M, Krayenbuehl HP: Improved late survival in patients with chronic aortic regurgitation by earlier operation. Circulation 1984;70:I-147-I-152.
16. Bonow RO, Lakatos E, Maron BJ, Epstein SE: Serial long-term assessment of the natural history of asymptomatic patients with chronic aortic regurgitation and normal left ventricular systolic function. Circulation 1991;84:1625-1635.
17. Klodas E, Enriquez-Sarano M, Tajik AJ, et al: Aortic regurgitation complicated by extreme left ventricular dilation: Long-term outcome after surgical correction. J Am Coll Cardiol 1996;27:670-677.
18. Byrne JG, Aranki SF, Cohn LH: Aortic valve operations under deep hypothermic circulatory arrest for the porcelain aorta: "No-touch" technique. Ann Thorac Surg 1998;65:1313-1315.

CHAPTER 10

AORTIC ROOT ENLARGEMENT TECHNIQUES

John R. Doty

Step 1. Surgical Anatomy

- The left ventricular outflow tract is best appreciated when viewed directly down into the aortic annulus. The aortic valve and pulmonary valve, although closely related, have different planes. The infundibular portion of the right ventricle elevates the plane of the pulmonary valve and trunk above the aortic valve, placing the pulmonary valve higher and more posterior. The aortic valve shares fibrous continuity with the anterior leaflet of the mitral valve (Fig. 10-1).

- The space between the fibrous attachments of the aortic valve leaflets is termed the *interleaflet triangle*. These triangles are more flexible than the other segments of the aortic root (Fig. 10-2). The commissure between the right and left coronary cusps is usually located directly across from the pulmonary artery, with a mirror-image configuration of the pulmonary valve cusps. The commissure between the right coronary cusp and the noncoronary cusp is located anteriorly and is closely related to the interventricular septum and the conduction system. The commissure between the left coronary cusp and the noncoronary cusp is located more posterior and to the right. This commissure is located opposite the middle portion of the anterior leaflet of the mitral valve (see Fig. 10-2).

- Various portions of the aortic valve are above, at, and below the true aortic annulus. The tops of the commissures rest above the aortic annulus, well into the sinus portion of the aorta. The central portions of the leaflets meet below the aortic annulus during diastole, within the left ventricular outflow tract. The true aortoventricular junction is between these two levels (Fig. 10-3).

- The right coronary artery arises from the right coronary sinus and courses rightward in the atrioventricular groove. The left main coronary artery is short and branches immediately into the left circumflex and left anterior descending arteries. The left circumflex artery courses laterally in the atrioventricular groove, being near the posterior mitral annulus. The left anterior descending artery lies posterior to the pulmonary artery in its proximal portion before coursing down the anterior interventricular groove. The first septal branch of the left anterior descending artery lies directly behind the posterior leaflet of the pulmonary valve (Fig. 10-4).

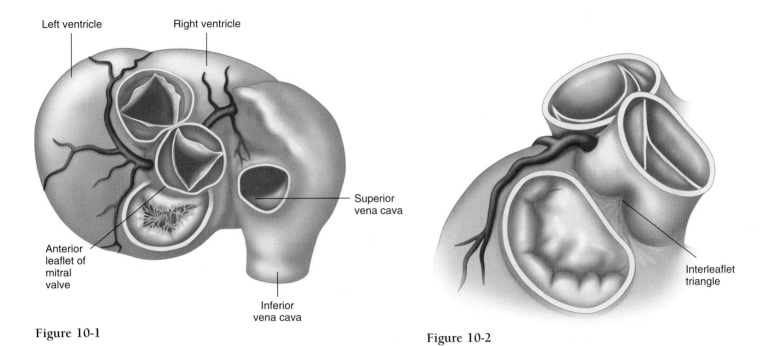

Figure 10-1

Figure 10-2

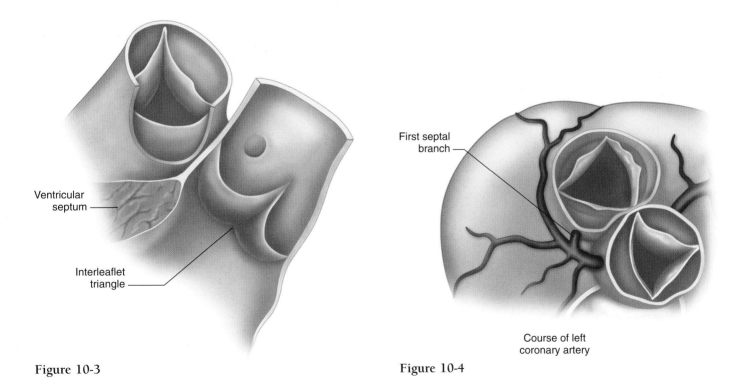

Figure 10-3

Figure 10-4

Step 2. Preoperative Considerations

- It is important to fully evaluate adult patients for concomitant coronary artery disease with stress testing and left heart catheterization. The coronary angiogram should be carefully studied for anomalous origin of either main coronary artery, and the location of the first septal branch of the left anterior descending artery should be identified if the pulmonary autograft operation is under consideration.
- The echocardiogram should be reviewed for evidence of left ventricular hypertrophy and to assess left ventricular function. Careful preoperative measurement of the aortic annulus can guide intraoperative valve sizing to avoid patient–prosthesis mismatch and to identify patients in whom aortic root enlargement is likely. Concomitant subaortic stenosis should be identified because this can be addressed with myotomy/myectomy if required.
- The echocardiogram can also demonstrate concomitant poststenotic dilation of the ascending aorta or true ascending aortic aneurysm. If the pulmonary autograft operation is under consideration, the pulmonary valve should be interrogated for insufficiency or other abnormalities. It is important to note mitral valve structure and degree of insufficiency on the preoperative echocardiogram because these may be altered with aortic root enlargement.
- Patients with more complex forms of aortic root disease, such as combined aortic stenosis and coarctation of the aorta or varying degrees of hypoplastic left heart syndrome, may require computed tomography or magnetic resonance imaging to delineate the aortic arch and descending thoracic aorta.
- A resting electrocardiogram should be reviewed to identify any preoperative conduction abnormalities. Patients should be evaluated for concomitant atrial fibrillation or other rhythm disturbance that can be addressed during the operation.

Step 3. Operative Steps

1. Left Ventricular Outflow Tract Exposure

- After establishment of cardiopulmonary bypass and cardioplegic arrest of the heart, the aorta is completely divided transversely approximately 1 cm above the sinotubular junction. Alternatively, a spiraling-type incision down into the noncoronary sinus may be used if extensive enlargement is not anticipated. The aortic valve is excised and the annulus is debrided. A careful determination is made as to the minimum size of prosthesis that would be acceptable for the patient's body size. If root enlargement is indicated to achieve an adequately sized prosthesis, the appropriate technique is used.

2. Root Enlargement

- Posterior enlargement of the aortic root is performed by either the Nicks-Nunez or the Rittenhouse-Manouguian technique (Fig. 10-5). The Nicks-Nunez method is a vertical incision through the commissure between the left coronary cusp and the noncoronary cusp, extending down into the interleaflet triangle. Limiting the incision to just the interleaflet triangle can enlarge the root sufficiently by 2 to 3 mm. If greater enlargement is required, the incision can be extended further into the anterior leaflet of the mitral valve and the roof of the left atrium.

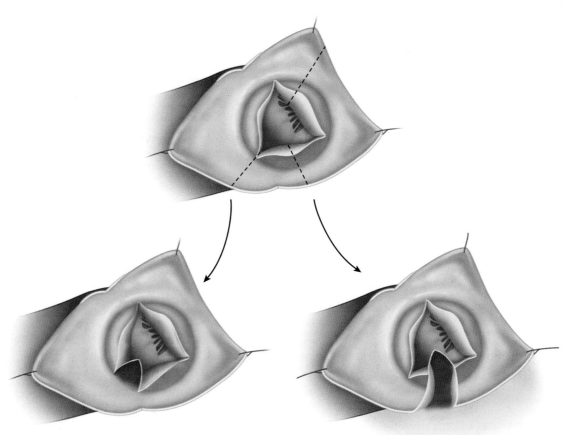

Nicks-Nunez technique

Rittenhouse-Manouguian technique

Figure 10-5

The Rittenhouse-Manouguian method is a vertical incision through the mid-portion of the noncoronary sinus through the aortic annulus and into the anterior leaflet of the mitral valve and roof of the left atrium. The incisions in the anterior leaflet of the mitral valve can be extended almost to the free edge of the leaflet, dramatically enlarging the outflow tract.

◆ Anterior enlargement of the aortic root, or aortoventriculoplasty, is performed according to the technique described by Konno and Rastan (Fig. 10-6). A vertical aortotomy is performed, and the incision is continued into the right coronary sinus well leftward of the right coronary artery. The incision is then extended through the aortic annulus, near the commissure between the right and left coronary leaflets. The incision is carried into the interventricular septum only as far as necessary to achieve the desired enlargement. Deep incisions place the first septal branch of the left anterior descending artery at risk for injury. A second incision is made on the right ventricular free wall to enlarge the right ventricular outflow tract.

3. Root Reconstruction

Nicks-Nunez Technique, Patch Reconstruction

◆ After the aortic root has been enlarged sufficiently, a diamond-shaped patch of autologous pericardium, prosthetic material, or a composite of both is fashioned. One end of the patch is inserted into the distal end of the enlargement at the level of aortic–mitral continuity if the incision is only into the interleaflet triangle. Interrupted sutures with pledgets are preferred because the interleaflet triangle lacks fibrous strength. The sutures are then passed through the sewing ring of the aortic valve prosthesis. The remainder of the valve sutures are placed through the aortic annulus in standard fashion (Fig. 10-7A through D).

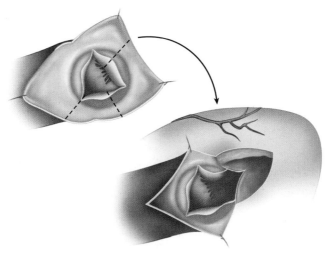

Konno-Rastan technique

Figure 10-6

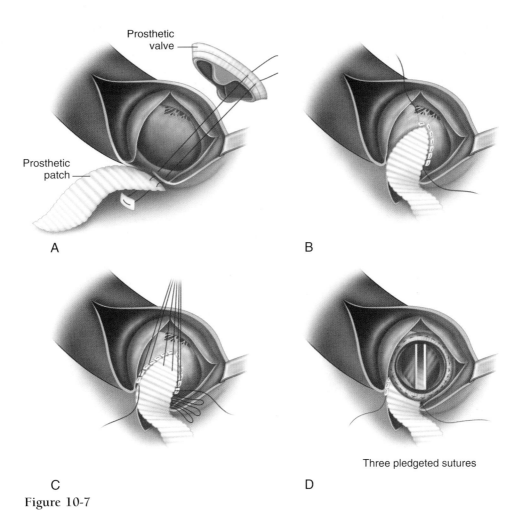

Prosthetic valve

Prosthetic patch

A

B

C

D

Three pledgeted sutures

Figure 10-7

- The patch is then tailored for closure of the aortotomy if a spiraled incision has been used, or it is transected flat at the level of the transverse aortotomy and incorporated as part of the reanastomosis of the aortic root to the ascending aorta (Fig. 10-8A and B).
- If the incision has been carried farther into the left ventricular outflow tract by crossing into the anterior leaflet of the mitral valve and the left atrium, reconstruction is begun by placing the patch into the deepest portion of the incision. The defect in the anterior leaflet is repaired with the patch. Interrupted sutures without pledgets are used for accuracy and strength (Fig. 10-9).
- At the level of the aortic annulus, interrupted sutures with pledgets are placed and passed first through the patch and then through the prosthetic valve. The remainder of the valve sutures are placed through the aortic annulus in standard fashion. If the left atrial wall is flexible and the defect is small, the left atrial wall can be approximated directly to the patch. Otherwise, a second patch is fashioned to reconstruct the left atrial defect (Fig. 10-10).
- The patch is then tailored for closure of the aortotomy or incorporated as part of the aortic reanastomosis, as previously described.

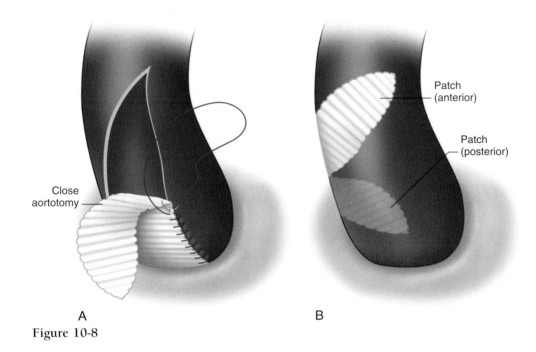

Close
aortotomy

Patch
(anterior)

Patch
(posterior)

A

B

Figure 10-8

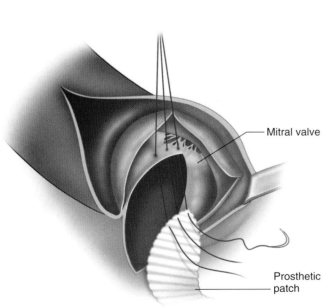

Mitral valve

Prosthetic
patch

Figure 10-9

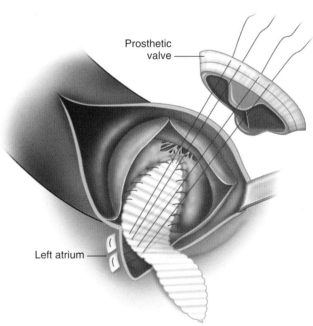

Prosthetic
valve

Left atrium

Figure 10-10

Rittenhouse-Manouguian Technique, Patch Reconstruction

- After enlargement of the root by extending the incision across the noncoronary portion of the aortic annulus into the anterior leaflet of the mitral valve and roof of the left atrium, a diamond-shaped patch of either autologous pericardium or prosthetic material (such as polytetrafluoro-ethylene [PTFE] or Dacron) is fashioned. As with the Nicks-Nunez method, reconstruction is begun by placing the patch into the deepest portion of the incision. The defect in the anterior leaflet is repaired with the patch, using interrupted or continuous sutures without pledgets for accuracy and strength (Fig. 10-11A and B).

- At the level of the aortic annulus, interrupted sutures with pledgets are placed and passed first through the patch and then through the prosthetic valve (Fig. 10-12A). The remainder of the valve sutures are placed through the aortic annulus in standard fashion (Fig. 10-12B). If the left atrial wall is flexible and the defect is small, it can be approximated directly to the patch. Otherwise, a second patch is fashioned to reconstruct the left atrial defect (Fig. 10-12C).

- The patch is then tailored for closure of the aortotomy if a spiraled incision has been used, or it is transected flat at the level of the transverse aortotomy and incorporated as part of the reanastomosis of the aortic root to the ascending aorta.

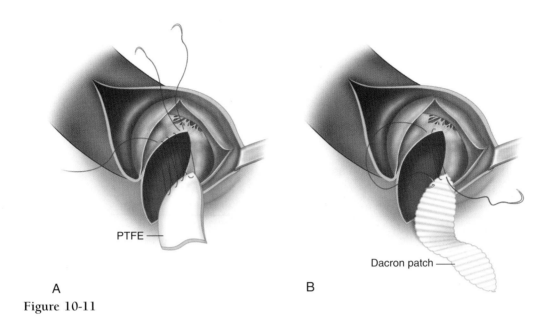

PTFE

A

Dacron patch

B

Figure 10-11

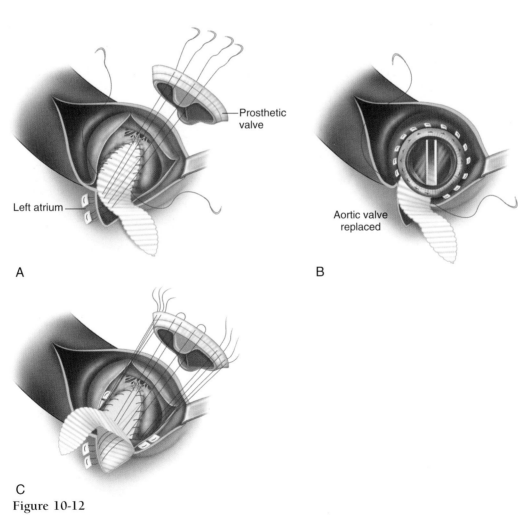

Prosthetic valve

Left atrium

A

Aortic valve replaced

B

C

Figure 10-12

Konno-Rastan Aortoventriculoplasty

◆ The aortic root is mobilized by careful dissection anteriorly between the right coronary sinus and the pulmonary artery. This dissection is performed to the left side of the right coronary artery and is carried down to the level of the aortic annulus. The aortic root is enlarged with an incision through the right coronary portion of the aortic annulus, near the commissure between the right and left coronary cusps. The incision is deepened into the interventricular septum, and a matching incision is made on the right ventricular free wall to enlarge the right ventricular outflow tract (Fig. 10-13).

◆ A diamond-shaped patch of prosthetic material is fashioned and placed deep into the interventricular septal incision. Continuous sutures are used to attach the patch to the ventricular muscle up to the level of the aortic annulus (Fig. 10-14). A second, triangular patch is fashioned. Interrupted sutures with pledgets are used to attach the base of the triangular right ventricular outflow tract patch to the junction of the diamond-shaped left ventricular outflow tract patch at the level of the aortic annulus; the sutures are then passed through the sewing ring of the prosthetic valve (Fig. 10-15). The remainder of the valve sutures are placed through the aortic annulus in standard fashion, and the prosthesis is secured into position.

◆ The right ventricular outflow tract patch is then folded over the right ventricular free wall defect, and continuous sutures are used to attach the patch to the ventricular muscle. The left ventricular outflow tract patch is tailored to close the defect in the aorta using continuous suture technique (Fig. 10-16A and B).

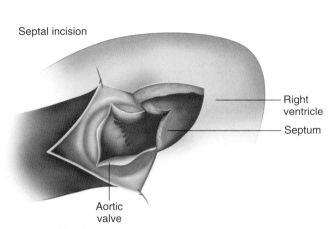

Septal incision

Right ventricle

Septum

Aortic valve

Figure 10-13

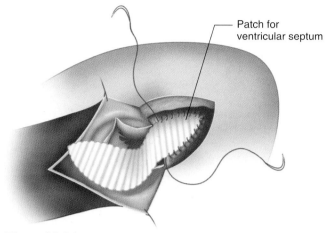

Patch for ventricular septum

Figure 10-14

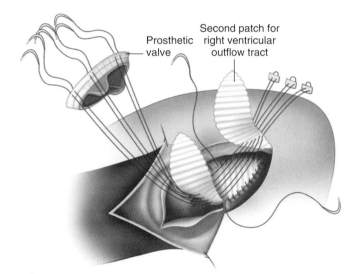

Prosthetic valve

Second patch for right ventricular outflow tract

Figure 10-15

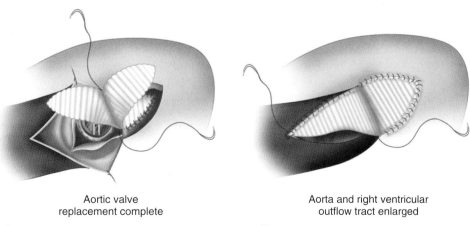

Aortic valve replacement complete

A

Aorta and right ventricular outflow tract enlarged

B

Figure 10-16

Aortic Allograft, Full Root Technique with Anterior Leaflet of Mitral Valve

◆ The aortic allograft is prepared with the attached, intact anterior leaflet of the mitral valve. A small rim of donor left atrial tissue is also usually present and should be retained on the allograft. The remnants of the chordae are removed from the allograft anterior leaflet. The allograft in this fashion can be used to reconstruct very large defects of the aortic root and also to enlarge the root substantially.

◆ The aortic valve and sinus tissue are removed. The coronary arteries are mobilized on generous buttons of sinus tissue. The left ventricular outflow tract is enlarged posteriorly with either a Nicks-Nunez or a Rittenhouse-Manouguian incision extending down into the anterior leaflet of the mitral valve (Fig. 10-17).

◆ The anterior leaflet of the allograft is inserted into the defect in the patient's anterior leaflet and attached using interrupted sutures without pledgets for accuracy and strength. Care and precision are used for this reconstruction to avoid distorting the mitral valve and causing undue tension (Figs. 10-18A and B and 10-19).

◆ The allograft is then attached to the left ventricular outflow tract using interrupted sutures for accuracy. This proximal suture line is then reinforced with biologic glue. If the left atrial wall is flexible and the defect is small, it can be approximated directly to the rim of the atrial wall of the allograft. Otherwise, a patch of autologous pericardium or allograft aorta is fashioned to reconstruct the left atrial defect (Fig. 10-20).

◆ The coronary artery buttons are attached in the appropriate position to the aortic allograft with continuous sutures. The allograft is attached to the ascending aorta with continuous sutures, and all suture lines are reinforced with biologic glue.

Ross-Konno Reconstruction

◆ Severe hypoplasia of the left ventricular outflow tract in young patients can be successfully managed with combined aortoventriculoplasty and pulmonary autograft replacement of the aortic valve.

◆ Bicaval cannulation and cardiopulmonary bypass are initiated, and a transverse aortotomy is performed after cardioplegic arrest. The aortic valve is excised and the annulus debrided. The sinus tissue is removed and the coronary arteries mobilized on generous buttons of sinus tissue. The pulmonary artery is carefully dissected off the aorta and top of the right ventricle until the ventricular muscle fibers are identified running in a perpendicular orientation. This portion of the dissection is begun at the commissure between the left and right coronary cusps and carried underneath the pulmonary artery. The pulmonary artery is transected near the bifurcation, and the pulmonary valve is carefully inspected.

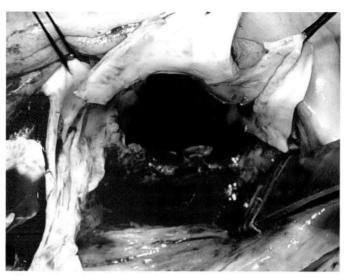

Figure 10-17

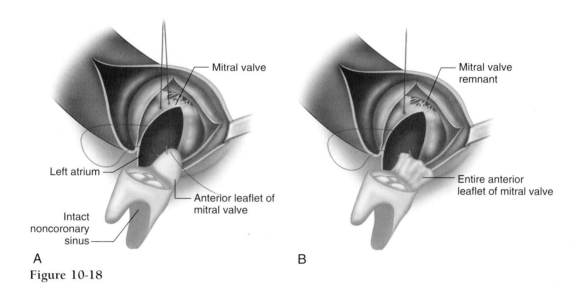

Figure 10-18

A — Mitral valve / Left atrium / Intact noncoronary sinus / Anterior leaflet of mitral valve

B — Mitral valve remnant / Entire anterior leaflet of mitral valve

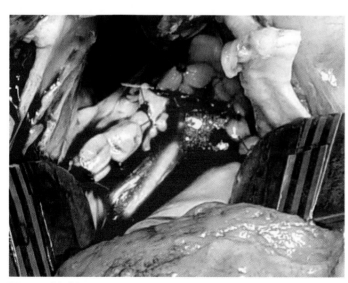

Figure 10-19

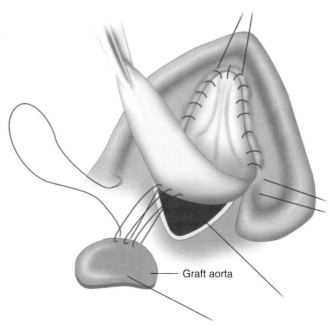

Graft aorta

Figure 10-20

- A small right-angled clamp is passed well below the pulmonary annulus along the line with the anterior commissure. The clamp is pushed out through the right ventricular free wall, and the right ventricle is divided well below the pulmonary annulus with direct visualization of the pulmonary valve leaflets. Scissors are used to divide the right ventricular outflow tract anteriorly, leaving a generous portion of the free wall with the autograft. Sharp dissection of the ventricular septum with a knife is used to separate the pulmonary trunk from the right ventricle to protect the first septal branch of the left anterior descending coronary artery.
- A vertical incision is made through the aortic annulus, near the commissure between the right and left coronary leaflets. The incision is carried into the interventricular septum to enlarge the left ventricular outflow tract (Fig. 10-21). The right ventricular muscle portion of the autograft is inserted deep into the left ventricular outflow tract (Fig. 10-22A), and interrupted sutures are used to attach it to the defect in the interventricular septum (Fig. 10-22B). The autograft is then attached to the aortic annulus with interrupted sutures. The sutures are secured and the suture line is reinforced with biologic glue.
- The coronary arteries are reimplanted onto the autograft in the appropriate position using continuous suture technique. The autograft is anastomosed to the ascending aorta with continuous suture technique, and the suture lines are reinforced with biologic glue.
- The right ventricular outflow tract is measured and an appropriately sized pulmonary homograft is selected. The distal end of the pulmonary homograft is attached to the bifurcation of the patient's pulmonary artery with continuous sutures. The proximal portion of the pulmonary homograft is attached to the right ventricular outflow tract using continuous sutures. Part of the suture line may include the pulmonary autograft. If additional enlargement of the right ventricular outflow tract is necessary, a patch of autologous pericardium is used to augment the right ventricular free wall.

Step 4. Postoperative Care

- Standard postoperative management in the intensive care unit includes ventilator support, continuous cardiac output monitoring with a pulmonary artery catheter, and other routine care for a cardiac surgical patient. Right and left atrial pressure lines are useful for direct, continuous measurement of atrial pressures.
- A judicious balance between fluid resuscitation and inotropic support is required. Many of these patients have left ventricular hypertrophy, and administration of relatively small amounts of intravenous fluids will drastically alter filling pressures. In addition, the thick ventricular myocardium is sensitive to inotropes and may be irritable after intraoperative myocardial ischemia.

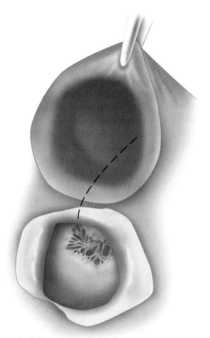
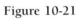

Incision into ventricular septum

Figure 10-21

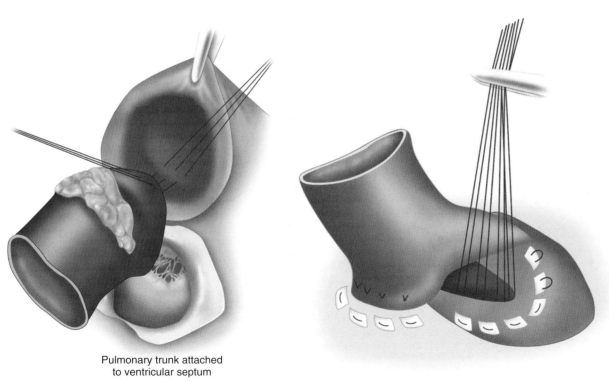

Pulmonary trunk attached
to ventricular septum

A

Figure 10-22

B

- Efforts should be made to avoid hypertension because this will place undue strain on the suture lines of the left ventricular outflow tract reconstruction. Placement of an intra-aortic balloon pump is preferable to high doses of inotropes and aggressive fluid resuscitation.
- A high index of suspicion for coronary insufficiency should be held for every patient, whether a full root replacement or simple aortic valve replacement was performed. Full root replacement with coronary reimplantation can result in kinking of a coronary artery. Prosthetic valve replacement can result in coronary ostial obstruction by a valve stent or sewing ring.
- The typical presentation of coronary insufficiency is the inability to wean from cardiopulmonary bypass. Intraoperative transesophageal echocardiography is essential to demonstrate impaired ventricular function, with or without electrocardiographic evidence of coronary ischemia. If a simple valve replacement was performed, the prosthesis should be removed and reinserted, or a different prosthesis selected. If a full root replacement was performed, the safest approach is to perform coronary artery bypass to the affected coronary artery.

Step 5. Pearls and Pitfalls

- Careful and thoughtful preoperative and intraoperative planning will avoid patient–prosthesis mismatch. In general, this is defined as a valve with an area that is insufficient relative to the patient's body surface area. It is calculated as (effective valve orifice area)/(body surface area). A value of less than 0.85 is indicative of patient–prosthesis mismatch and may result in reduced recovery of the left ventricle early and late after operation. Effort should be made to keep the ratio above 1.0 for all patients.
- Root enlargement and root replacement operations are extensive operations with multiple suture lines outside the heart exposed to systemic arterial pressure. The application of biologic glue can assist in control of intraoperative bleeding by sealing the needle holes. Biologic glue does not seal gaps in an anastomosis, and this feature allows identification of areas that require additional suture or pledgets to control hemostasis.
- The first septal branch of the left anterior descending artery should be meticulously preserved during pulmonary autograft harvest and pulmonary homograft implantation. Injury to the first septal branch can result in significant left ventricular dysfunction, which may not fully recover over time.
- The incisions described in this chapter for root enlargement are placed in areas of the aortic root that avoid the conduction system. Particular attention should be paid to the area below the commissure between the right and noncoronary leaflets, extending leftward under the right coronary artery ostium, to avoid injury to the conduction system. In addition, attempts to insert a rigid valve prosthesis tightly into a small aortic annulus can produce excessive pressure on the conduction system, resulting in dysfunction or heart block.

- The surgeon should be well versed in the long-term outcomes of the various valve prostheses that may be used in the operation. Reoperation after previous aortic root enlargement is challenging, and careful consideration should be given to the longevity of the intended prosthesis as well as to the patient's lifestyle and ability to withstand a future operation.
- Likewise, the surgeon should be prepared to perform extensive reconstruction of the aortic root and ascending aorta, as indicated during surgery. The best long-term outcomes can be expected by addressing all associated pathologic processes at the initial operation, rather than leaving behind conditions that may result in early reoperation.

Bibliography

Brown JW, Ruzmetov M, Vijay P, et al: The Ross-Konno procedure in children: Outcomes, autograft and allograft function, and reoperations. Ann Thorac Surg 2006;82:1301-1307.

Castro LJ, Arcidi JM, Fisher AL, Gaudiani VA: Routine enlargement of the small aortic root: A preventive strategy to minimize mismatch. Ann Thorac Surg 2002;74:31-36.

Doty DB: Cardiac anatomy (Chapter 1); Left ventricular outflow tract obstruction (Chapter 17); Aortic valve replacement (Chapter 31). In Cardiac Surgery: Operative Technique. St. Louis, Mosby-Year Book, 1997, pp. 6-7, 116-123, 230-231, 250-251.

Lamberti JJ: Patch aortoplasty for insertion of the porcine heterograft. J Thorac Cardiovasc Surg 1976;72:86-88.

Manouguian S, Seybold-Epting W: Patch enlargement of the aortic valve ring by extending the aortic incision into the anterior mitral leaflet: New operative technique. J Thorac Cardiovasc Surg 1979;78:402-412.

McKowen RL, Campbell DN, Woelfel GF, et al: Extended aortic root replacement with aortic allografts. J Thorac Cardiovasc Surg 1987;93:366-374.

Molina JE: Enlargement of the aortic annulus using a double-patch technique: A safe and effective method. Ann Thorac Surg 2002;73:667-670.

Najm HK, Coles JG, Black MD, et al: Extended aortic root replacement with aortic allografts or pulmonary autografts in children. J Thorac Cardiovasc Surg 1999;118:503-509.

Okuyama H, Hashimoto K, Kurosawa H, et al: Midterm results of Manouguian double valve replacement: Comparison with standard double valve replacement. J Thorac Cardiovasc Surg 2005;129:869-874.

Rastan H, Koncz J: Aortoventriculoplasty: A new technique for the treatment of left ventricular outflow tract obstruction. J Thorac Cardiovasc Surg 1976;71:920-927.

Reddy VM, Rajasinghe HA, Teitel DF, et al: Aortoventriculoplasty with the pulmonary autograft: The Ross-Konno procedure. J Thorac Cardiovasc Surg 1996;111:158-167.

Ross DB, Trusler GA, Coles JG, et al: Small aortic root in childhood: Surgical options. Ann Thorac Surg 1994;58:1617-1624.

Sakamoto Y, Hashimoto K, Okuyama H, et al: Prevalence and avoidance of patient-prosthesis mismatch in aortic valve replacement in small adults. Ann Thorac Surg 2006;81:1305-1309.

St. Rammos K, Ketikoglou DG, Koullias GJ, et al: The Nicks-Nunez posterior enlargement in the small aortic annulus: Immediate-intermediate results. Interact Cardiovasc Thorac Surg 2006;5:749-753.

Ullman MV, Gorenflo M, Sebening C, et al: Long-term results after reconstruction of the left ventricular outflow tract by aortoventriculoplasty. Ann Thorac Surg 2003;75:143-146.

CHAPTER 11

AORTIC VALVE–SPARING OPERATIONS

Tirone E. David

Step 1. Surgical Anatomy

- The aortic root is the anatomic segment between the left ventricle and the ascending aorta. From the surgical viewpoint, it consists of the aortic annulus, aortic cusps, aortic sinuses, and sinotubular junction.
- Although the term *aortic annulus* may be anatomically incorrect, it is often used in surgical anatomy and pathology to describe the aortoventricular junction.
- Approximately 45% of the circumference of the aortic root is attached to muscular interventricular septum and 55% is attached to fibrous tissue, as shown in Figure 11-1. This fibrous tissue is the membranous interventricular septum and the fibrous body that connects the anterior leaflet of the mitral valve to the aortic root.
- The aortic annulus is scalloped and attaches the aortic cusps to the aortic root and left ventricular outflow tract. The portion of the aortic annulus corresponding to the noncoronary cusp is attached entirely to fibrous tissue of the left ventricular outflow tract, whereas the portions corresponding to the left and right coronary cusps are partially attached to fibrous tissue and partially to cardiac muscle. The highest point of the aortic annulus where two cusps meet is the commissure. The anatomic arrangement of the aortic annulus creates a triangular space beneath the cusps, the *subcommissural triangle*.
- There are three commissures and three subcommissural triangles. The sinotubular junction lies immediately above the commissures and separates the aortic root from the ascending aorta. The arterial wall contained between the aortic annulus and sinotubular junction creates the aortic sinuses, or sinuses of Valsalva.
- The three aortic cusps have a crescent shape and often are of different sizes, but the length of the base of a cusp is always 1.5 times longer than the length of its free margin, as illustrated in Figure 11-2. Thus, a large cusp will have a proportionally longer base (aortic annulus [AA]), longer free margin (FM), longer intercommissural distance along the sinotubular junction (STJ), and larger aortic sinus. The noncoronary and right cusps and sinuses are often larger than the left cusp and sinus.
- The aortic annulus is a three-dimensional structure that evolves along three separate planes, as illustrated in Figure 11-3A through C. Each aortic cusp is inserted in the annulus along a horizontal plane (Fig. 11-3D). For practical purposes we usually refer to its diameter as the maximal distance at the level of its nadir.
- The relationship of the diameters of the aortic annulus at this level and at higher levels until reaching the commissures (sinotubular junction) varies with age. In children and young adults, the diameter of the aortic annulus is 15% to 20% larger than its diameter at the level of the commissures (sinotubular junction).

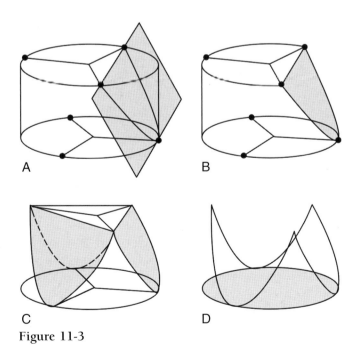

Figure 11-1

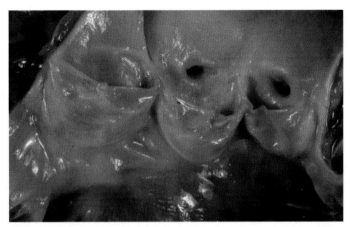

Figure 11-2

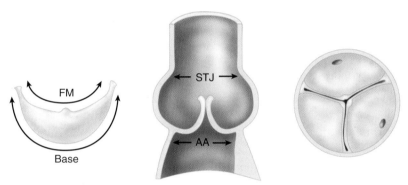

Figure 11-3

- As the elastic fibers of the arterial wall decrease with age, the sinotubular junction dilates and tends to become equal to the diameter of the lower aortic annulus in adults. However, the aortic annulus of each cusp evolves along a single horizontal plane (see Fig. 11-3).
- Ascending aortic aneurysms can cause aortic dissection or rupture when their transverse diameter exceeds 50 mm. Aneurysms of the ascending aorta can also cause dilation of the sinotubular junction with consequent aortic insufficiency due to lack of coaptation of the cusps, as illustrated in Figure 11-4.
- One or more aortic sinuses may also become dilated in patients with ascending aortic aneurysm, but the aortic annulus may remain unchanged.
- Patients with ascending aortic aneurysms and aortic insufficiency are usually in their sixth or seventh decade of life. If the aortic cusps are normal or minimally elongated along their free margins, it is possible to reconstruct the aortic root, repair the cusps if necessary, and reestablish aortic valve competence.
- Aortic root aneurysm starts at the level of the aortic sinuses and extends proximally into the aortic annulus and distally into the sinotubular junction and proximal ascending aorta.
- Patients with inherited connective tissue disorders such as Marfan syndrome or its forme fruste almost always develop dilation of the aortic annulus. The two subcommissural triangles of the noncoronary cusp flatten as the aortic annulus dilates, which decreases the coaptation area of the cusps (Fig. 11-5). This may lead to aortic insufficiency.
- Another cause of aortic insufficiency in these patients is concomitant dilation of the sinotubular junction and outward displacement of the commissures, as occurs in patients with ascending aortic aneurysm. Dilation of the sinotubular junction increases the tension on the cusps, and depending on the severity of the connective tissue disorder, the aortic cusps either may enlarge and develop stress fenestration along the commissure areas or may remain relatively unchanged.
- Patients with aortic root aneurysm are at risk of aortic dissection or rupture when the transverse diameter of the aortic sinuses exceeds 50 mm. Patients with aortic root aneurysm are often in their third or fourth decade of life when they require surgery. If the aortic cusps are normal or minimally enlarged, it is possible to reconstruct the aortic annulus, create new aortic sinuses with properly tailored tubular Dacron grafts, and repair the aortic cusps if necessary.
- This chapter reviews the operative techniques we have used to preserve the aortic valve in patients with ascending aortic aneurysm and aortic insufficiency, as well as in patients with aortic root aneurysm. The term *aortic valve–sparing operations* was introduced to describe these procedures.

Step 2. Preoperative Considerations

- Patients with ascending aortic aneurysm are usually asymptomatic even if they have aortic insufficiency. Although echocardiography often establishes the diagnosis of ascending aortic aneurysm and provides information regarding aortic valve function, computed tomography (CT) scan or magnetic resonance imaging (MRI) of the aorta is necessary to determine the extent of the aneurysm. The transverse arch is often involved in patients with aneurysm of the ascending aorta and aortic insufficiency.
- Most patients with aortic root aneurysm are asymptomatic and have only mild or no aortic insufficiency. Some patients complain of vague chest pain. Severe chest pain is suggestive of rapid expansion or intimal tear with dissection. Echocardiography establishes the diagnosis and gives information regarding the aortic valve function. CT scan or MRI of the aorta is also diagnostic and provides useful information on the remaining thoracic aorta.
- Transesophageal echocardiography is the best diagnostic tool to study the aortic valve and the mechanism of aortic insufficiency in patients with ascending aortic or aortic root aneurysms.
- Each component of the aortic root must be carefully interrogated, particularly the aortic cusps. The number of cusps, their thickness, the appearance of their free margins, and the excursion

Normal sinotubular junction   Dilated sinotubular junction

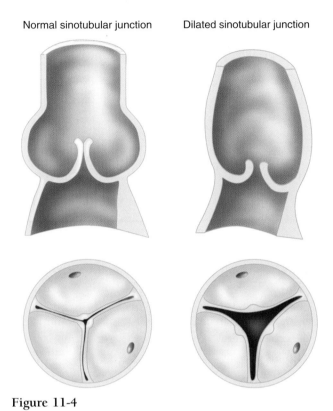

Figure 11-4

Normal aortic annulus   Dilated aortic annulus

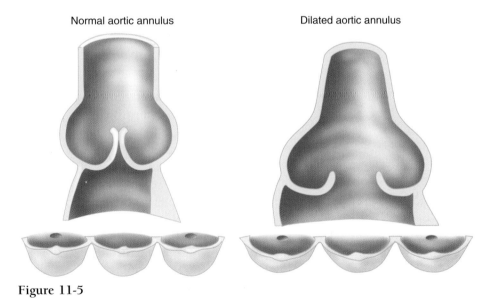

Figure 11-5

of each cusp during the cardiac cycle must be examined in multiple views. The lines of coapta tion of the aortic cusps should be interrogated by color Doppler imaging. The direction and size of the regurgitant jets should be recorded in many views. Information regarding the morphologic features of the aortic annulus, aortic sinuses, sinotubular junction, and ascending aorta should be obtained. Obviously, the aortic cusps are the most important determinant of aortic valve repair. If the cusps are thin and mobile and have smooth free margins, the feasibility of aortic valve repair is very high, including cases with bicuspid aortic valves.

Step 3. Operative Steps

- Aortic valve–sparing operations are usually performed through a full median sternotomy, but the procedure can also be done through a limited skin incision (8 to 10 cm) and partial or full median sternotomy.
- Cardiopulmonary bypass is established by inserting an arterial cannula into the proximal aortic arch if only the aortic root and proximal ascending aorta are involved, or into the right axillary or innominate artery if the aortic arch needs replacement.
- Venous drainage for cardiopulmonary bypass is usually done with a single double-stage cannula placed in the right atrium, or with bicaval cannulation when the mitral valve also needs repair.
- We protect the heart during aortic clamping by giving cold blood cardioplegia directly into the coronary arteries intermittently. We maintain the systemic temperature at around 34°C.
- If the aortic arch needs replacement, it is done first under moderate systemic hypothermia (22°C to 25°C) and continuous antegrade cerebral perfusion through the right axillary or innominate artery.
- A cannula is also inserted into the left carotid artery if the pressure in this artery is less than 50% that in the innominate artery.
- If the mitral valve needs repair, it is done before the aortic valve pathology is addressed.
- Intraoperative transesophageal echocardiography is indispensable in aortic valve–sparing operations for assessment of aortic valve function before and after repair of the valve.

1. Ascending Aortic Aneurysms with Aortic Insufficiency

- The ascending aorta is transected 6 to 8 mm above the sinotubular junction, and the aortic cusps are inspected. Although this inspection is largely to confirm what a preoperative transesophageal echocardiogram has already shown, stress fenestration close to the commissural areas and minor degrees of elongation of the free margins are not easily detected preoperatively.
- The aortic insufficiency is usually due to dilation of the sinotubular junction, and correction of the valve dysfunction is accomplished by reducing the diameter of the sinotubular junction by suturing a graft of appropriate diameter to it. The simplest method to determine the diameter of the graft is to approximate the three commissures until the cusps coapt centrally. Valve sizers such as the Toronto SPV (St. Jude Medical, St. Paul, Minn) or Medtronic Freestyle (Medtronic, Minneapolis, Minn) are metric and handy for this purpose. When in doubt between two sizes, it is safer to take the larger one because the sinotubular junction can be further reduced under echocardiographic guidance after completion of the operation by plication of the spaces between two commissures. In adult patients, grafts of small calibers may increase left ventricular afterload. Thus, if the estimated diameter of the sinotubular junction is 22 mm in a patient with a body surface area of 2 m^2, a larger graft (26 or 28 mm) should be used and reduced to 22 mm at the end of the procedure where is going to be used to correct the diameter of the sinotubular junction. Figure 11-6 illustrates this operative procedure. Before the graft is sutured to the sinotubular junction, the graft should be divided into thirds to correspond to each commissure.

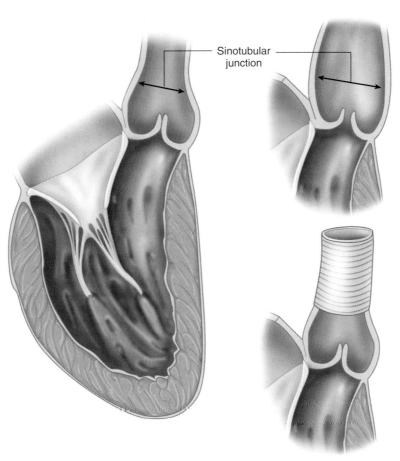

Figure 11-6

If one cusp is larger than the others, the third used for this sinus should be proportionately larger.

- If the noncoronary aortic sinus is excessively dilated or dissected (in cases of aortic dissection), it should be replaced. The graft is divided into thirds according to the spaces between commissures, and a neo-aortic sinus is fashioned, as illustrated in Figure 11-7A and B.
- The height of the tailored neo-aortic sinus should be approximately the same as the diameter of the graft. It actually is taller than the diameter because the graft is corrugated and stretches along its longitudinal axis.
- Next, the commissures of the noncoronary cusp are secured to the graft, and the neo-aortic sinus is sutured to the remnant of the arterial wall and aortic annulus with 4-0 polypropylene sutures. The remaining part of the graft is sutured to the sinotubular junction along the left and right aortic sinuses.
- If the noncoronary and right aortic sinuses are dilated or dissected, they should be replaced as described previously and illustrated in Figure 11-8. In this case, the right coronary artery should be reimplanted into its neo-aortic sinus.

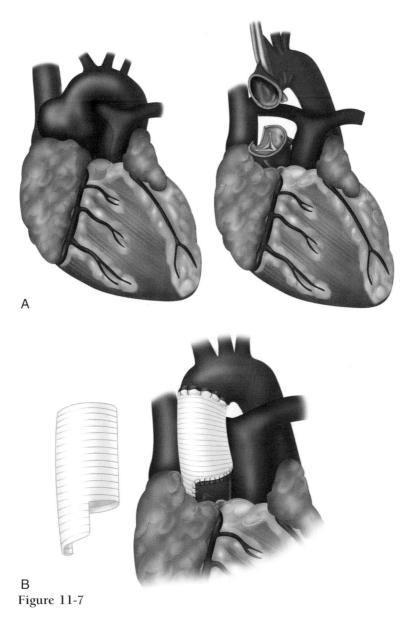

A

B
Figure 11-7

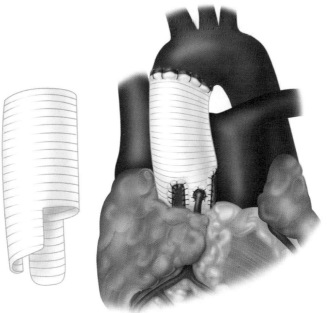

Figure 11-8

- Finally, if all three aortic sinuses are dilated, the sinuses are excised, leaving 5 mm of arterial wall attached to the aortic annulus. The coronary arteries are detached from their sinuses along with 5 mm of arterial wall around their orifices (Fig. 11-9A).
- The three commissures are suspended at the same level and positioned in such way as to allow the three cusps to coapt centrally (Fig. 11-9B). The diameter of the circle that includes all three commissures can be estimated with metric aortic valve sizers. As before, when in doubt between two sizes, it is safer to choose the larger one. Three neo-aortic sinuses are tailored in one of the ends of the graft, as illustrated in Figure 11-9C. The width of the neo-aortic sinuses is proportional to the size of the cusps and intercommissural distances.
- The arterial wall immediately above the commissures is secured to the graft, and the neo-aortic sinuses are sutured to the remnants of the native aortic sinuses and aortic annulus with continuous 4-0 polypropylene sutures (Fig. 11-9D).
- The coronary arteries are reimplanted into their respective sinuses (Fig. 11-9E). To avoid late aneurysm formation in the arterial buttons, the diameter of the openings in the neo-aortic sinuses should not exceed twice the diameter of the coronary arteries.

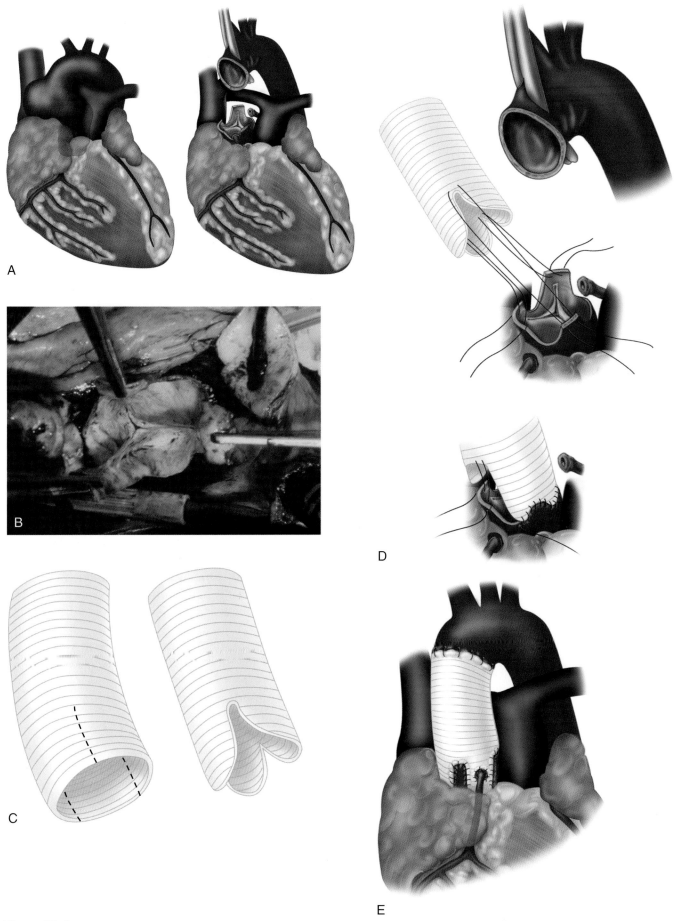

Figure 11-9

- The foregoing operative techniques are known as "remodeling of the aortic root." After correction of the dilated sinotubular junction and replacement of one or more aortic sinuses as described previously, the cusps should coapt well above the level of the nadir of the aortic annulus. If one or more cusps coapts at a lower level than the others, the free margin is elongated and should be shortened by plication along the nodule of Arantius, as illustrated in Figure 11-10. This is done with a 6-0 or 5-0 polypropylene suture, depending on the thickness of the cusp.
- A cusp with stress fenestration along its commissural edge can be reinforced by weaving a double layer of a fine (6-0 or 7-0) polytetrafluoroethylene along its free margin, as illustrated in Figure 11-11.
- After completion of the aortic root remodeling, valve competence is assessed by injecting cardioplegia into the graft under pressure. If the ventricle does not distend, there is no aortic insufficiency, or only trace.

2. Aortic Root Aneurysm

- Although the previously described aortic root remodeling procedure with replacement of all three aortic sinuses has been used to treat patients with aortic root aneurysm, we believe that the aortic annulus dilates in some patients late after surgery, limiting the durability of the valve repair. This is particularly true in young patients with Marfan syndrome or its forme fruste. Thus, in young adults with aortic root aneurysm the technique of reimplantation of the aortic valve may provide more durable results. This operation is more complicated than remodeling the aortic root because greater knowledge of the functional anatomy of the aortic valve is needed to reconstruct the aortic annulus, the sinotubular junction, the aortic sinuses, and sometimes the aortic cusps as well.
- Reimplantation of the aortic valve starts by freeing the aortic root from surrounding structures and excising the three aortic sinuses, as described earlier for the remodeling procedure (see Fig. 11-9A and B).
- Six to 8 mm of sinus wall is left attached to the aortic annulus all around. Stay sutures are placed immediately above each commissure for traction.
- The aortic root then is dissected free from the pulmonary artery and right ventricle down to a level immediately below the aortic annulus. On the right side of the aortic root, it may be difficult, if not impossible, to separate the subcommissural triangles of the noncoronary cusp from the right and left atria because their insertion in the root may be at a higher level than the base of those triangles. The dissection is extended down to the level of the insertion of the atria in the aortic root.

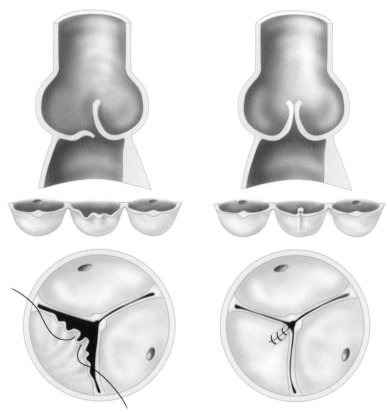

Figure 11-10

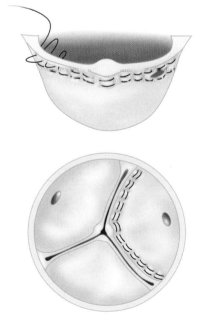

Figure 11-11

◆ Next, multiple horizontal mattress sutures of 2-0 or 3-0 polyester are passed from the inside to the outside of the left ventricular outflow tract, immediately below the nadir of the aortic annulus, through a single horizontal plane along the fibrous portion of the outflow tract, and along its scalloped shape in the interventricular septum, as illustrated in Figure 11-12A. These sutures are passed through the base of the subcommissural triangles of the noncoronary cusp, along a horizontal plane that corresponds to a level immediately below the nadir of the aortic annulus. These sutures may incorporate part of the right and left atria if their insertion is higher than that horizontal plane. If the membranous septum or anterior leaflet of the mitral valve is very thin, Teflon pledgets should be used in these sutures.

◆ The heights of the cusps are averaged and a tubular Dacron graft of diameter equal to the double of that average is selected for reconstruction of the root. Conversely, the diameter of the graft can be estimated as described for the remodeling technique and adding 5 to 6 mm.

◆ Three equidistant marks are placed in one end of graft to correspond to each commissure.

◆ A triangular segment of 5 to 6 mm is cut off along the mark that corresponds to the subcommissural triangle of the left and right cusps (see Fig. 11-12A).

◆ The sutures previously placed in the left ventricular outflow tract are now passed through the graft. The sutures should be spaced symmetrically if the aortic annulus is not dilated (Fig. 11-12B).

◆ If there is obvious dilation of the aortic annulus, the sutures should be spaced symmetrically along the muscular interventricular septum and the nadir of the aortic annulus, but closer together beneath the subcommissural triangles of the noncoronary cusp because that is where dilation occurs in patients with connective tissue disorders.

◆ The sutures are tied on the outside of the graft. Care must be exercised not to pursestring this suture line.

◆ The graft is then cut in a length of approximately 5 cm and pulled up gently, and the three commissures are also pulled vertically and temporarily secured to the graft with transfixing 4-0 polypropylene sutures, but they are not tied (Fig. 11-12C).

◆ Once the three commissures are suspended inside the graft, the commissures and the cusps are inspected to make sure they are all correctly aligned.

◆ Next, the sutures are tied on the outside of the graft and used to secure the aortic annulus into the graft. This is accomplished by passing the suture sequentially from the inside to the outside right at the level of the annulus, and from the outside to the inside at the level of the remnants of the arterial wall.

◆ We start at the level of the commissure and stop at the nadir of the aortic annulus, where the sutures are tied together on the outside of the graft. The coronary arteries are reimplanted into their respective sinuses.

◆ The coaptation of the aortic cusps is inspected. The coaptation level should be at least 5 mm above the nadir of the aortic annulus.

◆ If one or two cusps coapt at a lower lever, the free margin can be shortened, as illustrated in Figure 11-10 and Figure 11-12D.

◆ If fenestrations are present, the free margin can be reinforced with a double layer of 6-0 or 7-0 polytetrafluoroethylene suture (see Fig. 11-11).

◆ Finally, neo-aortic sinuses are created by plicating the graft between two commissures, as illustrated in Figure 11-12E. For every 3 mm of horizontal plication, the diameter of the graft is reduced by 1 mm.

◆ Valve competence can be assessed by injecting cardioplegia into the graft and inspecting the ventricle for distention, or by echocardiography.

◆ The mean graft size used in our patients for the reimplantation procedure with creation of neo-aortic sinuses has been 32 mm (range, 28 to 34 mm).

◆ We have also used reimplantation of the aortic valve in patients with bicuspid aortic valve and aortic insufficiency because they frequently have a dilated aortic annulus. Similarly, patients with acute type A aortic dissection who have a dilated aortic root are also good candidates for this type of aortic valve–sparing procedure.

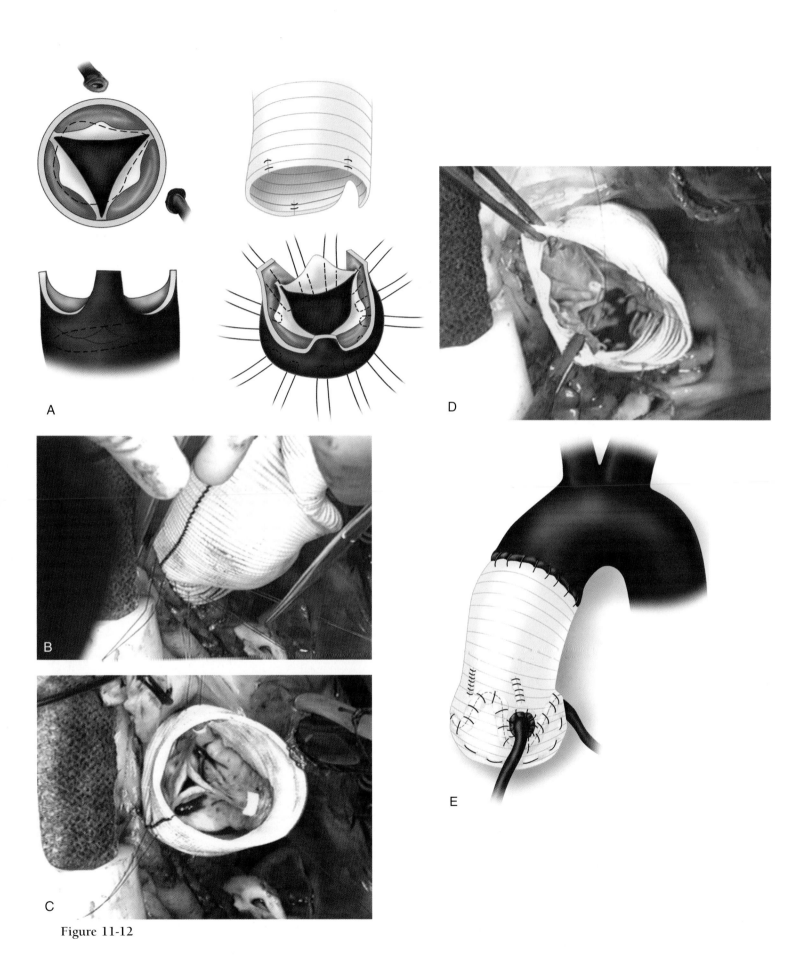

Figure 11-12

Step 4. Postoperative Care

- The operative mortality rate for aortic valve–sparing operations has been low in our experience (<2%), even in patients who require more extensive operations, including replacement of the aortic arch and myocardial revascularization. These patients do not require any procedure-specific care in the intensive care unit or ward.
- In our experience, patients with ascending aortic aneurysm and aortic insufficiency often have transverse arch and mega-aorta syndrome and require more extensive vascular surgery than those with aortic root aneurysm, with consequent higher rates of postoperative complications such as stroke, myocardial infarction, renal failure, and respiratory failure.
- However, over 90% of all patients experience no serious postoperative complication.
- Postoperative bleeding is relatively common and many require blood transfusion.
- Heart block has never occurred in over 350 patients who have had these operations in our unit. Atrial fibrillation occurs in approximately 20% of these patients and is managed pharmacologically.
- Patients with Marfan syndrome and those with acute type A aortic dissection are given a beta blocker if they tolerate it. No oral anticoagulation is given unless atrial fibrillation persists for more than 24 hours, in which case they receive heparin and warfarin.
- Echocardiographic studies to assess aortic valve function should be performed annually in all patients. In those with more extensive vascular disease or aortic dissection, annual CT scan or MRI of the aorta is also important during follow-up.

Step 5. Pearls and Pitfalls

- Aortic valve–sparing operations are complex procedures. A sound knowledge of the functional anatomy and pathology of the aortic root and technical expertise are needed for their performance.
- As with any other type of heart valve repair, it should not be performed if the aortic cusps are grossly abnormal.
- From the preoperative selection of patients by transesophageal echocardiography to the intra-operative analysis of the aortic cusps and root and what is needed to restore the functional anatomy of the aortic valve, every step is crucial.
- Sizing of the graft is difficult for the surgeon who is learning to do these operations. Sizing of the graft is easier for remodeling of the aortic root than for reimplantation of the aortic valve.
- The guidelines for sizing the graft for reimplantation of the aortic valve given in this chapter are based more on clinical experience than on scientific investigation of functional anatomy.
- The length of the free margins, the degree of scalloping of the aortic annulus, and the diameter of the sinotubular junction can all be altered during reconstruction of the root, but the height of the cusps cannot. For this reason, we use the average height of the cusps to estimate the appropriate diameter of the aortic annulus at the level of its nadir.
- By using grafts with a diameter equal to twice the average height of the cusps, the radius of the reconstructed aortic annulus becomes equal to the height minus the thickness of the aortic annulus, because it is sutured inside of the graft. This reduction in diameter of the annulus has proven effective in allowing the cusps to coapt well above the nadir of the annulus, and it provides a good seal of the aortic orifice during diastole.

◆ The height of coaptation of the aortic cusps has been shown to be important for the durability of these procedures. If the cusps coapt at the same level as the annulus, the probability of prolapse of a cusp with consequent aortic insufficiency is greatly increased, compared with cusps that coapt at least 5 mm above the lowest level of the aortic annulus. Thus, sizing of the graft and shortening the length of the cusps' free margins are extremely important determinants of late valve function.

◆ Aortic valve–sparing operations are extensive, and hemostatic anastomoses between the various components are of utmost importance. Coagulopathy at the end of long cardiopulmonary bypass is common, and every measure must be taken to avoid it. We often use antifibrinolytic agents in these cases.

Bibliography

Birks EJ, Webb C, Child A, et al: Early and long-term results of a valve-sparing operation for Marfan syndrome. Circulation 1999;100 (Suppl II):II29-II35.

David TE, Feindel CM, Webb GD, et al: Long term results of aortic valve sparing operations for aortic root aneurysms. J Thorac Cardiovasc Surg 2006;132:347-354.

de Oliveira NC, David TE, Ivanov J, et al: Results of surgery for aortic root aneurysm in patients with Marfan syndrome. J Thorac Cardiovasc Surg 2003;125:789-796.

Grande-Allen KJ, Cochran RP, Reinhall PG, Kunzelman KS: Re-creation of sinuses is important for sparing the aortic valve: A finite element study. J Thorac Cardiovasc Surg 2000;119:753-763.

Kunzelman KS, Grande J, David TE, et al: Aortic root and valve relationships: Impact on surgical repair. J Thorac Cardiovasc Surg 1994;107:162-170.

Yacoub MH, Gehle P, Chandrasekaran V, et al: Late results of a valve-preserving operation in patients with aneurysms of the ascending aorta and root. J Thorac Cardiovasc Surg 1998;115:1080-1090.

CHAPTER 12

BENTALL PROCEDURE

Richard J. Shemin

- In 1968, Bentall and De Bono[1] described a technique for composite aortic valve and root replacement with reimplantation of the coronary arteries. The coronary arteries were sewn to the graft as a side-to-side anastomosis, and the aneurysm wall was wrapped around the graft.
- During the ensuing years this technique underwent various modifications, primarily because of pseudoaneurysm formation at the side-to-side anastomosis of the coronary button to the graft.
- The Bentall operation currently uses a technique for treating combined disease of the aortic valve and aortic root with a button Bentall operation, a modification of the original technique described by Kouchoukos and coworkers in 1991.[2]
- All operations are performed by creating an open distal anastomosis when there is an inadequate cuff of normal aorta below the cross-clamp or by replacing the entire arch during a period of deep hypothermic circulatory arrest.
- The modified Bentall procedure is the procedure of choice in most centers when treating the aortic valve, aortic sinuses, and ascending aorta.

Step 1. Surgical Anatomy

- The pertinent anatomy consists of the aortic valve and related pathology, sinuses of Valsalva, coronary ostia, ascending aorta, and aortic arch. Specific pathologic processes present different challenges in a Bentall procedure. The more common situations are bicuspid aortic valve stenosis (AS) or aortic regurgitation (AR) with dilated ascending aorta; AR and ascending aortic aneurysm (e.g., Marfan syndrome); and acute or chronic aortic dissection.

Step 2. Preoperative Considerations

- The planning of the procedure requires a preoperative echocardiogram and cardiac catheterization with coronary angiography and aortic root angiography with panning into the aortic arch. A carotid artery Doppler examination may be useful. The use of a contrast magnetic resonance imaging or computed tomography scan can help measure the extent and size of the aneurysm.

- The choice of valve should be determined in consultation with the patient.
- If there is no associated coronary disease, the procedure can be performed through a minister-notomy. In this case, peripheral venous cannulation is often necessary because of limited access to the right atrial appendage.
- The need for circulatory arrest and possible electroencephalographic (EEG) monitoring should be determined if the arch is involved or if the aneurysm extends distally to the level of the innominate artery. When circulatory arrest is required, decisions about cerebral protection need to be made with regard to technique and cardiopulmonary bypass setup.
- A plan for cardioplegia administration is essential, especially if a ministernotomy is to be used.
- Special consideration is given to the treatment of postprocedure coagulopathy. Administration of aminocaproic acid (Amicar), platelets, and coagulation factors is often necessary.

Step 3. Operative Steps

- The Bentall procedure can be performed, through either a median sternotomy or a minister-notomy, with a 4-cm vertical skin incision over the upper sternum and the sternal split extending from the sternal notch to the right fourth interspace ("J"-shaped sternotomy).
- Cannulation for cardiopulmonary bypass can be through the ascending aorta, transverse arch, or femoral artery in most patients. Often it is best, especially in cases of aortic dissection, to establish perfusion through the right axillary artery after attaching a side graft (8-mm Gore-Tex). This is a safe and effective technique.
- The site chosen for cannulation depends on the anatomy, extent of pathology, and indications for the operation. For example, the femoral or axillary artery is preferred for aortic dissections. The upper ascending aorta or arch is a safe and convenient site in aneurysmal disease. If the replacement extends into the aortic arch, the arterial perfusion cannula will be removed during the circulatory arrest period with subsequent recannulation of the graft, directly or through a side limb. Venous cannulation is through the right atrial appendage, with a double-stage cannula or occasionally with a femoral venous cannula, inserted by cut-down or percutaneously with a Seldinger technique. The position of the cannula in the right atrium is confirmed with trans-esophageal echocardiography.
- To protect the heart, cold blood cardioplegia solutions are infused antegrade directly into the coronary ostia or retrograde through the coronary sinus. Topical cold saline can augment myocardial cooling. Systemic cooling to a temperature of 34°C is sufficient for routine replacement of the aortic root, but a temperature of 12°C to 18°C is necessary during the period of circulatory arrest. An isoelectric tracing on the EEG monitor can be a biologic guide to circulatory arrest. Antegrade and retrograde cerebral perfusion techniques should be used.
- A vent inserted into the right superior pulmonary vein and placed into the left ventricle or a pulmonary artery vent allows decompression of the heart. With severe aortic insufficiency, the heart will distend in spite of venting the left ventricle, especially during fibrillation induced during the cooling period.
- Cardiac distention during cooling will require cross-clamping the aorta and the initiation of cardioplegic arrest. As cooling continues, the proximal portion of the procedure can be performed (valve replacement and coronary button reimplantation). As soon as the goal temperature is achieved in circulatory arrest cases, the proximal portion of the procedure is stopped and the arch replacement performed. Antegrade cerebral perfusion can extend the safe circulatory arrest time, and retrograde perfusion is most effective in preventing debris and air from embolizing into the cerebral circulation. After the arch replacement is completed the graft can be cannulated or, if the axillary artery has been used, antegrade perfusion and de-airing of the arch are initiated. Rewarming is begun, and the proximal portion of the procedure is completed.

1. Proximal Portion of the Procedure

◆ The aorta is transected below the cross-clamp, leaving a cuff of aorta for the distal anastomosis. The proximal aorta is opened with a longitudinal incision. The incision is extended toward the noncoronary sinus to avoid the right coronary artery ostia, which may have migrated high owing to the aneurysm. Buttons of aortic tissue around the ostia of the coronary arteries are created and mobilized (Fig. 12-1).

◆ The right coronary artery must be adequately mobilized to prevent later torsion after reanastomosis to the graft (Fig. 12-2).

◆ The aortic valve is excised and the annulus debrided of all calcium. After sizing of the aortic annulus, a series of pledgeted mattress sutures are placed (Fig. 12-3A and B).

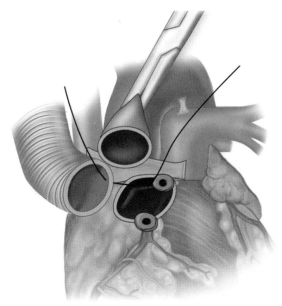

Figure 12-1

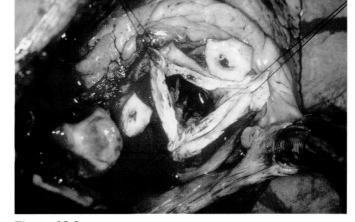

Figure 12-2

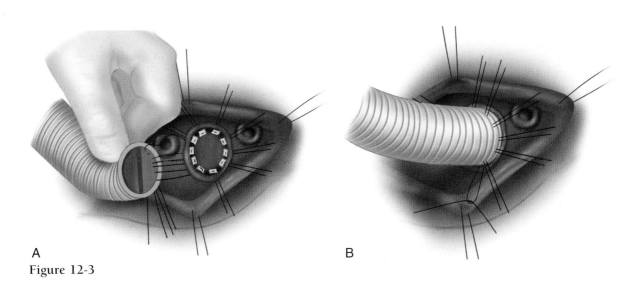

A

B

Figure 12-3

- If a bioprosthetic valve is to be used, the suture needle is passed from the ventricular to the aortic aspect of the annulus for fixation of a heterograft in a supra-annular position.
- For a mechanical prosthetic valve, the sutures are placed from the aortic to the ventricular aspect of the annulus to effect intra-annular fixation of the valve (Fig. 12-4A and B).
- Figure 12-4A and B shows details of the intra-annular everting technique for valve implantation. Visualization of this anastomosis for hemostasis will not be possible until the heart is ejecting, and inspection of the annular areas beneath the coronary buttons will be almost impossible. These sutures must be placed close together and tied tightly to create a hemostatic seal.
- If the annulus is small and a larger valve is desired, a mechanical valve can be placed in a supra-annular position using the technique for the bioprosthetic valve.
- A composite graft consisting of a St. Jude valve (St. Jude Medical, St. Paul, Minn) and a Hemashield graft (Boston Scientific Corp., Wayne, NJ) is used in cases for which a mechanical valve is indicated (Fig. 12-5).
- In cases in which a biologic valve is chosen, a homemade composite, consisting of a stented pericardial valve (Edwards Lifesciences LLC, Irvine, Calif) or porcine valve (Medtronic, Inc., Minneapolis) and a Hemashield graft, is used. The size of the Hemashield graft should equal the outer diameter of the valve sewing cuff. A running 4-0 polypropylene suture is used to attach the graft to the sewing cuff.
- A homograft and an autograft (Ross procedure) are composite biologic conduits. The Freestyle porcine valve (Medtronic) is a valve-and-aorta composite biologic device.
- After the valve suture line is completed, the buttons including the coronary ostia are prepared. Minimal mobilization of the left coronary artery is necessary. The first centimeter of the right coronary artery is mobilized. The buttons are implanted in an end-to-side fashion with a running 6-0 suture, incorporating a polytetrafluoroethylene (Teflon) felt strip to reinforce the adventitial surface of the coronary arteries (Fig. 12-6A and B).

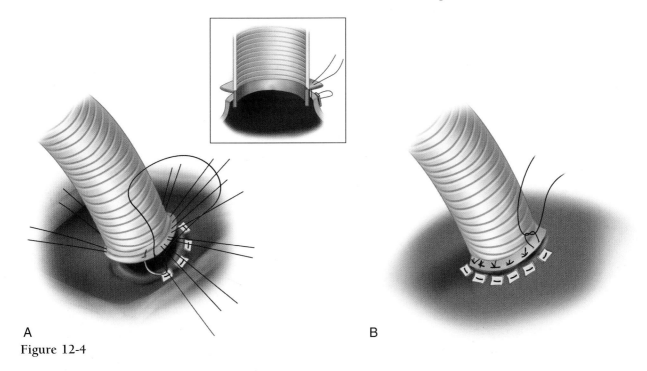

A

Figure 12-4

B

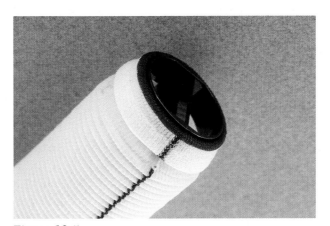

Figure 12-5

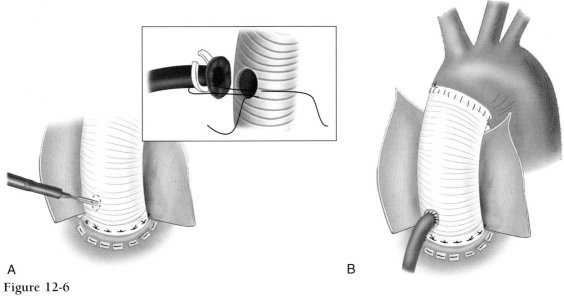

A

Figure 12-6

B

- The valve is tied down and the reattachment of the left coronary artery is completed. The length of the graft is determined by clamping the distal end of the graft and stretching the graft by distending it with antegrade cardioplegia. The left main suture line is tested for leaks during this maneuver. Excess graft material is removed with the ophthalmic cautery to prevent fraying of the Dacron material. The distal graft-to-aorta or graft-to-graft (if an arch replacement was performed) anastomosis is completed with 4-0 polypropylene running suture that can be reinforced with Teflon felt.
- Cardioplegia is readministered antegrade into the graft. With the graft distended, the correct position to anastomose the right coronary button can be accurately determined to avoid tension and torsion (Fig. 12-7). The right coronary artery is sewn (6-0 polypropylene) to the graft. Warm cardioplegia is administered retrograde and then antegrade into the graft, allowing a final check of the suture lines for bleeding, before completing the air maneuvers and removal of the cross-clamp.
- Rarely, the coronary arteries cannot be mobilized to reach the prosthetic aortic graft. Dacron graft extensions are a possible option (Fig. 12-8A and B).
- The Cabrol technique using a simple Dacron graft is illustrated in Figure 12-9. The ends of the tubular graft are sewn end-to-end to the coronary arteries. The length and orientation of the graft should be carefully planned. The body of the graft is sewn side-to-side to the aortic graft, providing inflow and distribution to the coronary arteries.

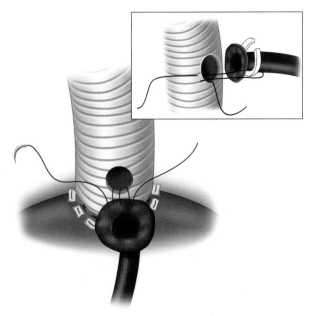

Figure 12-7

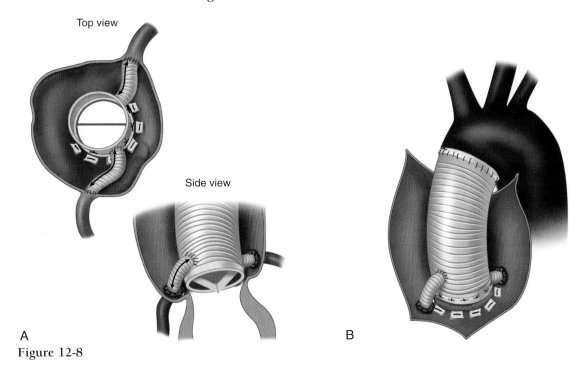

Top view

Side view

A
Figure 12-8

B

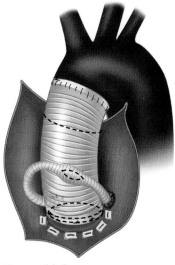

Figure 12-9

2. Bentall with Arch Replacement

- To allow open distal anastomosis or total aortic arch reconstruction, the patient's head is placed downward, cardiopulmonary bypass is discontinued, and the aorta is trimmed appropriately for the extent of the replacement. The anastomosis between the trimmed Dacron graft and the aorta is performed with a 4-0 polypropylene running suture, reinforced by an outer Teflon felt strip. Before cardiopulmonary bypass is resumed, the head vessels are carefully aspirated to remove air and particulate debris. Selective cerebral perfusion is discontinued, and in cases with an especially high risk of embolization, a brief period of retrograde perfusion through the superior vena cava, at a pressure of 20 mm Hg, can be useful to further flush out air and debris.
- The heart is reperfused and allowed to resume sinus rhythm. Defibrillation is used if necessary. Atrial and ventricular bipolar pacing wires are placed. Adequacy of air removal from the cardiac chambers is monitored with transesophageal echocardiography.
- Cardiopulmonary bypass is discontinued when a bladder temperature of 37°C is reached. Hemostasis often requires transfusion of clotting factors and platelets. Appropriate drainage tubes are placed in the mediastinum.
- A variety of biologic glues are available. It is often helpful to seal the suture lines with glue when they are dry. When used, the glues should be applied sparingly. Overapplication of glues may prevent observation of important surgical leaks that require suture repair. In most cases, I do not routinely use glues. Only when the aorta is very friable, thin, or dissected do I apply a biologic glue.

Step 4. Postoperative Care

- The basic principles of hemodynamic monitoring of the cardiac surgical patient after aortic valve replacement apply. Specific considerations relate to the extent of root and arch replacement. Neurologic assessment is important. Close monitoring for excessive bleeding or tamponade is essential and may prompt urgent return to the operating room for exploration and evacuation of hematoma. Monitoring for myocardial ischemia or right ventricular dysfunction can indicate a problem with the coronary buttons, most commonly the right button.
- If a mechanical composite conduit was implanted, anticoagulation with warfarin can be started on the first postoperative day. I do not use heparin unless the international normalized ratio (INR) has not responded by the fourth or fifth postoperative day. The target INR is 2.5.
- The recent introduction of home testing of coagulation status offers a new opportunity for improved follow-up of patients undergoing mechanical valve replacement. Data suggest that the ability to monitor the INR at home results in improved maintenance of in-range values compared with a laboratory-based testing regimen[3] and may translate into a lower frequency of bleeding and thrombotic complications.[4] Furthermore, Schmidtke and coworkers[5] demonstrated that self-management of anticoagulation leads to a superior quality of life after mechanical valve replacement compared with conventional physician-monitored anticoagulation.

- If a bioprosthetic composite valve was used, I do not prescribe warfarin, only aspirin.
- An echocardiogram before discharge is helpful to ensure normal valve and myocardial function and to evaluate residual pericardial hematoma. As in any group of patients with aneurysms or dissections, a significant number of patients in this series required subsequent operations for aneurysms elsewhere in the aorta. This reinforces previous observations indicating that conscientious postoperative follow-up of patients with disease in the ascending aorta is mandatory.
- The practice of monitoring patients with yearly computed tomographic scans is necessary when an aneurysm has been resected as part of the procedure.
- Bentall failures are rare during long-term follow-up. The Bentall technique is safe and durable, with a low incidence of postoperative complications in a population with disease of the ascending aorta and aortic valve.
- The lower frequency of reoperation is a major advantage compared with the results of valve-sparing approaches, in which significant aortic insufficiency develops in a variable proportion of patients.
- Because the Bentall operation is associated with excellent short- and long-term results, aggressive use of this operation is appropriate if aortic valve surgery is necessary in a patient with even mild ascending aortic dilation.
- The Bentall operation is considered the standard procedure against which to measure the outcomes of newer valve-sparing approaches to aortic root disease.

Step 5. Pearls and Pitfalls

- "Cut well and sew well and the patient will do well."
- "The right operation, for the right indication, that is well executed helps ensure clinical success."
- Preoperative planning is very important. Understanding the extent of the pathologic process involving the valve, aorta, and coronary arteries is essential. Three-dimensional reconstructions of the aortic contrast-enhanced computed tomography scan provide very helpful information.
- Proper creation and mobilization of the coronary buttons will prevent kinking and twisting. If the coronary arteries are adequately mobilized, especially the right coronary artery, it is rarely necessary to use graft extensions or the Cabrol technique. Redo Bentalls, as well as endocarditis and other inflammatory diseases involving the base of the aortic root, are situations in which adequate mobilization of the arteries may not be possible.
- Secure suturing of the valve to the annulus is essential. This anastomosis cannot be tested. Any leaks under the left or right coronary arteries are impossible to visualize if a repair suture is necessary.
- The graft should be distended with cardioplegia to test the left coronary anastomosis after it is performed, because this is a location that will be difficult to visualize later. With the graft distended, the length to the distal aorta can be determined. I perform the distal end-to-end anastomosis and redistend the graft with cardioplegia to accurately determine the exact location for the right coronary anastomosis. This technique, along with proper mobilization of the right coronary, prevents technical errors leading to inadequate flow through the coronary artery.
- Do not leave the operating room without achieving good hemostasis.

References

1. Bentall H., De Bono A: A technique for complete replacement of the ascending aorta. Thorax 1968;23:338-339.
2. Kouchoukos NT, Wareing TH, Murphy SF, Perrillo JB: Sixteen-year experience with aortic root replacement: Results of 172 operations. Ann Surg 1991;214:308-320.
3. Rosengart TK: Anticoagulation self-testing after heart valve replacement. J Heart Valve Dis 2002;11(Suppl 1):S61-S65.
4. Kortke H, Korfer R: International normalized ratio self-management after mechanical heart valve replacement: Is an early start advantageous? Ann Thorac Surg 2001;72:44-48.
5. Schmidtke C, Huppe M, Berndt S, et al: Quality of life after aortic valve replacement: Self-management or conventional anticoagulation therapy after mechanical valve replacement plus pulmonary autograft. Z Kardiol 2001;90:860-866.

Bibliography

Birks EJ, Webb C, Child A, et al: Early and long-term results of a valve-sparing operation for Marfan syndrome. Circulation 1999;100(19 Suppl):II-29-II-35.

David TE, Armstrong S, Ivanov J, Webb GD: Aortic valve sparing operations: An update. Ann Thorac Surg 1999;67:1840-1856.

Ehrlich MP, Ergin MA, McCullough JN, et al: Favorable outcome after composite valve-graft replacement in patients older than 65 years. Ann Thorac Surg 2000;71:1454-1459.

Ergin MA, Griepp EB, Lansman SL, et al: Hypothermic circulatory arrest and other methods of cerebral protection during operations on the thoracic aorta. J Card Surg 1994;9:525-537.

Hagl C, Ergin MA, Galla JD, et al: Neurologic outcome after ascending aorta-aortic arch operations: Effect of brain protection technique in high-risk patients. J Thorac Cardiovasc Surg 2001;121:1107-1121.

Hagl C, Galla JD, Spielvogel D, et al: Diabetes and evidence of atherosclerosis are major risk factors for adverse outcome after elective thoracic aortic surgery. J Thorac Cardiovasc Surg 2003;126:1005-1012.

Harringer W, Pethig K, Hagl C, et al: Ascending aortic replacement with aortic valve reimplantation. Circulation 1999;100(19 Suppl):II-24-II-28.

Kallenbach K, Karck M, Leyh RG, et al: Valve-sparing aortic root reconstruction in patients with significant aortic insufficiency. Ann Thorac Surg 2002;74(Suppl):S1765-S1799.

Luciani GB, Casali G, Tomezzoli A, Mazzucco A: Recurrence of aortic insufficiency after aortic root remodeling with valve preservation. Ann Thorac Surg 1999;67:1849-1852.

Schafers HJ, Langer F, Aicher D, et al: Remodeling of the aortic root and reconstruction of the bicuspid aortic valve. Ann Thorac Surg 2000;70:542-546.

Yacoub MH, Gehle P, Chandrasekaran V, et al: Late results of a valve-preserving operation in patients with aneurysms of the ascending aorta and root. J Thorac Cardiovasc Surg 1998;115:1080-1190.

Yotsumoto G, Moriyama Y, Toyohira H, et al: Congenital bicuspid aortic valve: Analysis of 63 surgical cases. J Heart Valve Dis 1998;7:500-503.

Zehr KJ, Thubrikar MJ, Gong GG, et al: Clinical introduction of a novel prosthesis for valve-preserving aortic root reconstruction for annuloaortic ectasia. J Thorac Cardiovasc Surg 2000;120:692-698.

CHAPTER 13

AORTIC HOMOGRAFTS

Nahush A. Mokadam and Edward D. Verrier

- An aortic homograft describes a cadaveric aortic root that has been procured and preserved using a variety of techniques. Also known as an *allograft*, the first aortic homograft was implanted in 1956 by Gordon Murray in the descending aorta for the treatment of severe aortic insufficiency. Over the next several years, techniques were established such that orthotopic implantation was both practical and successful. The first series using aortic homografts was reported in 1964 by Barratt-Boyes, in which 41 of 44 patients experienced fair to good results. Homograft procurement and preservation has evolved over the last 40 years. Initially, homografts were implanted shortly after procurement. This technique was quickly replaced with procedures consistent with modern tissue banking. Chemical preservation, freeze-drying, and antibiotic sterilization were all used, but the most consistently used technique for tissue banking today remains cryopreservation, first introduced in 1975.

- In the United States, the majority of aortic homografts are obtained from beating-heart donors whose hearts are not suitable for transplantation. The secondary source is from cadavers less than 24 hours old. Because modern tissue banking is now regionalized into specialized centers, the majority of homografts are implanted at an average interval of 3.9 days, using cryopreservation.

- Finally, it should be noted that the implantation techniques described here can be applied to the implantation of stentless bioprostheses, such as the Toronto SPV valve and the Medtronic Freestyle valve.

Step 1. Surgical Anatomy

- It is critical during any aortic valve procedure to have a thorough understanding of the three-dimensional relationships of the aortic valve to the other heart chambers, the coronary arteries, the other valves, and the conduction system (Fig. 13-1A).
- The aortic root separates the left ventricular outflow tract from the aorta. The aortic root is a complex structure, consisting of the aortic annulus, the aortic cusps, the sinuses of Valsalva, and the sinotubular junction.
- The aortic annulus attaches the aortic cusps and sinuses of Valsalva to the left ventricle. Like the subaortic apparatus, the majority of the annular circumference is fibrous tissue consisting of the anterior leaflet of the mitral valve and the membranous septum. The bundle of His courses through the right fibrous trigone, along the posterior edge of the membranous septum. The remainder of the annular circumference is composed of left ventricular myocardium in the form of the ventricular septum.
- The aortic cusps are semilunar and termed the right, left, and noncoronary cusps, corresponding to the sinuses of Valsalva immediately above and obviously related to the right and left coronary ostia. The aortic root typically has a leftward rotation, making the right coronary ostium anterior and the left coronary ostium posterior. The right coronary ostium tends to emerge farther from the annulus than does the left coronary ostium. Anomalous coronary anatomy is an important factor to consider in the treatment of aortic valvular disease but is beyond the scope of this discussion.
- The aortic cusps attach to the annulus and meet at the commissures. The commissures are located immediately below the sinotubular junction, which defines the distal limit of the aortic root. The sinuses of Valsalva are defined as the spaces between the aorta and the aortic cusps.
- The circumferential anatomy of the aortic root is equally critical to these operations (Fig. 13-1B). The commissure between the left and noncoronary cusps overlies the area of so-called aortic–mitral continuity and the fibrous subaortic curtain. Below the noncoronary cusp is the right atrial wall. Starting under the noncoronary cusp and across the commissure between it and the right coronary cusp lies the membranous septum. Within it is the conduction system, consisting of the atrioventricular node, the bundle of His, and the left and right bundle branches. The commissure between the left and right coronary cusps is immediately related to the corresponding commissure in the pulmonary valve; the right ventricular infundibulum lies beneath.
- The dynamic relationships of the aortic root structures collectively contribute to the overall function of the valvular apparatus. Because the free edges of the aortic leaflets are about 50% longer than their bases, the leaflets can coapt during diastole and allow unobstructed flow during systole. Indeed, for effective hemodynamics, the additive length of the free edges must exceed the diameter of the aortic orifice. Without this relationship intact, both insufficiency and stenosis become evident. Also important is the diameter of the sinotubular junction, which is typically 15% to 20% smaller than that of the aortic annulus. Because the commissures are intimately related to the sinotubular junction, changes in diameter can profoundly affect valve competency. Finally, the sinuses of Valsalva do not directly contribute to valvular competence, but instead are thought to minimize mechanical stress on the leaflets.

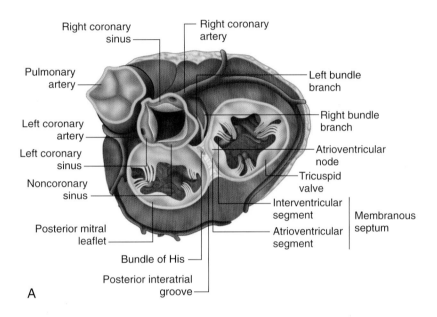

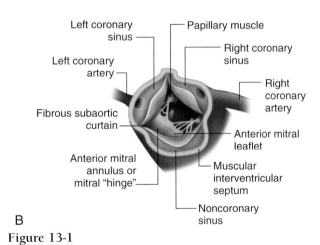

Figure 13-1

Step 2. Preoperative Considerations

1. Indications and Contraindications

- The use of a homograft for aortic valve replacement has a number of theoretical and realized advantages, including an excellent hemodynamic profile with low transvalvular gradient, no need for systemic anticoagulation and therefore a low thromboembolic risk, low risk of prosthetic valve endocarditis, and enhanced remodeling of left ventricular hypertrophy. It is particularly advantageous when endocarditis has left an infected field and, more important, when endocarditis has resulted in tissue destruction due to abscess.
- One disadvantage of a homograft is the difficulty with its implantation, as both valve and root replacement. Not only is the procedure itself technically demanding (see later), but subtle errors in implantation may alter the geometric relationships critical to valvular competence and longevity. In addition, the homograft tissue is more fragile than prosthetic material. Another disadvantage is the durability of the grafts. Like other bioprosthetic valves, homograft durability may be limited; however, as with other bioprosthetic valves, recent advances in preservation techniques may allow for improved durability.
- Because of the overall limited availability of homografts, the indications for their use should remain narrow. Homograft implantation should be considered for the treatment of active endocarditis of a native or prosthetic valve; in patients 30 to 60 years of age, with at least a 10-year life expectancy, who have contraindications for anticoagulation; in patients with small aortic annuli; and in patients who require aortic root replacement. Homografts are contraindicated in patients with a heavily calcified noncompliant aortic root and in patients less than 20 years of age because of the likelihood of valve degeneration, requiring early replacement.

2. Preoperative Echocardiography

- For any patient undergoing an aortic valve operation, a transthoracic echocardiogram is of paramount importance. It describes valvular morphology and function, may elucidate the etiology of valvular dysfunction, and can evaluate ventricular function and the presence of additional lesions. Furthermore, the transthoracic echocardiogram can measure aortic annular diameter, allowing the surgeon to ensure availability of an appropriately sized homograft.
- There are data to support the increased use of transesophageal echocardiography to estimate aortic annular diameter, but these must be considered in light of the additional invasiveness of the procedure.

Step 3. Operative Steps

1. Incision

- A full median sternotomy is performed. We prefer to resect residual thymic tissue and clip large thymic vessels to aid in wide exposure of the superior mediastinum. A pericardial well is created.
- Cardiopulmonary bypass is established through aortic cannulation at the level of the innominate artery and two-stage cannulation of the right atrial appendage. Alternatively, if ascending aortic replacement is necessary, axillary or femoral cannulation may be required in certain circumstances. Cardioplegia is delivered antegrade and retrograde, and a left ventricular vent is placed through the right superior pulmonary vein.

2. Dissection

- The aortotomy begins approximately 4 to 5 cm above the coronary ostia in a reverse "lazy-S" configuration (Fig. 13-2). The proximal portion of the incision should extend to the center of the noncoronary sinus.
- After three stay sutures are placed, the aortic valve is excised and annular debridement of calcific deposits is performed with a rongeur forceps. The aortic root and annulus are then evaluated for suitability for homograft placement: most notably, the overall morphology, symmetry, and degree of calcification may lend toward specific repairs. The aortic annulus is directly measured with standard valve-sizing instruments, with special care taken not to stretch the annulus. Because this size represents the external diameter of the homograft, a homograft 2 to 4 mm smaller is selected (homograft size is based on the aortic orifice, not the external diameter). Furthermore, there is obligate minor shrinkage of the homograft tissues after implantation. Thawing procedures should have commenced when preoperative transthoracic or transesophageal measurements were taken; if they have not, thawing procedures should commence immediately when the annulus is sized.
- During homograft procurement, a variable amount of ventricular muscle, mitral valve, and aortic arch is included with the specimen. Depending on the technique of implantation to be used, tailoring the homograft appropriately is critical. After the mitral leaflet and ventricular septum are trimmed, a straight lower suture line approximately 2 to 3 mm below the nadir of each aortic cusp is fashioned. The aortic tissue is trimmed appropriately depending on the technique for insertion.
- A number of implantation techniques have been developed over the years, and these techniques continue to evolve. Currently, there are four principal methods used: 120-degree rotation scalloped technique, free-hand intact noncoronary sinus scalloped technique, aortic root inclusion cylinder technique, and aortic root replacement with free-standing (interposition) graft. Advantages and disadvantages of each are discussed in the following.

120-Degree Rotation Scalloped Technique

- The aortic sinuses are trimmed within 5 mm of the commissures and within 3 mm of the cusp bases, leaving only aortic valve (Fig. 13-3A).
- Before implantation, the homograft is rotated 120 degrees counterclockwise, such that the original homograft right coronary sinus underlies the patient's left coronary ostium (Fig. 13-3B). This is a crucial maneuver for this technique because it attaches the weaker muscular portion of the homograft posteriorly, adjacent to the patient's fibrous trigone and anterior leaflet of the mitral valve.
- Two suture lines are used. The proximal suture line can be a continuous running suture of 4-0 or 5-0 polypropylene; alternatively, it can be performed using either simple or mattress interrupted sutures, also 4-0 or 5-0 polypropylene. If a running suture line is used, the homograft can be inverted into the ventricle to ease suture placement. The distal suture line is performed in a running fashion using 4-0 polypropylene. Starting at the commissure between the (neo) noncoronary and left coronary sinuses, the suture line is completed beneath the left coronary ostium. Next, the suture line beneath the right coronary ostium is completed, starting at the noncoronary commissure and continuing to the commissure between the left and right cusps. Finally, the noncoronary suture line is completed.
- Great care must be taken not to injure or incorporate the cusps into the suture line. In addition, care must be taken not to distort the coronary ostia. Proper alignment of the commissures within the aortic root is absolutely critical for both short- and long-term valve function. Over the short term, commissural malalignment leads to improper leaflet coaptation and valvular regurgitation. Over the long term, even slight malalignment leads to premature structural deterioration because of increased mechanical stress.

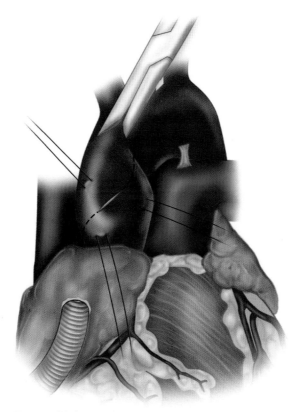

Figure 13-2

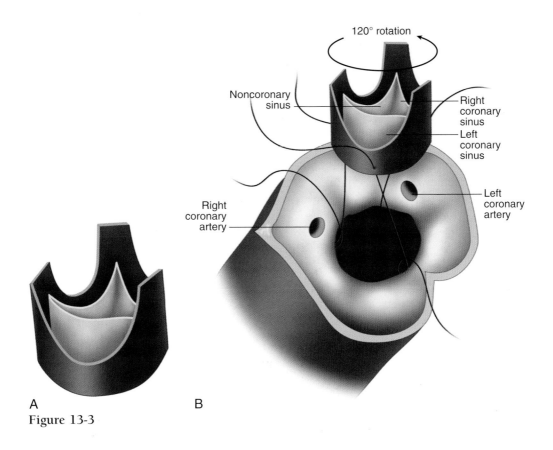

A   B

Figure 13-3

♦ The 120-degree rotation scalloped technique is considered more demanding than the other homograft implantation techniques, and technical errors may compromise its long-term results. On the other hand, the technique is advantageous in patients with relatively small aortic roots and nondilated sinotubular junctions. It is a poor choice in patients with asymmetric roots or annuloaortic ectasia.

Free-hand Intact Noncoronary Sinus Scalloped Technique

♦ The free-hand intact noncoronary sinus scalloped technique is a minor modification to the 120-degree rotation scalloped technique. Homograft preparation is similar—the aortic tissue of the left and right sinuses is resected to within 5 mm of the commissures and within 3 mm of the nadir of each cusp, whereas the noncoronary sinus is preserved (Fig. 13-4A).

♦ While maintaining anatomic alignment, the homograft is inserted into the aortic root, using either an interrupted or continuous technique (Fig. 13-4B). Next, the left coronary sinus is attached to the native aorta with a 4-0 polypropylene suture, followed by the right coronary sinus (Fig. 13-4C). The sutures are tied over the commissure between the left and right coronary cusps. Then, the sutures are continued along the preserved noncoronary sinus and tied. Finally, the space between the homograft outside the noncoronary sinus and the native aorta is obliterated with several mattress sutures (Fig. 13-4D).

♦ The primary objective of this modification is to improve stability of the homograft and therefore maintain its symmetry. In addition, this procedure has decreased risk of noncoronary cusp prolapse, particularly in patients with dilated sinotubular junctions. This technique is reasonable for patients with mild annuloaortic ectasia.

Aortic Root Replacement Techniques

♦ Aortic root replacement should be considered in patients in whom anatomic distortion due to scar, calcium deposits, or other factors precludes the likelihood of a successful free-hand technique reconstruction. Root replacement techniques are technically less demanding than the free-hand techniques previously described. In addition, a 2- to 3-mm disparity in donor–recipient root size is tolerated reasonably well, which increases the effective donor pool and reduces the probability of not having a homograft available.

♦ Current experience with aortic root replacement has rendered this strategy both safe and effective, despite earlier concerns regarding perioperative morbidity. Root replacement techniques have become the most commonly used techniques for placement of a homograft in the aortic position. Homograft preparation is minimal, leaving intact the periannular tissue and the aortic root with coronary ostia.

♦ Aortic root inclusion cylinder technique
  ▲ The aortic root inclusion cylinder technique was originally described by Ross. After debridement and sizing maneuvers, an appropriately sized homograft is inserted *within* the native aortic root. The proximal suture line is performed using interrupted sutures in a manner routine to aortic valve implantation. Depending on the degree of patient–prosthesis mismatch, the homograft can be implanted in an infra-annular or a supra-annular fashion.
  ▲ Next, the coronary ostia are anastomosed to the homograft. Depending on their height, the homograft ostia may be used, or new ostia can be created using an appropriately sized coronary punch. The coronary ostia are anastomosed to the homograft using a 5-0 polypropylene suture (Fig. 13-5). Conversely, if the overall homograft height is sufficiently small, minimal scalloping of the sinuses may allow the homograft to remain below the native coronary ostia, ensuring adequate flow.

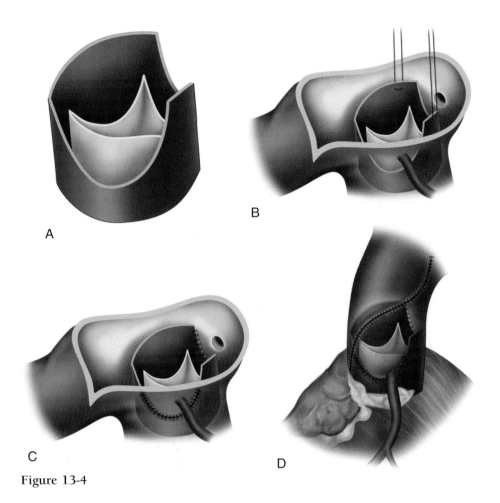

Figure 13-4

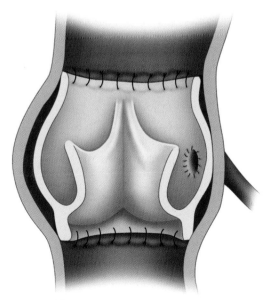

Figure 13-5

▲ Using a 4-0 polypropylene suture, the distal suture line is completed in a running fashion. The advantage of this technique lies in its simplicity. It is more challenging than a standard aortic valve replacement in that the coronary arteries need to be addressed, but it does not require understanding of the significant three-dimensional relationships between the cusps, sinuses, and annulus. Once the appropriate coronary height and location within the sinus is selected, the anastomosis is easily completed. The main disadvantage of this technique is the obligate loss—up to 3 mm—of effective aortic orifice.

♦ Aortic root replacement with free-standing (interposition) graft

▲ The most common application of a homograft in the aortic position is as a free-standing interposition graft (Fig. 13-6A). Coronary artery anomalies should have been noted on pre-operative catheterization studies and carefully studied before proceeding to the operating room.

▲ The coronary arteries are carefully dissected approximately 1 cm distal to the coronary ostia, with care taken to avoid injury to the arteries to the sinus node (right coronary system) and the first septal perforator (left coronary system). Although these arteries can be sacrificed if necessary for mobilization, unrecognized injury can lead to difficult-to-control bleeding and malperfusion.

▲ After coronary mobilization, the aortic root is carefully excised to the level of the annulus, with the coronary ostia preserved as buttons (Fig. 13-6B). Distally, the aorta is divided just above the sinotubular junction.

▲ An appropriately sized homograft is selected. Using an interrupted or continuous suturing technique, the proximal anastomosis is fashioned as previously described.

▲ Next, the coronary buttons are attached to the homograft. In most cases, a punch is used to create a new ostium; however, if the native coronary ostia are appropriately placed, they can be used after excising the residual coronary arteries. Finally, the distal aortic suture line is completed using a 4-0 polypropylene suture in a running fashion (Fig. 13-6C).

▲ The main advantage of this technique is that it is familiar to most surgeons. It is generally fast and, like the inclusion technique, does not involve significant three-dimensional aortic root relationships. Further, this technique can maximize the aortic outflow diameter without aortic root enlargement.

3. Intraoperative Assessment

♦ Intraoperative assessment of the homograft by transesophageal echocardiography is critical to a successful outcome. Supplemental views can be obtained with a hand-held epiaortic probe, if necessary. Adjunctive Doppler color flow measurement further enhances the ability of the surgeon to determine the adequacy of repair and the need for re-repair or replacement.

♦ The primary determinants of aortic insufficiency, as determined by echocardiography, include the transvalvular pressure gradient, the valvular orifice area, and the duration of diastole; these should be carefully evaluated after a complete wean from cardiopulmonary bypass. With appropriate loading conditions, moderate to severe aortic insufficiency warrants reinstitution of cardiopulmonary bypass, cardioplegic arrest, and inspection and revision of the allograft, as needed. Most surgeons believe that mild aortic insufficiency is well tolerated and should not independently mandate reexploration.

Step 4. Postoperative Care

1. Postoperative Management

♦ Postoperative management after these procedures is largely predicated on the patient's presenting pathophysiology. The noncompliant left ventricular hypertrophy resulting from aortic stenosis requires adequate preload and therefore benefits greatly from maintenance of normal sinus

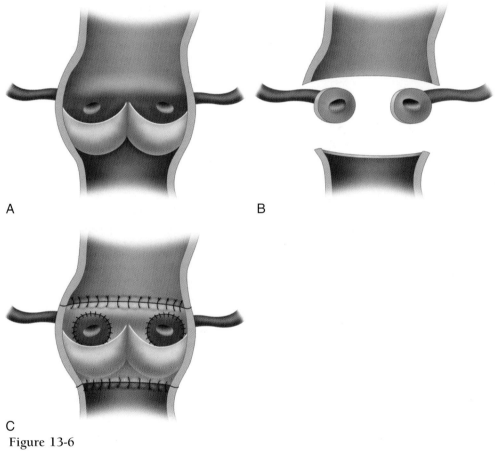

A

B

C

Figure 13-6

rhythm. The dilated, hypertrophied left ventricle associated with aortic insufficiency is managed similarly.

- Patients with aortic insufficiency are frequently maintained on substantial afterload reduction and may require vasoconstriction after cardiotomy.
- As with any patient with an aortic suture line, systemic hypertension is avoided.
- If heart block persists after several days, a permanent implantable pacemaker is indicated.
- Although not yet borne out by randomized, prospective data, it is our practice to keep patients on statins on the theory that graft longevity is increased.
- Finally, systemic anticoagulation is not beneficial; aspirin (81 mg per day) should suffice.

2. Perioperative Complications

- In the absence of endocarditis, the reported operative mortality rate ranges from 1% to 5%, consistent with mortality rates in patients undergoing aortic valve replacement. Although root replacement strategies were thought to increase mortality, numerous groups have refuted this. Endocarditis increases the operative mortality substantially, ranging from 8% to 16%, depending on the series.
- Other factors predicting mortality include cardiogenic shock and prosthetic (as opposed to native) valve endocarditis.

3. Results

- Structural homograft degeneration occurs in all cases, with rates reported as high as 38% at 10 years and 82% at 20 years. Extremes in age of donor and recipient appear to worsen homograft deterioration.
- Homograft deterioration has obvious consequences for the initially excellent hemodynamic profile. Although homograft deterioration is predictable and progressive, it does not always lead to repeat aortic valve replacement; the percentage of homograft recipients who remain free from aortic valve re-replacement is about one-half the reported degeneration rate.
- The rate of homograft infection is low, with a 2% to 7% rate of endocarditis at 10 years. Even in patients with active endocarditis requiring aortic valve replacement, recurrent endocarditis occurs in less than 4% of patients at 4 years.
- The thromboembolism rate also is low, with rates of 8% at 15 years and 17% at 20 years reported. Neither preservation nor implantation techniques appear to affect the long-term results using aortic homografts.

4. Note on Reoperation

- The structural degeneration of aortic homografts affects both the aortic valve complex and the aortic wall. The homograft becomes almost entirely calcified, resulting in a loss of leaflet competence. Unfortunately, the homograft wall not infrequently incorporates into the posterior sternal table (Fig. 13-7).
- In patients requiring reoperation, this represents an incredibly hazardous situation. Preoperative imaging with computed tomographic angiography may aid in planning. It is our practice to ensure rapid groin access for peripheral bypass by either preemptive cut-down or placement of a percutaneous line.

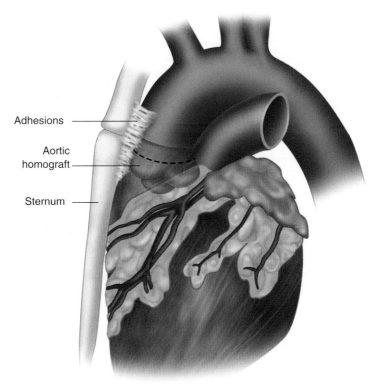

Adhesions

Aortic
homograft

Sternum

Figure 13-7

♦ This process is particularly worrisome in patients with severe aortic insufficiency because peripheral bypass can result in unrecognized and potentially catastrophic left ventricular distention. Under these circumstances, exposure of the right atrium for a retrograde cardioplegia cannula along with placement of a percutaneous aortic occlusive balloon may be the only options for safe dissection.

Step 5. Pearls and Pitfalls

♦ The conduction system lies along the membranous septum—sutures should be kept as superficial as possible to avoid heart block.

♦ Placing tension on either coronary ostium can produce ischemia that is not readily apparent. Have a low threshold to revise an ostium by several techniques: rotation of root, raising or lowering the button, creating a patch ostium, and, ultimately, coronary artery bypass grafting.

♦ Prefashioned pledgeted, braided valve sutures are usually not used for homografts because the suture material tends to tear the homograft tissue and their needles tend to be larger than those on polypropylene sutures.

♦ Inadequate or excessive coronary artery mobilization can lead to kinking.

♦ Coronary buttons should be fashioned in an upside-down bullet shape, with the flat end indicating the distal aspect of the aorta. In cases of extensive mobilization, it is worthwhile to mark the anterior aspect of the coronary artery with a surgical marker to prevent twisting.

♦ Division of the artery to the sinus node during right coronary artery mobilization may result in atrial arrhythmia.

Bibliography

Dearani JA, Orszulak TA, Daly RC, et al: Comparison of techniques for implantation of aortic valve allografts. Ann Thorac Surg 1996;62:1069-1075.

Dearani JA, Orszulak TA, Schaff HV, et al: Results of the allograft aortic valve replacement for complex endocarditis. J Thorac Cardiovasc Surg 1997;113:285-291.

Hasegawa J, Kitamura S, Taniguchi S, et al: Comparative rest and exercise hemodynamics of allograft and prosthetic valves in the aortic position. Ann Thorac Surg 1997;64:1753-1756.

Langley SM, McGuirk SP, Chaudhry MA, et al: Twenty-year follow-up of aortic valve replacement with antibiotic sterilized homografts in 200 patients. Semin Thorac Cardiovasc Surg 1999;11:28-34.

Lund O, Chandrasekaran V, Grocott-Mason R, et al: Primary aortic valve replacement with allografts over twenty-five years: Valve related and procedure related determinants of outcome. J Thorac Cardiovasc Surg 1999;117:77-91.

Maselli D, Pizio R, Bruno LP, et al: Left ventricular mass reduction after aortic valve replacement: Homografts, stentless and stented valves. Ann Thorac Surg 1999;67:966-971.

McGiffin DC, O'Brien MF: A technique for aortic root replacement by an aortic homograft. Ann Thorac Surg 1989;47:623-627.

Murray G, Roschlau W, Lougheed W: Homologous aortic-valve-segment transplants as surgical treatment for aortic and mitral insufficiency. Angiology 1956;7:466-471.

O'Brien MF, Harrocks S, Stafford EG, et al: The homograft aortic valve: A 29-year, 99.3% follow up of 1,022 valve replacements. J Heart Valve Dis 2001;10:334-344.

O'Brien MF, Stafford EG, Gardner MA, et al: A comparison of aortic valve replacement with viable cryopreserved and fresh allograft valves, with a note on chromosomal studies. J Thorac Cardiovasc Surg 1987;94:812-823.

Yacoub M, Rasmi NRH, Sundt TM, et al: Fourteen-year experience with homovital homografts for aortic valve replacement. J Thorac Cardiovasc Surg 1995;110:186-194.

CHAPTER 14

ROSS PROCEDURE

Craig J. Baker and Vaughn A. Starnes

- The Ross procedure replaces the aortic valve with a viable pulmonary autograft and uses a cryopreserved pulmonary homograft to reconstruct the right ventricular outflow tract (RVOT).
- As initially described, the autograft was placed as a scalloped subcoronary implant. The complexity of the operation and concerns regarding autograft insufficiency limited widespread adoption of the procedure. The subsequent use of the full-root technique, in addition to increasing availability of homografts, has increased interest in the operation.
- More recent concerns regarding autograft dilation and neo-aortic insufficiency have led to further refinements.

Step 1. Surgical Anatomy

- Relevant surgical anatomy centers on proper enucleation of the pulmonary valve and undistorted implantation into the left ventricular outflow tract (LVOT). In adults, we currently place the pulmonary autograft within an appropriately sized Dacron conduit to prevent pulmonary autograft root dilation and subsequent neo-aortic insufficiency. This technique also stabilizes the sinotubular junction.
- A thorough understanding of the anatomic relationships between the pulmonary and aortic valves is critical (Fig. 14-1A and B).

Step 2. Preoperative Considerations

- The growth potential of the autograft, favorable hemodynamics, and avoidance of anticoagulation have made the Ross procedure the operation of choice in infants, children, and adolescents with aortic valve disease requiring aortic valve replacement. It should also be considered in young adults who wish to avoid anticoagulation or who have endocarditis requiring valve replacement.
- We have had excellent results using the Ross procedure in adults with bicuspid aortic valves requiring replacement. Recent evidence suggests a low rate of RVOT stenosis in older patients, which may extend popularity of the operation in patients up to the sixth decade.
- It is important to inform patients about the possibility of autograft failure. Avoiding the Ross operation when a significant geometric discrepancy between the pulmonary and aortic annuli is detected preoperatively should minimize this complication. If a moderate size discrepancy exists between the aortic and pulmonary roots, a number of techniques to minimize mismatch have been developed; the surgeon should be familiar with them before performing the procedure.
- Patients with an abnormal pulmonary valve, a connective tissue disease, or an immune complex–mediated disease with known valvular sequelae should be excluded.

Step 3. Operative Steps

- A standard median sternotomy is performed. The pericardium is incised and pericardial stay sutures are placed. Bicaval cannulation is used, which facilitates exposure and avoids venous air entrapment. Antegrade and retrograde cardioplegia cannulae are placed except when aortic sufficiency is present, in which case hand-held cannulae may be used. The patient is placed on cardiopulmonary bypass and cooled to 32°C. A vent is placed through the right superior pulmonary vein (Fig. 14-2).

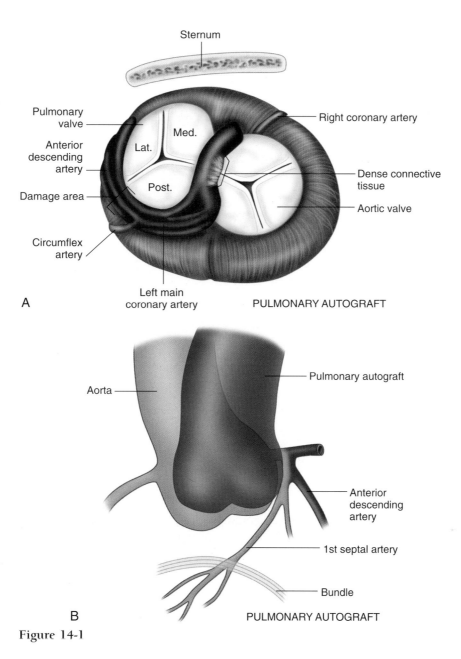

Figure 14-1

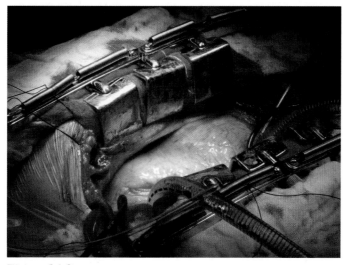

Figure 14-2

- The aorta is divided at the sinotubular junction, and the aortic valve is inspected. If no repair option is available, generous coronary buttons are harvested and the aortic valve is excised. The pulmonary artery is transected below the branch pulmonary artery (Fig. 14-3).
- After visual inspection of the pulmonary valve leaflets, the pulmonary root and contained valve leaflets are excised from the RVOT. The incision is initiated in the RVOT across the infundibulum approximately 4 mm below the pulmonary valve leaflets. A right-angled clamp can be placed through the pulmonary valve to identify the proper site to begin the ventriculotomy. The pulmonary root should be excised with a 3- to 4-mm rim of myocardium (Figs. 14-4 and 14-5).
- Aberrant coronary arteries coursing across the RVOT should be identified. The dissection extends along the septal myocardium, avoiding the first septal perforator and the left anterior descending artery. The dissection continues along the course of the left anterior descending artery posteriorly, avoiding injury to the left main coronary artery (Figs. 14-6 and 14-7).

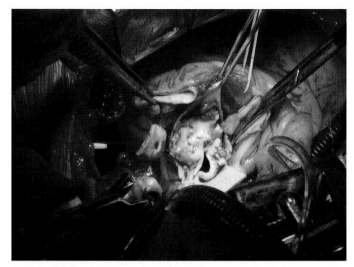

Figure 14-3

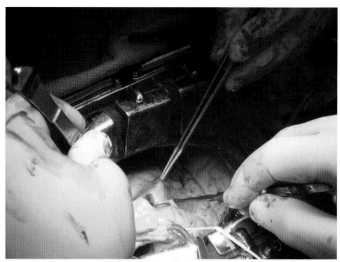

Figure 14-4

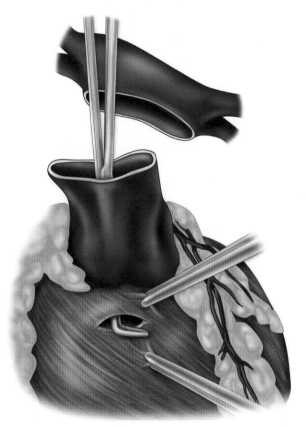

Figure 14-5

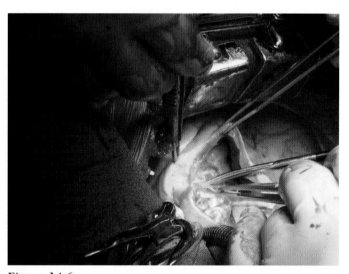

Figure 14-6

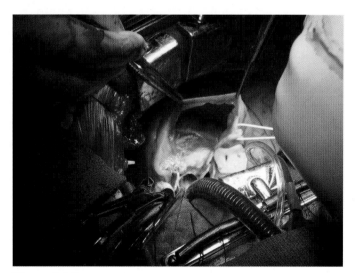

Figure 14-7

♦ After the autograft is harvested, excessive myocardium is excised from the explanted pulmonary root to avoid LVOT obstruction after implantation (Fig. 14-8).

♦ A Hegar dilator is gently passed through the pulmonary valve to select an appropriate-size Dacron tube. We usually pick a tube graft 2 mm larger than the sizer to avoid distortion and narrowing. The autograft is secured within the tube graft using a running 4-0 polypropylene suture passed through the myocardium just below the valve leaflet (Fig. 14-9).

♦ After the pulmonary root is secured, the graft is cut at the top of the commissures and the distal autograft is sutured using 4-0 polypropylene (Fig. 14-10). Once the autograft is completely implanted within the graft, a saline test can confirm leaflet patency (Fig. 14-11).

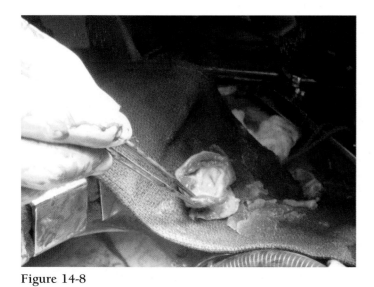

Figure 14-8

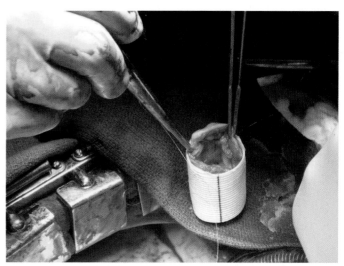

Figure 14-9

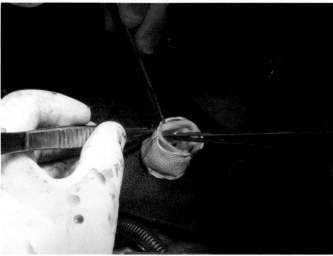

Figure 14-10

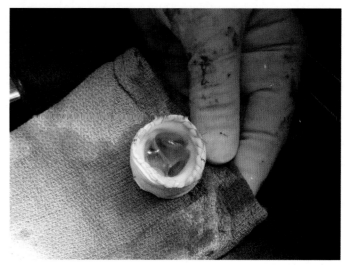

Figure 14-11

◆ The tubularized autograft is sutured to the LVOT using 3-0 polypropylene (Figs. 14-12 and 14-13). After the proximal anastomosis is complete, the coronary buttons are reimplanted. A portion of the Dacron conduit and the corresponding internal autograft sinus are excised after determining the proper location for coronary reimplantation (Fig. 14-14). The left and right coronary button anastomoses are performed with 5-0 polypropylene. The coronary buttons create structural support to the right and left sinuses of the autograft by stabilizing them to the tube graft. Because of concerns regarding the nonsupported noncoronary sinus, we suture a piece of homograft inside the noncoronary sinus to the corresponding wall of the Dacron conduit (Fig. 14-15).

◆ An appropriately sized pulmonary homograft is used to reconstruct the RVOT. The distal anastomosis is performed below the bifurcation. The proximal suture line is completed with 4-0 polypropylene (Fig. 14-16).

◆ The distal suture of the tubularized autograft is completed (Fig. 14-17).

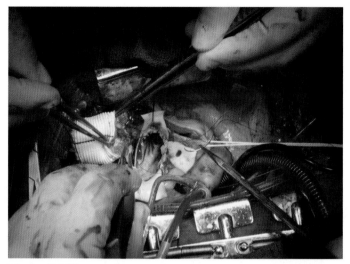

Figure 14-12

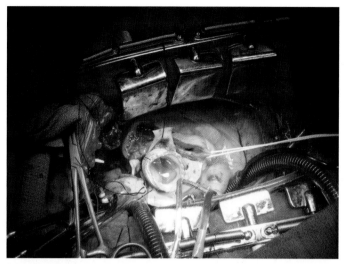

Figure 14-13

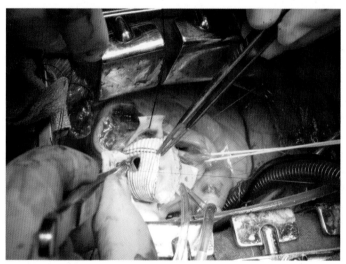

Figure 14-14

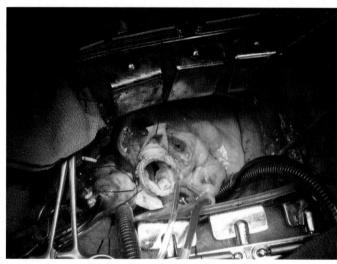

Figure 14-15

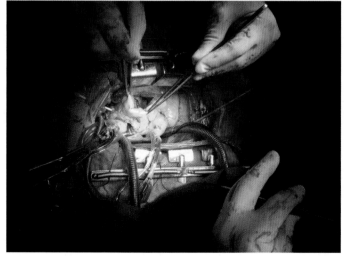

Figure 14-16

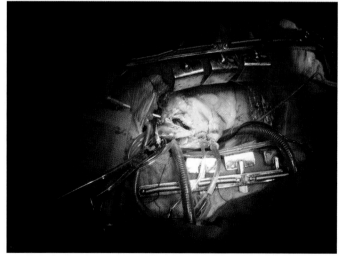

Figure 14-17

Step 4. Postoperative Care

- Good postoperative care mandates ensuring excellent hemostasis before leaving the operating room. Any bleeding, especially from the LVOT suture line or coronary buttons, should be repaired, if necessary on cardiopulmonary bypass using cardioplegic arrest.
- Placement of blind sutures at the proximal suture line should be avoided because autograft leaflets may be injured.
- Transesophageal echocardiography should confirm good valve function and no evidence of an LVOT gradient.
- Avoidance of hypertension should be emphasized in the intensive care unit. Generally, myocardial function is good and inotropic support is not necessary.

Step 5. Pearls and Pitfalls

- Meticulous technique is imperative to avoid bleeding.
- When enucleating the autograft, a definite tissue plane can be identified between the pulmonary root and surrounding structures. This is most easily identified by initiating the enucleation on the right (aortic) side of the autograft.
- Proper alignment of the autograft in the LVOT is mandatory for a successful outcome.

Bibliography

Chambers JC, Somerville J, Stone S, Ross DN: Pulmonary autograft procedure for aortic valve disease: Long-term results of the pioneer series. Circulation 1997;96:2206-2214.

Elkins RC, Knott-Craig CJ, Ward KE, Lane MM: The Ross operation in children: 10-year experience. Ann Thorac Surg 1998;65:496-502.

Hampton CR, Chong AJ, Verrier ED: Stentless aortic valve replacement: Homograft/autograft. In Cohn LH, Edmunds LH Jr (eds): Cardiac Surgery in the Adult, 2nd ed. New York, McGraw-Hill, 2003, pp 867-888.

Luciani GB, Favaro A, Casali G, et al: Ross operation in the young. Ann Thorac Surg 2005;80:2271-2277.

Ross DN: Replacement of the aortic and mitral valves with pulmonary autograft. Lancet 1967;2:956-958.

CHAPTER 15

REPAIR OF THE MYXOMATOUS DEGENERATED MITRAL VALVE

Lawrence H. Cohn

- Repair of the myxomatous degenerated mitral valve has become the most common reparative operation for mitral valve disease in the United States and the Western world. Although the incidence of surgical repair in rheumatic disease in general has diminished, the ability to repair the myxomatous degenerated prolapsed mitral valve has increased with case recognition and definition of simplified surgical techniques to ensure long-term valve competency.

- Reparative procedures for the myxomatous degenerated mitral valve have become standardized over the past 25 years and are reproducible in many surgical centers specializing in valvular heart surgery. This chapter presents simplified techniques that allow even the relatively inexperienced surgeon to perform mitral valve repair for the myxomatous degenerated prolapsed mitral valve.

- Despite more than 20 years of experience with and dissemination of reparative procedures, the most recent survey by the Society of Thoracic Surgeons indicated that of the mitral valves that *could* be repaired in the United States, less than 50% of these valves *were* repaired, suggesting a lack of knowledge, experience, or understanding of the reparative treatment of myxomatous degenerated mitral valves.[1] In reviewing their own data, all surgeons should calculate their personal "reparability index"—that is, of those patients with myxomatous degenerated mitral valves with severe mitral regurgitation presenting for operation, what is the percentage of valve repair versus valve replacement.

- This chapter presents techniques that allow improvement of that reparability index for most surgeons who treat patients with myxomatous degenerated prolapsed mitral valves.

Step 1. Surgical Anatomy

- The bicuspid mitral valve is one of the most complex structures of the human heart, with a multifaceted anatomy whose several parts play a role in closure during systole and opening during diastole (Fig. 15-1A). There are five discrete components of the mitral valve complex: the annulus; the two leaflets, anterior and posterior; the aortic root superiorly; and the atrioventricular node superomedially. The posterior annulus, whatever the disease affecting the mitral valve, is the area that dilates significantly. Previous dicta suggested that the anterior annulus, the area between the two trigone points, does not dilate, but recent imaging data suggest that it may dilate a limited amount.[2]

- The anterior leaflet of the mitral valve (AML) is in continuity with the left and noncoronary cusps of the aortic valve and is located directly beneath, forming a part of the left ventricular outflow tract. It accounts for over 40% of the circumference of the annulus, with the posterior leaflet accounting for the rest. In effect, the anterior leaflet of the mitral valve plus the septum form the left ventricular outflow tract, and they account for obstruction in diseases such as idiopathic hypertrophic subaortic stenosis.

- The crescent-shaped posterior leaflet of the mitral valve (PML) is associated with the part of the annulus that may significantly dilate in degenerative disease. For the purposes of clarification in surgical decision making, valve analysis, and surgical repair techniques, both the AML and the PML are divided into three parts corresponding to the typical scalloped areas of each leaflet: A1, A2, and A3 for the AML, and P1, P2, and P3 for the PML. A1/P1 refers to the leftmost or lateral scallop near the anterolateral commissure, A2/P2 is the middle scallop, and A3/P3 is the rightmost scallop, which forms part of the posteromedial commissure (Fig. 15-1B).

- The two papillary muscles, the anterolateral and the posteromedial, are shown in Figure 15-1A. Each muscle is attached to both leaflets by the chordae tendineae, cords of stringlike fibrous connective tissue. The primary cords are attached to the edge of the leaflet, and the secondary cords are attached to the undersurface of the leaflet directly from the ventricular wall instead of from the papillary muscles; these are found only on the PML. The anterolateral papillary muscle receives blood supply from both the left anterior descending and the circumflex coronary arteries, whereas the posteromedial papillary muscle receives blood supply usually from the posterior descending coronary artery or a branch of the circumflex artery. Thus, because of its more tenuous coronary blood supply, the posteromedial papillary muscle is more susceptible to infarct than is the anterolateral papillary muscle.

- Finally, the left ventricle acts in concert with papillary muscles through the chordae to pull in the leaflet edges during systole, therefore maintaining the line of coaptation and valve competency. If the left ventricle dilates, the competency of the valve is affected by the papillary muscle's being drawn downward and outward, thus opening the leaflets and causing regurgitation.

Step 2. Preoperative Considerations

- The underlying etiology of degenerative mitral valve disease is a genetic structural defect in the fibroelastic connective tissue of the valve leaflets and chordae.[3] The defect leads to abnormal elongation and redundancy of valve tissue and chordae tendineae.

- In the presence of the underlying fibroelastic connective tissue disorder, secondary annular dilation ensues, obliterating the normal coaptation line between the AML and PML. The dilation is primarily posterior because the anterior annulus is relatively constrained by the aortomitral curtain.

- Leaflet redundancy results in a movement of the redundant leaflet back into the left atrium during diastole and leads to further compromise of the coaptation line. Elongation of the chordae causes leaflet tissue to move into the atrium during diastole, further complicating leaflet coaptation.

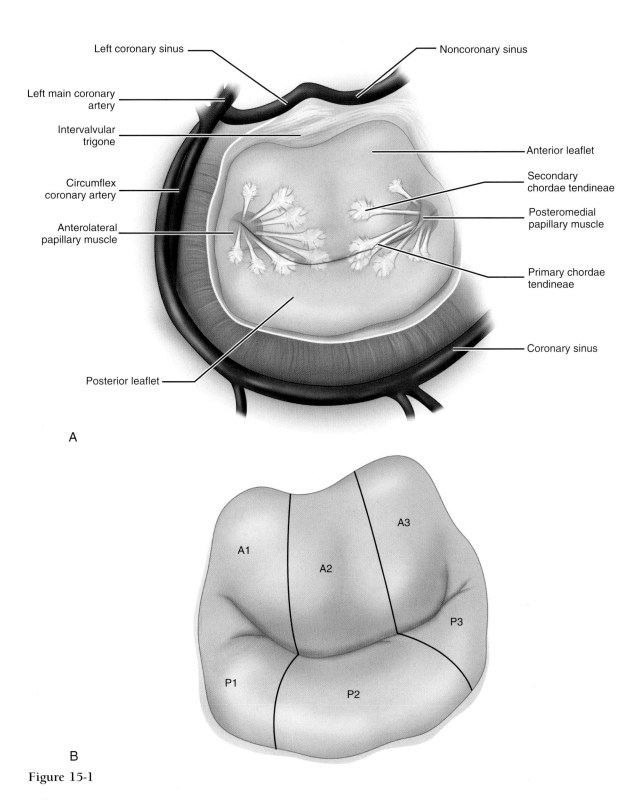

A

B

Figure 15-1

- A ruptured leaflet, or flail leaflet, one of the most common pathologic scenarios, is the result of systolic stresses' fracturing weakened and stretched chordae, resulting in severe regurgitation. Mitral regurgitation represents pure volume overload for the left ventricle, and a vicious cycle is perpetrated whereby the excessive volume load, over time, results in ventricular failure, which causes more annular dilation, which in turn causes more mitral regurgitation: hence the well-known scenario of "mitral regurgitation begets more mitral regurgitation."[4]
- Echocardiography is the mainstay clinical tool with which patients with mitral valve prolapse are followed. Patients with mild to moderate amounts of mitral regurgitation and normal left ventricular volumes are followed at yearly intervals, but at the point where left atrial or left ventricular dilation begins to appear along with moderately severe to severe mitral regurgitation, even in symptomatic patients, surgery is recommended.
- The threshold for referral for surgery often depends on surgeons' ability to perform reparative operations in patients with myxomatous degeneration a high percentage of the time. Most large valve surgery centers have a "reparability index" of better than 90%. This will lower the threshold for patient referral.
- Regardless of atrial or ventricular dilation, any person with symptoms, including shortness of breath, fatigue, or intermittent atrial fibrillation, is a candidate for surgical intervention. This philosophy of early referral to valve repair centers has been codified in the new American College of Cardiology/American Heart Association valvular disease management guidelines.[5]
- In the typical preoperative work-up, coronary angiography is necessary in all patients older than 40 years of age. It is of interest that the incidence of coronary disease in patients with myxomatous degenerated valves appears to be relatively low. In our experience, 5% of these patients require a concomitant coronary bypass. In fact, even in patients older than 70 years of age with valve disease, in whom the incidence of coronary disease might be expected to be quite high, we have observed that the incidence is decreasing.[6]
- Patients older than 70 years of age are excellent candidates for mitral valve repair provided that it can be done relatively efficiently. Some cardiologists believe that patients older than 70 years may be better served by a rapid mitral valve replacement, but physiologically this approach is not nearly as beneficial as a valve repair, and therefore these patients should be encouraged to have valve repair whenever possible.

Step 3. Operative Steps

1. Incision

- Ordinarily, in full-sternotomy cases, cardiopulmonary bypass is achieved with bicaval cannulation, with the inferior vena cava cannula placed low down in the right atrium and the superior vena cava cannula placed above the superior vena cava–right atrial junction, so that when the left atrium is retracted there are no tubes to retract (Fig. 15-2).
- Our version of minimally invasive mitral valve surgery[7] entails a lower ministernotomy with percutaneous peripheral venous cannulation of the right atrium through the right femoral vein. If placed in the proper spot in the superior vena cava, the long, flexible cannula from the femoral vein can serve as a drainage port for both the superior and inferior venae cavae, freeing the operative field of any further cannulae.
- The ascending aorta in the minimally invasive mitral valve procedure is also approached for cannulation by the Gensini needle technique, passing first a needle, then a wire, then a dilator, and then the perfusion cannula. Cardiac protection is effected primarily by antegrade cardioplegia but in many instances by retrograde cardioplegia; retrograde cardioplegia is used in every patient who requires combined mitral valve repair and coronary bypass. Potassium-enriched cold blood cardioplegia is used. Regardless of approach, exposure of the mitral valve is facilitated by developing Sondergaard's plane separating the right atrium from the left atrium[8] (see Fig. 15-2A).

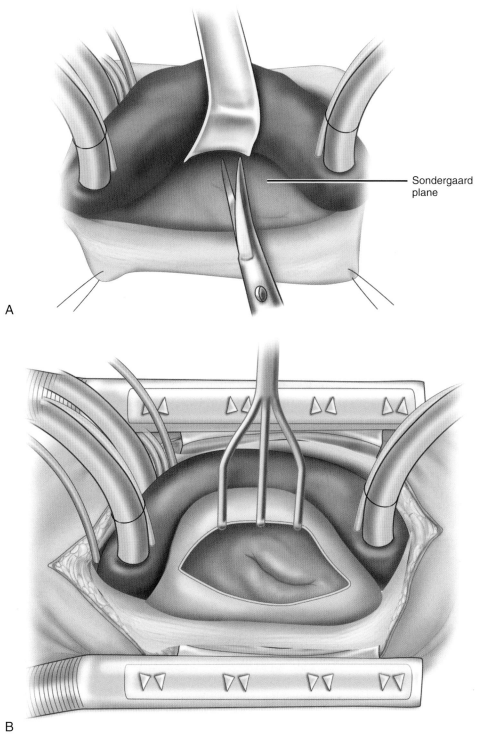

A

Sondergaard
plane

B

Figure 15-2

2. Operative Technique

- The operative philosophy of mitral valve repair has changed considerably over the years. Beginning in the 1980s, the classic repair techniques were developed by Carpentier[9] and Duran and colleagues.[10] These included leaflet resection, sliding annuloplasty,[9] and sliding valvuloplasty[10] and an annuloplasty ring or band to reshape the deformed, dilated annulus.

- As experience with mitral valve repair has increased, we have shown that there are many simplified techniques that can be used to repair the myxomatous mitral valve, producing a competent valve and a long-lasting operative result. As described in the following paragraphs, simplified techniques, particularly for PML repair, can be successful even when a surgeon performs them only occasionally. My basic philosophy has centered on doing the obvious reparative procedure, such as fixing a ruptured cord in the PML or AML, then, as a second step, implanting the annuloplasty band or ring to refashion and stabilize the distorted annulus. We have found that this approach allows for maintenance of competency without resorting to unnecessary techniques, particularly in repairs to the AML.

- Once the ring or band has been placed, the need for additional procedures (e.g., commissuroplasty, cleft closure, artificial cord placement) can be determined.

- Correctly sizing the annuloplasty band or ring based on the size of the AML is also very important, because the size of the annuloplasty ring determines the likelihood of the patient's developing systolic anterior motion (SAM) if the ring is sized too small.

- This operative philosophy applies in a variety of reparative scenarios depending on the extent of the pathologic process, from isolated small sections of P2 with a ruptured cord to the patient with Barlow syndrome in whom every segment of the mitral valve is prolapsed.

- The most common pathologic scenarios are ruptured cords of an isolated segment of the PML, usually the middle segment (P2); a prolapsed segment of P2 without ruptured chordae; a generalized prolapsed condition with every segment of the PML enlarged with redundant, elongated chordae; and finally, prolapse of P3 or P1 at either commissure.

- The classic mitral valve repair procedure consists of resection of the middle segment of the PML (P2) and a leaflet advancement technique, known as a *sliding valvuloplasty*, which involves incising the PML off the annulus to each commissure and resuturing it back on to the annulus, thus "sliding" the remaining segments of the valve to cover the area previously occupied by the resected P2 (Fig. 15-3). This technique, although effective, is somewhat forbidding to the inexperienced mitral valve repair surgeon. In the case of Barlow syndrome, in which every segment is markedly elongated, this technique may be preferred.

- In most other situations, however, more simplified techniques can be used to obtain complete, long-lasting resolution of mitral regurgitation: (1) resection of a limited area of the PML segment (P2) using a modified folding leaflet advancement to bridge the gap left by the resected leaflet; (2) for the prolapsed segment with intact cords, a folding valvuloplasty imbricating the leading edge of the leaflet back to the annulus, cutting the height of this leaflet by half; and (3) for markedly prolapsed or ruptured cords in P1 or P3, simply obliterating the commissure and adjacent valve segments by commissuroplasty.

- Figure 15-3 shows the classic sliding valvuloplasty: the PML is incised and the residual P1 and P3 are slid toward each other for completion of the valvuloplasty. In the procedures shown in Figures 15-2 and 15-3, the leaflet is assembled with running 4-0 polypropylene, first as a running mattress suture and then using a running over-and-over technique.

- Figure 15-4 shows the resection of a limited area of the PML with ruptured cords and the modified folding leaflet advancement technique to fill the space left by the resected leaflet. In this technique, the leaflet is folded on itself for a short distance, reducing the height substantially and filling the gap left by the small area of resected leaflet without incising the PML off the annulus.

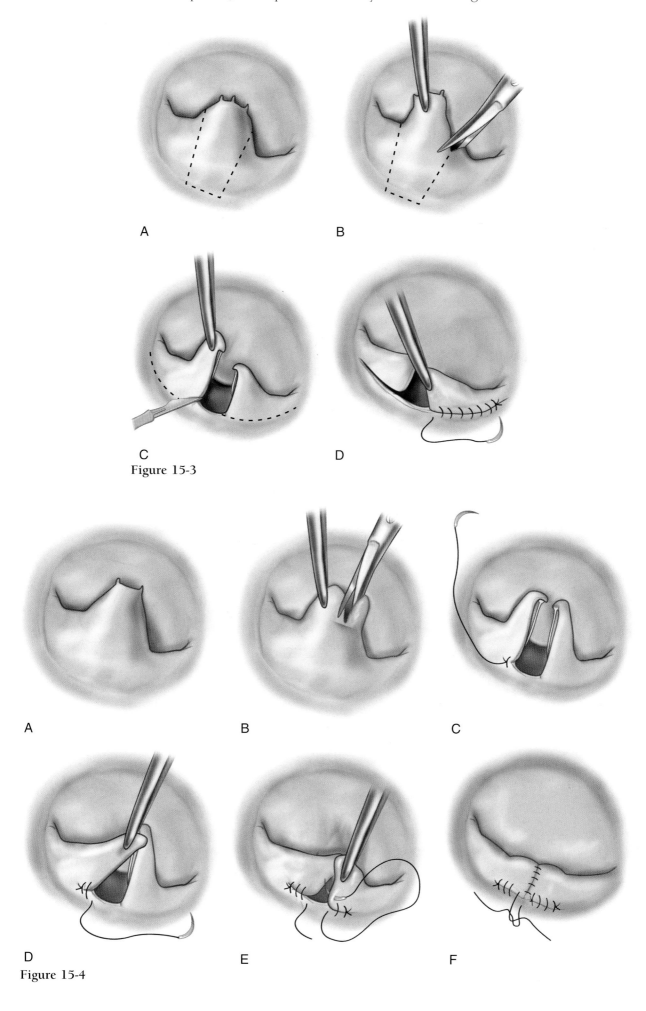

A

B

C   D

Figure 15-3

A   B   C

D   E   F

Figure 15-4

- Figure 15-5 shows a folding valvuloplasty in a patient with a prolapsed P2 section of the PML with intact cords. A 4-0 polypropylene suture is passed through the tip of the central leading edge of the leaflet, brought underneath the leaflet and back to the annulus in a mattress fashion, and tied down, thus reducing the height of the enlarged leaflet by 50%. We have used this technique in over 200 patients.
- Figure 15-6 shows the simple commissuroplasty technique for obliterating P3 when there is a ruptured cord or severely prolapsed A3/P3 commissure.
- True AML pathology is relatively uncommon, occurring in less then 15% of cases of mitral valve prolapse. As indicated in the previous section, many cases of so-called bileaflet prolapse may be corrected once the height of the posterior ring has been placed to establish normal annular anatomy, an observation noted by others.[11]

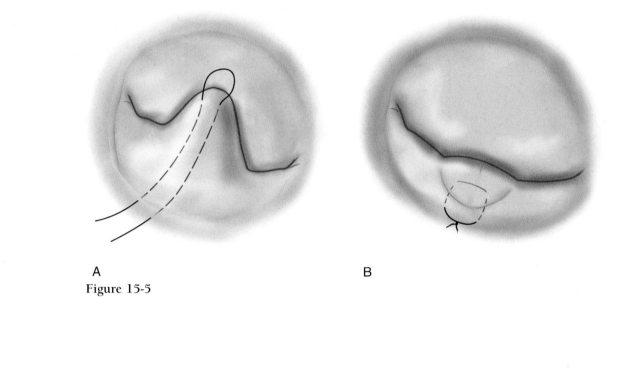

A

B

Figure 15-5

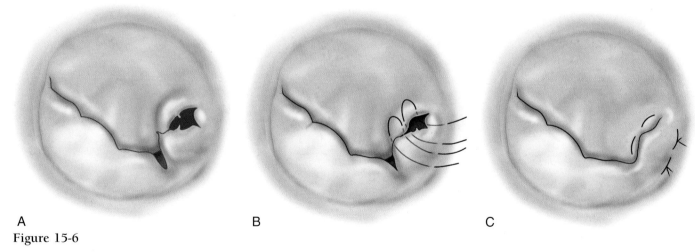

A

B

C

Figure 15-6

◆ True AML pathology consisting of very elongated or ruptured cords can be handled in a variety of ways. The original technique of lowering the AML cords by incising the papillary muscles and dropping the cords into the resulting so-called papillary muscle trench (Fig. 15-7) has been largely abandoned because the scissoring effect of the papillary muscle trench on the cords with cardiac contraction led to cord rupture.[12] A limited leaflet resection can be carried out as shown in Figure 15-8.

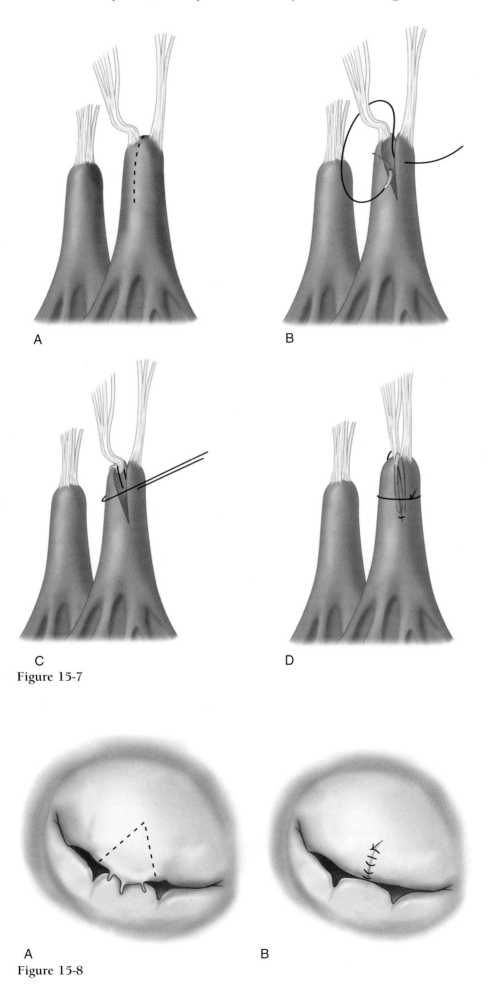

Figure 15-7

Figure 15-8

◆ A more consistent way to repair the pathologic AML is use of artificial chordae, promulgated by a number of surgeons beginning with Frater and colleagues in the 1980s.[13] In this technique, polytetrafluoroethylene (Gore-Tex) cords are sutured to the papillary muscle in a mattress fashion anchoring the artificial cord with a Teflon pledget on the nearest papillary muscle and then putting the two needles of a mattress suture through the leading edge of the section of leaflet that contains the pathologic cords. A variety of techniques have been used to lower the height of these cords,[14] but whatever the technique, the AML height should be related to the maximum height of the PML during cardiac systole. Papillary muscle mattress sutures may also be used to replace a variety of different cordal pathologies. Figure 15-9 demonstrates one technique for lowering AML height with Gore-Tex cords.

◆ A third technique to repair the AML is cordal transfer from the PML to the AML, the "flip-over" technique[15,16] (Fig. 15-10). In this technique the surgeon incises an uninvolved portion of the PML with normal-length cords and "flips over" this segment to the AML, suturing it to the pathologic segment of the AML and thus limiting AML excursion by the length of the posterior cords. The only disadvantage of this technique is that it uses an uninvolved area of the PML that is otherwise normal.

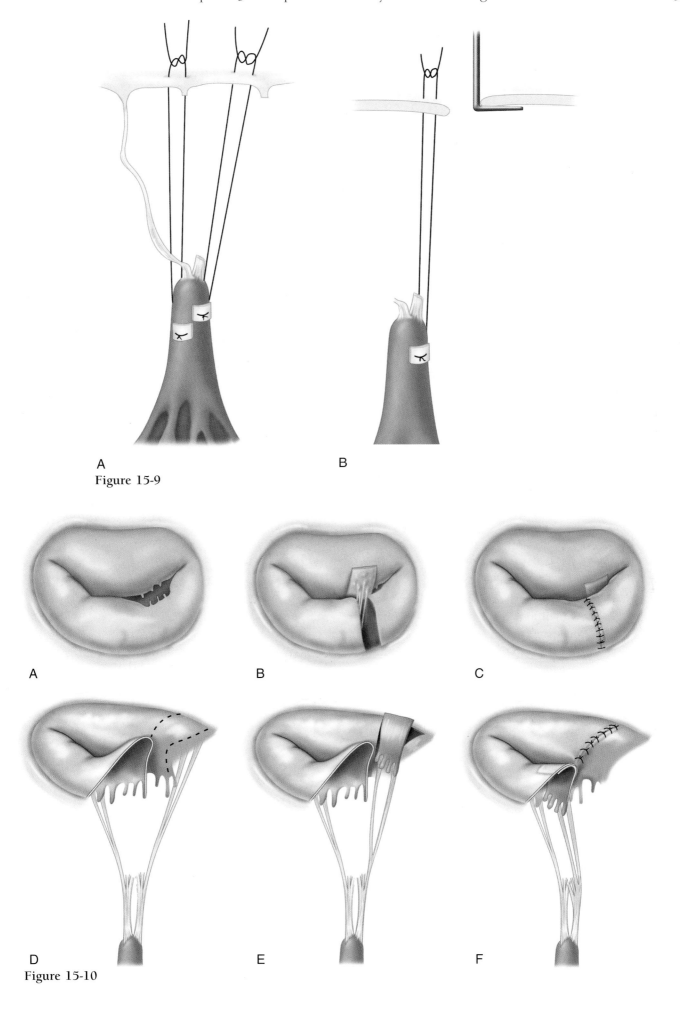

A   B

Figure 15-9

A   B   C

D   E   F

Figure 15-10

- Finally, in patients with severe disease for whom time is of the essence, particularly those with an enlarged AML and severe left ventricular dysfunction, the edge-to-edge technique popularized by Alfieri and coworkers has proved useful.[17] In this technique, a multifilament figure-of-eight suture attaches the flail segment of the AML to the corresponding part of the PML, thus making a double-orifice mitral valve (Fig. 15-11).
- Commissuroplasty is another effective technique for the prolapsed valve when there is cordal rupture or severe elongation of A1 or A3.[18] This is the simplest form of mitral valve repair and can be accomplished by placing polypropylene mattress sutures, obliterating the commissure at each side wherever the lesion exists, thus stabilizing leakage through the AML defect. This has little or no effect on the overall surface area of the mitral valve, thus allowing for easy redirection of the AML.
- Another technique for repairing the AML is to resect part of it to foreshorten the large, billowing leaflet[19] (Fig. 15-12).
- One of the mains concerns with mitral valve repair surgery is production of SAM after repair of an enlarged myxomatous mitral valve causing left ventricular outflow obstruction. This is a relatively common outcome if the PML is not reduced in height, the AML pathologic process is not addressed, or the annuloplasty ring is not large enough.
  - ▲ Recently published observations by our group[20] suggest that in certain patients the AML is enlarged disproportionately so that the left half of the leaflet is larger than the right half (Fig. 15-13), and that this may be a major risk factor for SAM despite adherence to all the general techniques for avoidance of SAM, as noted previously.
  - ▲ As mentioned, the first intervention to prevent SAM is to reduce the height of the PML. Next, the sizing of the annuloplasty ring is extremely important. Many cases of chronic SAM have been created by downsizing the annuloplasty ring by using either intercommissural or trigone area measurements. The correct manner of sizing the annuloplasty ring is by measurement of the AML, not the intertrigonal distance. The latter measurement is used for ischemic or myopathic mitral regurgitation but is incorrect for myxomatous valve surgery.

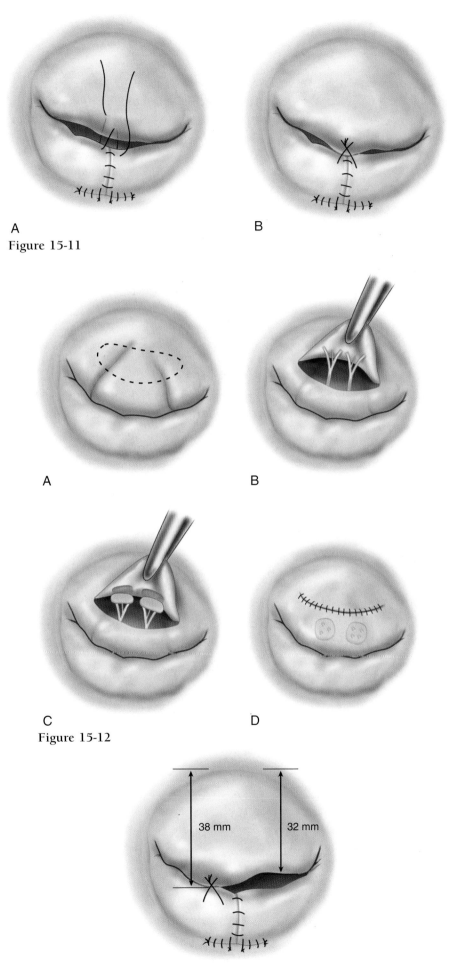

A

B

Figure 15-11

A

B

C

D

Figure 15-12

38 mm

32 mm

Figure 15-13

▲ In patients in whom there has been disproportionate enlargement of the left side of the AML, we have advocated use of the edge-to-edge Alfieri repair.[20] This allows for prevention of SAM providing a large double orifice in the valve with a low left ventricular outflow tract pressure gradient. An annuloplasty ring is always included with the edge-to-edge repair (Fig. 15-14).

▲ If all precautions have been addressed and SAM is still present after bypass is terminated, the operative team observes this for several minutes, ensuring that the patient's heart is completely filled, avoiding the use of positive inotropic agents and supporting blood pressure with α-adrenergic agents to increase left ventricular resistance. These simple steps are necessary before any further work is considered.

▲ After the blood volume has been brought to normal levels, blood pressure has been verified as adequate, and all the aforementioned physiologic adjustments have been made, if the patient still has severe left ventricular outflow tract obstruction, the best technique is to reestablish bypass, open the left atrium, and apply the edge-to-edge repair to guarantee obliteration of the left ventricular outflow tract gradient. One must ensure that there are two adequate valve orifices after the edge-to-edge repair. In the worst-case scenario, mitral valve replacement maybe necessary, but this has been extremely rare in our experience.

▲ To emphasize the point about correctly sizing the annuloplasty ring, our mitral valve re-repair experience[21] has mostly consisted of patients with myxomatous mitral valves in whom the original annuloplasty ring was downsized, and the re-repair merely upsized the ring, which obliterates SAM.

◆ An annuloplasty ring is required in every mitral valve repair. Previous work by our group showed that in a nonrandomized group of repair operations using an annuloplasty ring the recurrence rate was 3% over a 3-year period, compared with a 15% rate in those without an annuloplasty ring.[22]

◆ There are a variety of annuloplasty rings for the myxomatous degenerated valve, varying from the full circular, rigid ring to the totally flexible C-ring. Size is critical, and in most repairs of the myxomatous mitral valve, a large ring, regardless of type, is desirable because of the huge expanse of the AML and dilated annulus (see Fig. 15-14A).

◆ Once correct sizing is obtained, braided sutures are placed circumferentially, extending medially for the AML and posteriorly for the PML (see Fig. 15-14B). We are careful to place these sutures precisely at the annulovalvular junction and not beyond, to prevent injury to the circumflex coronary artery. Any deviation from this, particularly when the circumflex artery anatomy is uncertain, can be dangerous.

◆ Once the sutures have been placed into the annulus, they are placed into the ring, and the ring is lowered and the sutures tied.

◆ For flexible rings, we leave the mandrel in place until the last two sutures have been placed, and then remove it so as not to distort the trigone sutures (see Fig. 15-14C). The valve should then be tested by infusion of saline into the left ventricle to maximum left ventricular volume, noting leakage through any part of the valve.

◆ Most patients undergoing mitral valve repair have little or no calcium deposit in the leaflets or annulus of the valve.

◆ In some individuals, particularly the elderly, the presence of subannular calcification may make it difficult to carry out repair unless some or all of the calcium is removed.

◆ Carpentier's group[23] advocated radical excision of the entire calcified bar, which is unrelated to the leaflets per se, and then reattaching the left ventricle to the right atrium by figure-of-eight sutures.

◆ We have taken a different approach, using pituitary rongeurs to carefully chip away enough of the calcified deposits that the leaflets can be brought together, thus allowing for performance of the techniques described previously, but without separating the atrium from the ventricle.[24]

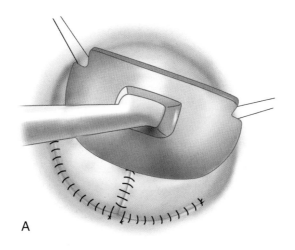

A

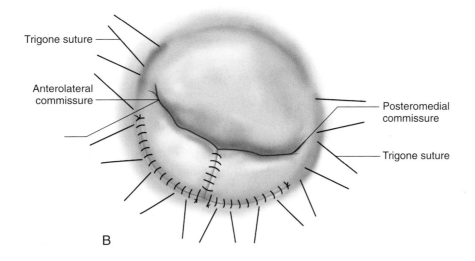

Trigone suture

Anterolateral
commissure

Posteromedial
commissure

Trigone suture

B

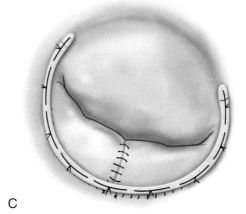

C

Figure 15-14

◆ In a consecutive group of 100 patients, 98 were reparable (a reparability index of 98%). All patients left the operating room with only trace or no mitral regurgitation.

Step 4. Postoperative Care

◆ Postoperative care is routine for cardiac surgery, but with special attention to arrhythmia prevention and maintaining afterload reduction.

Step 5. Pearls and Pitfalls

◆ Using the simplified techniques described in this chapter, with an annuloplasty ring used in all cases of myxomatous valve repair, mitral valve repair should be possible in over 90% of patients.
◆ Conditions prohibiting valve repair include extensive calcification of parts of the leaflets or sometimes the annulus, and previous multiple bouts of endocarditis, which may cause severe scarring and contraction of leaflet tissue.
◆ Use of complex techniques in every case is unnecessary; many of the simplified modifications described in this chapter should aid the surgeon in deciding what techniques to use based on the pathologic process encountered.

References

1. Savage EB, Ferguson TB Jr, DiSesa VJ: Use of mitral valve repair: Analysis of contemporary United States experience reported to the Society of Thoracic Surgeons National Cardiac Database. Ann Thorac Surg 2003;75:820-825.
2. Parish LM, Jackson BM, Enomoto Y, et al: The dynamic anterior mitral annulus. Ann Thorac Surg 2004;78:1248-1255.
3. Grande-Allen KJ, Griffin BP, Ratliff NB, et al: Glycosaminoglycan profiles of myxomatous mitral leaflets and chordae parallel the severity of mechanical alterations. J Am Coll Cardiol 2003;42:271-277.
4. Enriquez-Sarano M, Avierinos JF, Messika-Zeitoun D, et al: Quantitative determinants of the outcome of asymptomatic mitral regurgitation. N Engl J Med 2005;352:875-883.
5. Bonow RO, Carabello BA, Chatterjee K, et al: ACC/AHA 2006 guidelines for the management of patients with valvular heart disease: A report of the American College of Cardiology/American Heart Association Task Force on Practice Guidelines (Writing Committee to revise the 1998 guidelines for the management of patients with valvular heart disease) developed in Collaboration with the Society of Cardiovascular Anesthesiologists, endorsed by the Society for Cardiovascular Angiography and Interventions and the Society of Thoracic Surgeons. J Am Coll Cardiol 2006;48:e1-e148.
6. Gogbashian A, Sepic J, Soltesz EG, et al: Operative and long-term survival of elderly is significantly improved by mitral valve repair. Am Heart J 2006;151:1325-1333.

7. Greelish JP, Cohn LH, Leacche ML, et al: Minimally invasive mitral valve repair suggests earlier operations for mitral valve disease. J Thorac Cardiovasc Surg 2003;126:365-371.
8. Larbalestier RI, Chard RB, Cohn LH: Optimal approach to the mitral valve: Dissection of the interatrial groove. Ann Thorac Surg 1992;54:1186-1188.
9. Carpentier A: Cardiac valve surgery: "The French correction." J Thorac Cardiovasc Surg 1983;86:323-337.
10. Duran CG, Pomar JL, Revuelta JM, et al: Conservative operation for mitral insufficiency: Critical analysis supported by postoperative hemodynamic studies of 72 patients. J Thorac Cardiovasc Surg 1980;79:326-337.
11. Gillinov AM, Cosgrove DM, Wahi S, et al: Is anterior leaflet repair always necessary in repair of bileaflet mitral valve prolapse? Ann Thorac Surg 1999;68:820-824.
12. Smedira NG, Selman R, Cosgrove DM, et al: Repair of anterior leaflet prolapse: Chordal transfer is superior to chordal shortening. J Thorac Cardiovasc Surg 1996;112:287-292.
13. Frater RW, Vetter HO, Zussa C, Dahm M: Chordal replacement in mitral valve repair. Circulation 1990;82(5 Suppl):IV125-IV130.
14. Duran CM, Pekar F: Techniques for ensuring the correct length of new mitral chords. J Heart Valve Dis 2003;12:156-161.
15. Duran CG: Repair of anterior mitral valve leaflet chordal rupture or elongation (the flip-over technique). J Card Surg 1986;1:161-166.
16. Uva MS, Grare P, Jebara V, Fuzelier JF, et al: Transposition of chordae in mitral valve repair. Circulation 1993;88:35-38.
17. Alfieri O, Maisano F, De Bonis M, et al: The double-orifice technique in mitral valve repair: A simple solution for complex problems. J Thorac Cardiovasc Surg 2001;122:674-681.
18. Gillinov AM, Shortt KG, Cosgrove DM: Commissural closure for repair of mitral commissural prolapse. Ann Thorac Surg 2005;80:1135-1136.
19. Duran CM: Surgical techniques for the repair of anterior mitral leaflet prolapse. J Card Surg 1999;14:471-481.
20. Brinster DR, Unic D, D'Ambra MN, et al: Midterm results of the edge-to-edge technique for complex mitral valve repair. Ann Thorac Surg 2006;81:1612-1617.
21. Shekar PS, Couper GS, Cohn LH: Mitral valve re-repair. J Heart Valve Dis 2005;14:583-587.
22. Cohn LH, Couper GS, Aranki SF, et al: The long-term results of mitral valve reconstruction for the "floppy" valve. J Cardiac Surg 1994;9:278-281.
23. el Asmar B, Acker M, Couetil JP, et al: Mitral valve repair in the extensively calcified mitral valve annulus. Ann Thorac Surg 1991;52:66-69.
24. Bichell DP, Adams DH, Aranki SF, et al: Repair of mitral regurgitation from myxomatous degeneration in the patient with a severely calcified posterior annulus. J Cardiac Surg 1995;10:281-284.

CHAPTER 16

MINIMALLY INVASIVE MITRAL VALVE REPLACEMENT: PARTIAL STERNOTOMY APPROACH

Tomislav Mihaljevic, Jason O. Robertson, Amir K. Durrani, and A. Marc Gillinov

Step 1. Surgical Anatomy

- Mitral valve dysfunction can be caused by pathologic processes affecting any component of the valve or subvalvular apparatus, including the valve leaflets, the annulus, the papillary muscles, the chordae tendineae, and the left ventricular wall.
- The anterior portion of the mitral valve annulus is positioned posterior to the aortic annulus and is bordered by the left and right fibrous trigones. Both the atrioventricular node and the bundle of His are adjacent to the right trigone. The circumflex artery runs along the posterior annulus of the mitral valve and is at risk for injury during mitral valve repair or replacement (Fig. 16-1).
- Chordae tendineae extend from the anterior and posterior papillary muscles to both leaflets of the mitral valve. Primary chordae tendineae attach along the free margin of the leaflet, whereas secondary and tertiary chordae tendineae attach progressively closer to the annulus.

Step 2. Preoperative Considerations

- The most common indications for mitral valve replacement are rheumatic mitral stenosis and infective endocarditis. Mitral valve replacement is less commonly performed in patients with degenerative mitral valve disease and functional mitral regurgitation.
- Long-standing, severe mitral stenosis results in pulmonary hypertension and right ventricular dysfunction with a variable degree of tricuspid valve regurgitation. If severe, this can result in secondary hepatic and renal dysfunction, with a resultant increase in operative risk.
- Mitral annular calcifications are frequently present in elderly patients, most commonly in those with rheumatic mitral stenosis. Calcification typically involves the posterior aspect of the mitral annulus and in some cases can extend into the base of the posterior leaflet and the base of the left ventricle. In the most extreme cases, calcification can involve the bases of the papillary muscles. Severe calcification of the mitral annulus appears as a "horseshoe sign" on the preoperative chest radiograph or coronary angiogram.

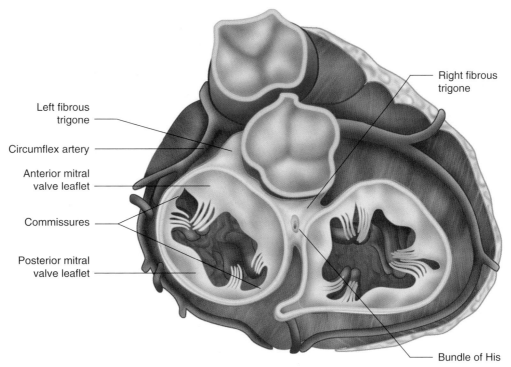

Left fibrous trigone

Circumflex artery

Anterior mitral valve leaflet

Commissures

Posterior mitral valve leaflet

Right fibrous trigone

Bundle of His

Figure 16-1

- Standard preoperative assessment of mitral valve disease is performed by transthoracic or transesophageal echocardiography. Transesophageal echocardiography allows more precise assessment of the anatomy and function of the mitral valve and represents the gold standard in preoperative assessment.
- Mechanical prostheses are indicated in patients younger than 65 years of age. Biologic prosthses are commonly used for the elderly, although improved performance of newer-generation bioprostheses has resulted in their expanded use in younger patients.

Step 3. Operative Steps

1. Incision

- Selection of the surgical approach depends on the etiology of the mitral valve disease, the presence of concomitant coronary or valvular disease, and the body habitus of the patient. Most patients who require isolated mitral valve replacement are candidates for a minimally invasive approach. Relative contraindications to the described minimally invasive approach include morbid obesity and the presence of extensive mitral annular calcifications.
- The standard incision for traditional minimally invasive mitral valve repair is a 6- to 8-cm skin incision and partial upper sternotomy, extending into the left fourth intercostal space. This is the approach described in this chapter (Fig. 16-2).
- Alternatively, minimally invasive mitral valve replacement can be performed through a partial lower sternotomy that preserves the xiphoid and extends into the right second intercostal space.
- A right anterolateral thoracotomy through the fourth intercostal space represents another possible approach and is particularly suitable for patients who have had prior coronary artery bypass grafting or who have undergone prior aortic or mitral valve surgery.

2. Dissection

- A small sternal retractor with removable blades (Baxter Healthcare Corporation, Deerfield, Ill) is used to retract the sternum before proceeding with the dissection. The thymic remnants are then divided and ligated with nonabsorbable suture, and the upper pericardium is divided along the midline.
- The retractor is then removed and a pericardial cradle is formed by placing stay sutures in the skin, using 2-0 silk sutures. Transient hypotension may occur when the edges of the pericardium are pulled toward the skin owing to the displacement of the superior mediastinum and an associated decrease in venous return to the right atrium.
- The sternal retractor is reinserted to expose the great vessels and the right atrium. Cardiopulmonary bypass is then instituted by cannulation of the ascending aorta and the superior and inferior venae cavae. The ascending aorta is cannulated by a flexible aortic cannula (21F), whereas bicaval cannulation is accomplished by placing flexible venous cannulae (24F) into the distal superior vena cava (SVC) and through the right atrial appendage into the inferior vena cava (IVC). Vacuum-assisted venous drainage is used in all cases. Finally, an antegrade cardioplegia cannula is placed in the proximal ascending aorta (Fig. 16-3).

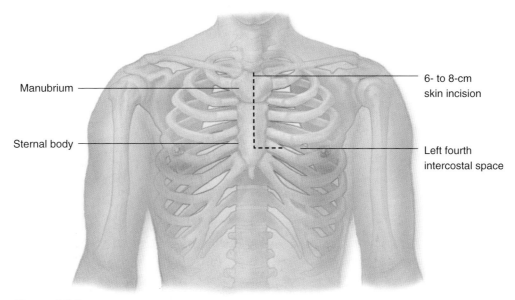

Manubrium

6- to 8-cm
skin incision

Sternal body

Left fourth
intercostal space

Figure 16-2

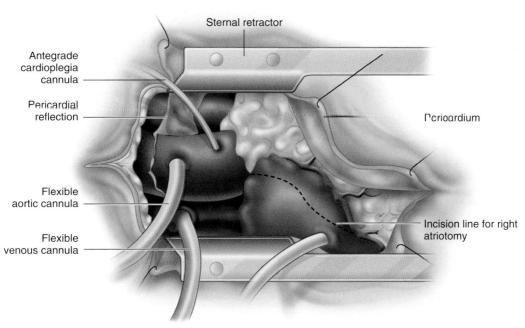

Sternal retractor

Antegrade
cardioplegia
cannula

Pericardial
reflection

Pericardium

Flexible
aortic cannula

Flexible
venous cannula

Incision line for right
atriotomy

Figure 16-3

♦ After initiation of bypass, the right atrium is isolated by encircling both the SVC and IVC using flexible vessel loops. To place these loops, the pericardial reflections around the vessels must be dissected. The isolation of the IVC is facilitated by use of a semicircular Favaloro clamp (Fig. 16-4).

♦ Cross-clamping of the aorta is performed with a Cosgrove Flex Clamp (Allegiance Healthcare Corporation, V. Mueller, McGraw Park, Ill) such that there is minimal obstruction of the surgical field, and a modified Buckberg solution is administered as the main component of cold, antegrade blood cardioplegia.

♦ 2-0 silk sutures are placed into the right atrial appendage medial to the insertion site of the inferior venous cannula to ensure retraction of the atrial wall edges. A right atriotomy is then performed with the incision extending between the SVC and aorta superiorly and the base of the right atrium inferiorly. A cannula for retrograde cardioplegia can be inserted directly into the coronary sinus at this point (see Fig. 16-3).

♦ A trans-septal incision is performed through the mid-portion of the fossa ovalis and extended superiorly across the roof of the left atrium between the SVC and the aortic root (Fig. 16-5).

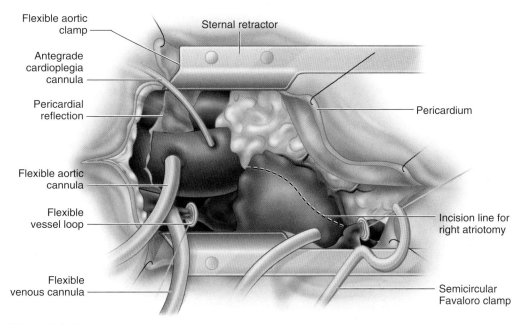

Flexible aortic clamp

Antegrade cardioplegia cannula

Pericardial reflection

Flexible aortic cannula

Flexible vessel loop

Flexible venous cannula

Sternal retractor

Pericardium

Incision line for right atriotomy

Semicircular Favaloro clamp

Figure 16-4

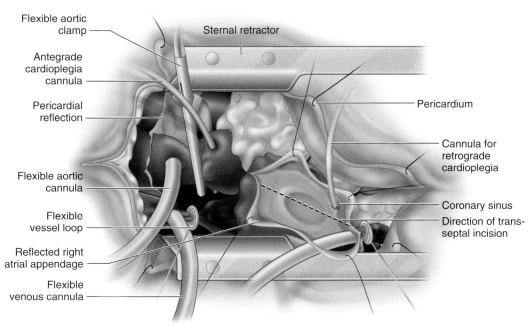

Flexible aortic clamp

Antegrade cardioplegia cannula

Pericardial reflection

Flexible aortic cannula

Flexible vessel loop

Reflected right atrial appendage

Flexible venous cannula

Sternal retractor

Pericardium

Cannula for retrograde cardioplegia

Coronary sinus

Direction of trans-septal incision

Figure 16-5

♦ Exposure of the mitral valve is achieved by placing two or three pledgeted 3-0 polypropylene stay sutures into the medial aspect of the incised septum. Further retraction of the interatrial septum is provided by two low-profile hand-held retractors (Fig. 16-6).

♦ Once the mitral valve is exposed, the anterior leaflet is incised, leaving a residual rim of approximately 5 mm, and the two small areas of the leaflet that contain the chordae from the anterior and posterior papillary muscles are retained. Gentle traction on the partly detached anterior leaflet allows excellent visualization of the anterior portion of the mitral annulus and secure placement of everted pledgeted sutures (2-0 Ethibond; Fig. 16-7).

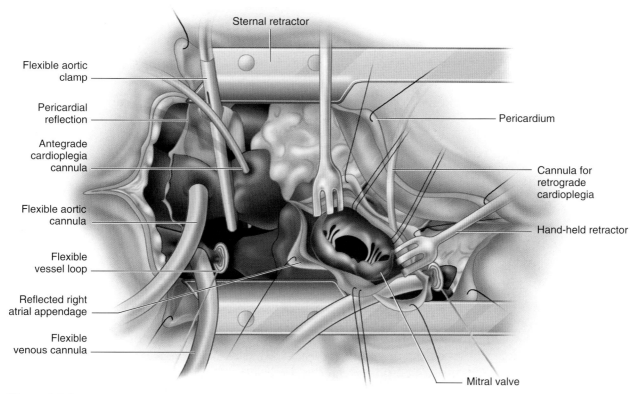

Sternal retractor

Flexible aortic clamp

Pericardial reflection

Antegrade cardioplegia cannula

Flexible aortic cannula

Flexible vessel loop

Reflected right atrial appendage

Flexible venous cannula

Pericardium

Cannula for retrograde cardioplegia

Hand-held retractor

Mitral valve

Figure 16-6

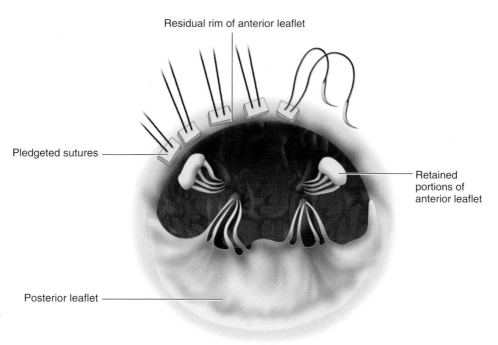

Residual rim of anterior leaflet

Pledgeted sutures

Posterior leaflet

Retained portions of anterior leaflet

Figure 16-7

◆ The retained areas of the anterior leaflet containing the chordae are attached to the lateral and medial annulus with pledgeted 2-0 Ethibond sutures (Fig. 16-8A). This placement preserves the chordae and ensures that they will not obstruct the left ventricular outflow tract or cause uneven heaping of tissue on the posterior leaflet. An alternative approach to preserve the chordae is simply to incise a portion of the anterior leaflet and fold the rest of the leaflet onto the posterior aspect of the annulus (Fig. 16-8B).

◆ Next, pledgeted sutures are placed along the posterior annulus by running a needle through the annulus and then into the body of the leaflet around any annular calcification (Fig. 16-9A through C).

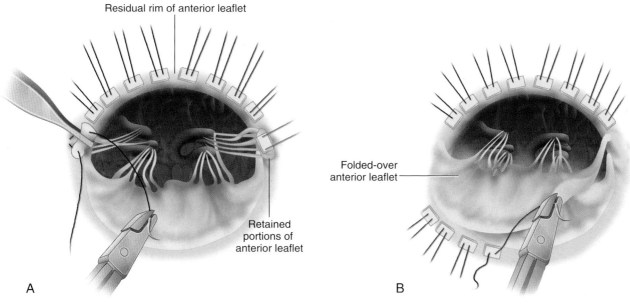

Residual rim of anterior leaflet

Folded-over anterior leaflet

Retained portions of anterior leaflet

A

B

Figure 16-8

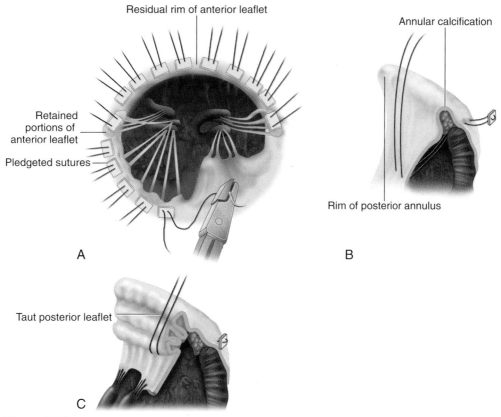

Residual rim of anterior leaflet

Retained portions of anterior leaflet

Pledgeted sutures

Annular calcification

Rim of posterior annulus

A

B

Taut posterior leaflet

C

Figure 16-9

- Calcification of the posterior leaflet should be debrided (Fig. 16-10A). In cases where extensive decalcification is needed, the annulus is instead reconstructed with a strip of autologous pericardium (Fig. 16-10B).
- Biologic prostheses are most commonly used for mitral valve replacement. Approximately 12 sutures are placed into the valve sewing ring, and the valve is lowered into place and secured. The valve should be oriented in such a way as to keep the struts from obstructing the left ventricular outflow tract (Fig. 16-11).

3. Closure

- Air must be displaced from the left ventricle to the left atrium before the aortic cross-clamp is removed, either by filling the left ventricle with saline or by administrating antegrade cardioplegia. Running 4-0 polypropylene sutures are then used to sequentially close the interatrial septum and the right atrium.
- Mediastinal and right pleural chest tubes are placed, and pacing wires are inserted in the anterior surface of the right ventricle. This is done while the heart is still decompressed and on cardiopulmonary bypass, which allows better visualization of the operative field and safe placement. Once chest tubes and pacing wires have been placed, and once all intracardiac air has been removed, the patient is weaned from cardiopulmonary bypass.
- Simple stainless steel sternal wires are used for the sternal closure in usual fashion.

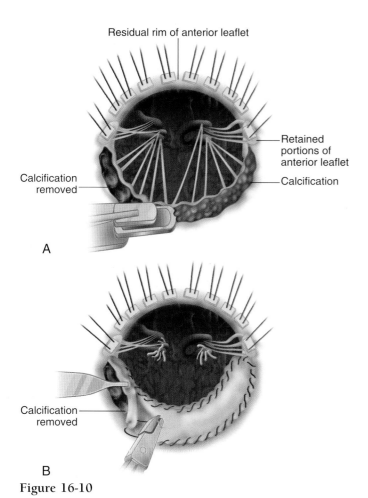

Residual rim of anterior leaflet

Retained portions of anterior leaflet

Calcification

Calcification removed

A

Calcification removed

B

Figure 16-10

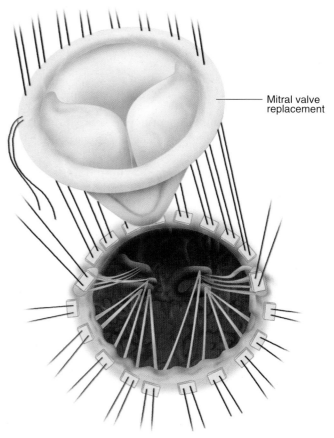

Mitral valve replacement

Figure 16-11

Step 4. Postoperative Care

- Patients who underwent uncomplicated, minimally invasive mitral valve replacement can be extubated in the operating room. Early extubation allows for faster recovery and a shorter intensive care unit stay.
- Patients with long-standing mitral stenosis and severe pulmonary hypertension with right ventricular dysfunction often benefit from inotropic support with phosphodiesterase inhibitors (milrinone) and pulmonary vasodilators (nitric oxide, sildenafil).
- Long-term warfarin anticoagulation with an ideal international normalized ratio of 2.5 to 3.5 is indicated for patients receiving mechanical prostheses, with consideration given to the use of low-dose aspirin in addition to warfarin.
- Patients in normal sinus rhythm who have received a biologic prosthesis may be adequately managed with aspirin alone, without including short-term anticoagulation, barring the presence of other risk factors for thromboembolism.
- Patients with atrial fibrillation who have undergone mitral valve replacement with a biologic prosthesis may be maintained on anticoagulation for the first 6 to 9 weeks, or as long as they remain in atrial fibrillation and are not contraindicated for anticoagulation.
- Emergency cardioversion is seldom successful in patients with a long history of atrial fibrillation who have undergone mitral valve replacement.

Step 5. Pearls and Pitfalls

- Transesophageal echocardiography is the essential diagnostic tool in the preoperative and intra-operative assessment of patients requiring minimally invasive mitral valve replacement.
- A partial upper sternotomy allows excellent access to the aortic and tricuspid valves, as well as allowing performance of minimally invasive multivalve surgery.
- The operative field should be flooded with continuous CO_2 to reduce intracardiac air and peripheral embolization, because CO_2 dissolves more readily in blood than do other components of air.
- Extension of the partial upper sternotomy into the left fourth intercostal space should be conducted with care not to injure the left internal thoracic artery and vein.
- A trans-septal incision provides excellent exposure of the mitral valve but may cause transient postoperative dysfunction of the sinus node. However, the incidence of permanent postoperative sinus node dysfunction is not different from that in patients operated on through a conventional, complete sternotomy.
- The superior part of the trans-septal incision should be at least 1 cm lateral to the base of the aortic root to avoid injury to the aortic valve during closure of the incision.
- Sutures along the lateral aspect of the mitral annulus should be placed with care to avoid injury to the circumflex artery.

Bibliography

Byrne JG, Mitchell ME, Adams DH, et al: Minimally invasive direct access mitral valve surgery. Semin Thorac Cardiovasc Surg 1999;11:212-222.

Gillinov AM, Banbury MK, Cosgrove DM: Hemisternotomy approach for aortic and mitral valve surgery. J Cardiac Surg 2000;15:15-20.

Gillinov AM, Cosgrove DM: Minimally invasive mitral valve surgery: Mini-sternotomy with extended transseptal approach. Semin Thorac Cardiovasc Surg 1999;11:206-211.

Gillinov AM, Cosgrove DM III: Mitral valve repair. In Cohn LH, Edmunds LH Jr (eds): Cardiac Surgery in the Adult. New York, McGraw-Hill, 2003, pp 933-950.

Mihaljevic T, Cohn LH, Unic D, et al: One thousand minimally invasive valve operations: Early and late results. Ann Surg 2004;240:529-534; discussion 534.

Nair RU, Sharpe DA: Limited lower sternotomy for minimally invasive mitral valve replacement. Ann Thorac Surg 1998;65:273-274.

CHAPTER 17

PERCUTANEOUS MITRAL VALVE REPAIR TECHNIQUES

William E. Cohn

Step 1. Surgical Anatomy

- In any percutaneous intervention for mitral valve disease, it is essential to appreciate the pathologic process of the valve so that an appropriate therapy can be selected.
- Patients with central, discrete regurgitant jets with relatively narrow bases and single-leaflet prolapse or flail may benefit from percutaneous edge-to-edge repair.
- Patients with enlarged hearts, annular dilation, minimal tenting, and central jets may benefit from percutaneous transvenous mitral annuloplasty (PTMA).
- Because several of the coronary sinus–based devices must be positioned distally in the coronary venous system, it is helpful if patients have a large coronary sinus, a large great cardiac vein with minimal tortuosity, and a generous anterior interventricular vein adjacent to the left anterior descending coronary artery. Furthermore, it is preferable if the coronary sinus and great cardiac vein lie in the same plane as the mitral annulus because close proximity is essential for efficacy (Fig. 17-1).
- In many patients with heart failure and left atrial enlargement, the coronary venous structures may lie closer to the base of the heart than to the annulus. These patients are less likely to benefit from implantation of a transvenous device.
- A computed tomogram with three-dimensional reconstruction (3DCT) is helpful in identifying patients with unsuitable geometry, and 3DCT may prove to be an essential step in identifying patients who are well suited for PTMA. Similarly, the relationship between the coronary sinus and the circumflex coronary artery and its branches is readily shown by 3DCT, which may reveal whether a patient is at risk for coronary compromise and ischemia after percutaneous annuloplasty.

Step 2. Preoperative Considerations

1. Percutaneous Treatment of Mitral Stenosis

- Until recently, the only percutaneous intervention performed on the mitral valve was balloon mitral valvuloplasty (BMV), a simple and effective means of treating mitral stenosis, which usually results from rheumatic heart disease.

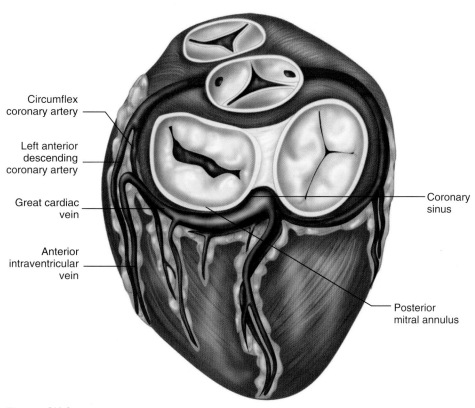

Circumflex
coronary artery

Left anterior
descending
coronary artery

Great cardiac
vein

Anterior
intraventricular
vein

Coronary
sinus

Posterior
mitral annulus

Figure 17-1

- ◆ Preprocedural analysis of the stenotic valve is essential in determining whether a patient is likely to benefit from BMV. Patients with extensive irregular calcification may be at increased risk of embolic complications and may be better served by a surgical procedure. Similarly, patients with mitral stenosis and concomitant mitral regurgitation are at increased risk of worsening regurgitation after the procedure, so BMV is usually contraindicated in these patients.

2. Percutaneous Treatment of Mitral Regurgitation

- ◆ The percutaneous tools for mitral valve repair introduced to date are designed to emulate a specific geometric manipulation of the diseased valve that has been shown to be effective during open surgical mitral valve repair. Just as BMV is a means of performing a catheter-based mitral valve commissurotomy of the stenotic valve, so the newer catheter-based technologies emulate aspects of the surgical reconstruction of the regurgitant valve. These new tools include catheter technology for performing edge-to-edge leaflet repair, and percutaneous tools for performing annular plication or reduction, either by manipulating the coronary sinus or by directly inserting subannular tissue anchors into the left ventricle.

Percutaneous Edge-to-Edge Leaflet Repair

- ◆ At this time, the largest clinical experience in percutaneous mitral repair is with the MitraClip by Evalve (Menlo Park, Calif). The clip is used to affix the midpoint of the anterior leaflet to the midpoint of the posterior leaflet to create a dual-orifice mitral valve. This type of leaflet repair was first described and popularized by Alfieri (Fig. 17-2).
- ◆ Edge-to-edge repair is especially effective in cases of segmental flail or prolapse involving only one leaflet. When performed surgically, it is usually done in conjunction with an annuloplasty; however, reports of small series of cases in which this type of repair was performed without annuloplasty suggest that this treatment strategy might be effective in carefully selected patients.

Percutaneous Transvenous Mitral Annuloplasty: Coronary Sinus–Based Cinching

- ◆ Of the several catheter-based annuloplasty technologies currently undergoing clinical evaluation, the largest experience is with the Monarch device (Edwards LifeScience, Irvine, Calif). The device consists of two self-expanding stents connected by a collapsible bridge: in essence, a superelastic spring made from Nitinol that is held in an elongated state by multiple bioabsorbable spacers wedged between adjacent coils. After 3 to 4 weeks in the bloodstream, the spacers dissolve, allowing the bridge to shorten. By this time, the self-expanding stents have become firmly fixed to the coronary venous wall by the investing neointima. When the bridge shortens, traction is applied between the coronary sinus os and the confluence of the anterior interventricular vein and great cardiac vein. This traction results in compression and anterior displacement of the posterior annulus and a decrease in the septal-lateral dimension of the mitral valve (Fig. 17-3), thus improving coaptation and reducing regurgitation in appropriately selected patients.

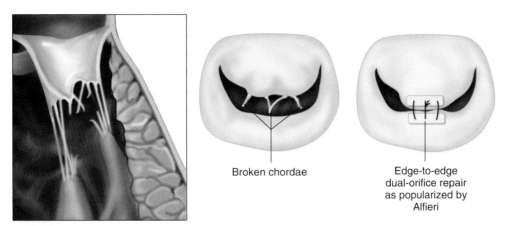

Figure 17-2

Broken chordae

Edge-to-edge
dual-orifice repair
as popularized by
Alfieri

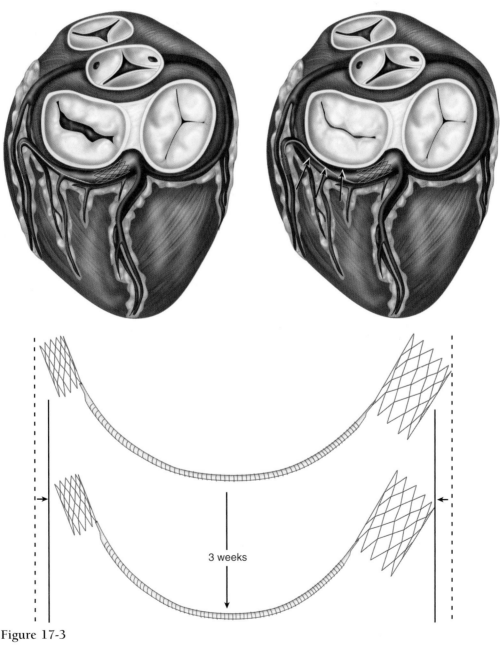

3 weeks

Figure 17-3

- Careful patient selection is necessary to ensure the efficacy of this treatment. Currently, it is unclear how widely applicable coronary sinus–based technologies will be for the treatment of mitral regurgitation. At present, it seems that those best suited to this intervention are patients with secondary or myopathic mitral regurgitation with preserved leaflet mobility and geometry. Therapeutic efficacy has been demonstrated in patients with both ischemic and nonischemic cardiomyopathy, and those with isolated annular dilation and without excessive tenting of the leaflets seem to respond well. With currently available tools, the septal-lateral dimension of the mitral orifice can be decreased by up to 1 cm; patients with regurgitant valves that would benefit from such a shortening may be well suited for this procedure.
- Patients with significant prolapse or flail leaflet do not seem well suited for coronary sinus–based interventions.

Percutaneous Transvenous Mitral Annuloplasty: Coronary Sinus–Based Straightening

- There is preliminary European clinical experience with the PTMA device developed by Viacor, Inc. (Wilmington, Mass).
- The same considerations apply to this procedure as apply to coronary sinus–based cinching.

Step 3. Operative Steps

1. Percutaneous Treatment of Mitral Stenosis

- The procedure is performed by introducing a long, specially curved, retractable needle-in-a-sheath through the femoral vein into the right atrium and puncturing the atrial septum at the fossa ovalis to gain access to the left atrium (Fig. 17-4A). One or two large, high-pressure balloon catheters are then positioned across the stenotic mitral orifice (Fig. 17-4B) and inflated until the orifice is stretched or adhesions between leaflets are torn, thus increasing the valve area and decreasing the transvalvular pressure gradient (Fig. 17-4C).

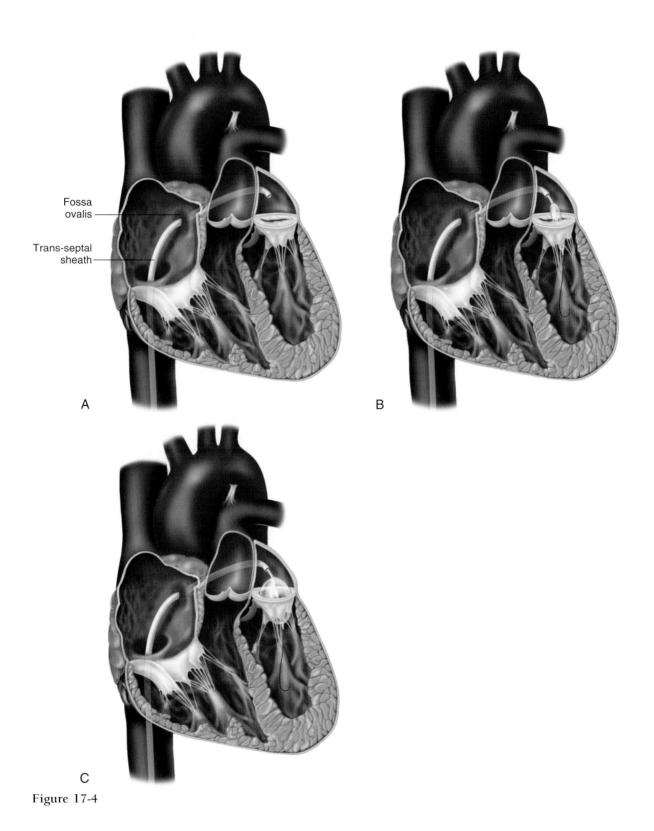

Fossa
ovalis

Trans-septal
sheath

A

B

C

Figure 17-4

2. Percutaneous Treatment of Mitral Regurgitation

Percutaneous Edge-to-Edge Leaflet Repair

◆ To position the clip, a large deflectable sheath is introduced through the femoral vein and passed up the inferior vena cava, through the right atrium, and into the left atrium across the atrial septum (Fig. 17-5). The clip is then passed up the sheath at the end of a deflectable catheter (Fig. 17-6) and passed across the mitral valve into the left ventricular cavity under fluoroscopic and echocardiographic guidance. The clip is then slowly withdrawn toward the left atrium until it grasps the edges of both leaflets.

◆ Color Doppler ultrasonography is used to assess the clip's effect on mitral regurgitation (Fig. 17-7). If the result is suboptimal, the clip is repositioned until an acceptable reduction in regurgitation is obtained. The clip is then fastened to the leaflets and released from the sheath (Fig. 17-8).

Percutaneous Transvenous Mitral Annuloplasty: Coronary Sinus–Based Cinching

◆ The device is inserted percutaneously through the subclavian vein (preferably the left), down the superior vena cava, and into the right atrium and coronary sinus. The distal stent is deployed in the proximal anterior interventricular vein, and the proximal stent is released adjacent to the coronary sinus os.

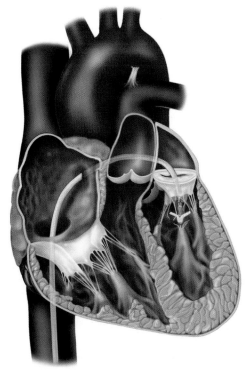

Figure 17-5

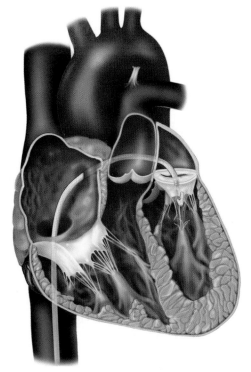

Figure 17-6

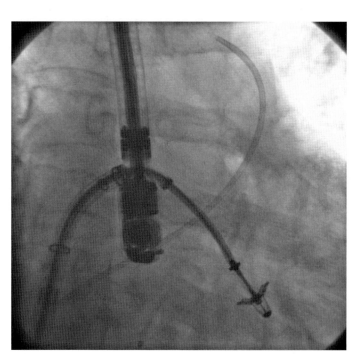

Figure 17-7

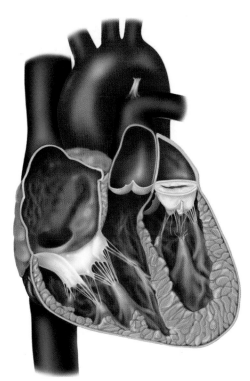

Figure 17-8

Percutaneous Transvenous Mitral Annuloplasty: Coronary Sinus–Based Straightening

- Like the Monarch, the Viacor PTMA device is inserted through the left subclavian vein into the coronary sinus and great cardiac vein. The Viacor system has separate diagnostic and implant catheters; each is a flexible 7F, three-lumen catheter that, when in position, surrounds the posterior mitral annulus.
- Once the catheter is in place, progressively stiff Nitinol rods are passed down each of the three lumens of the catheter while mitral geometry and regurgitation are observed echocardiographically. The progressive stiffening of the catheter gradually straightens the coronary sinus and great cardiac vein and displaces the posterior mitral annulus anteriorly. In properly selected patients, this change in geometry results in a decrease in the septal-lateral dimension of the mitral valve, an improvement in leaflet coaptation, and reduction in regurgitation (Fig. 17-9).
- If a desirable reduction in regurgitation is achieved, the diagnostic catheter is removed and replaced with an implant catheter that has a sealable titanium hub at its proximal end. The rods identified as being most efficacious during the diagnostic portion of the procedure are then threaded down the three lumens of the implant catheter, and the hub is sealed. The hub is placed in a subcutaneous pocket below the left clavicle, where it can be readily accessed later if the device needs to be removed or if it is deemed desirable to exchange the Nitinol rods for stiffer or longer ones.

Step 4. Postoperative Care

1. Percutaneous Treatment of Mitral Stenosis

- Patients are monitored for the return of mitral stenosis. Specifically, transesophageal echocardiograms are obtained, and patients are monitored for symptoms of pulmonary edema and low cardiac output.

2. Percutaneous Treatment of Mitral Regurgitation

Percutaneous Edge-to-Edge Leaflet Repair

- Physical examinations and serial echocardiograms are performed to assess the robustness of the reduction in mitral regurgitation.
- Patients receive routine cardiac care, including optimization of intravascular volume and afterload reduction, as well as beta blockers and other treatments for heart failure. Patients in whom mitral regurgitation returns are evaluated for other possible therapies.
- It is currently thought that anticoagulation is not needed for patients with percutaneously implanted devices, but current experience is limited. As it increases, so will our sophistication in postprocedural management.

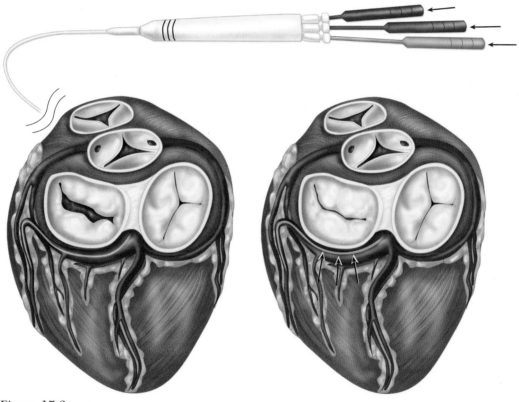

Figure 17-9

Percutaneous Transvenous Mitral Annuloplasty: Coronary Sinus–Based Cinching

- ◆ Serial echocardiograms and fluoroscopic images are obtained over the next several weeks to verify bridge contraction and assess its impact on mitral regurgitation.
- ◆ The postoperative care regimen is otherwise the same as that for percutaneous edge-to-edge leaflet repair.

Percutaneous Transvenous Mitral Annuloplasty: Coronary Sinus–Based Straightening

- ◆ The postoperative care regimen is the same as that for percutaneous edge-to-edge leaflet repair.

Step 5. Pearls and Pitfalls

1. Percutaneous Treatment of Mitral Stenosis

- ◆ Although the increase in valve area is usually not as great as that produced by surgical valve repair or replacement, and although the results are occasionally short lived, BMV can be repeated multiple times. In many patients, BMV allows surgery to be delayed for decades or avoided altogether.
- ◆ Careful patient selection is necessary because performing BMV on some valves will result in the development of problematic mitral regurgitation or systemic emboli.

2. Percutaneous Treatment of Mitral Regurgitation

Percutaneous Edge-to-Edge Leaflet Repair

- ◆ Of the first 170 patients we treated with percutaneous mitral repair (in March 2007), 25% required surgery for return or worsening of regurgitation within the first 18 months after the original procedure; 85% of these operations were successful. Mitral regurgitation was decreased on average by 1.7 grades on a 0 to 4+ scale. Twenty-four months or more after placement of the clip, more than 50% of patients had residual regurgitation of 2+ or less. A randomized trial comparing the edge-to-edge clip with open surgical mitral valve repair is ongoing.

Percutaneous Transvenous Mitral Annuloplasty: Coronary Sinus–Based Cinching

◆ To date, 59 patients at our institution have undergone implantation of the Monarch device. Mitral regurgitation progressively decreased during the first 6 months of observation, suggesting favorable geometric remodeling with time. At the end of the 6-month observation period, patients with 3 to 4+ mitral valve regurgitation at baseline experienced, on average, a 1.8-grade reduction in regurgitation. In this series, there were two cases of pericardial tamponade (caused by coronary sinus perforation) that were managed successfully with percutaneous drainage. In addition, there was one diagonal territory infarct. There were no other device-related major adverse cardiac events.

Percutaneous Transvenous Mitral Annuloplasty: Coronary Sinus–Based Straightening

◆ At this time, the results of this procedure are preliminary but promising, and plans for a pilot study in the United States are underway.

◆ Several other coronary sinus–based technologies for mitral valve repair are currently in various stages of development. Several have shown promise in preclinical evaluation.

Bibliography

Block PC: Percutaneous mitral valve repair: Are they changing the guard? Circulation 2005;111:2154-2156.

Block PC: Percutaneous transcatheter repair for mitral regurgitation. J Interv Cardiol 2006;19:547-551.

Cohn WE: Percutaneous valve interventions: Where we are and where we are headed. Am Heart Hosp J 2006;4:186-191.

Daimon M, Gillinov AM, Liddicoat JR, et al: Dynamic change in mitral annular area and motion during percutaneous mitral annuloplasty for ischemic mitral regurgitation: Preliminary animal study with real-time 3-dimensional echocardiography. J Am Soc Echocardiogr 2007;20:381-388.

Daimon M, Shiota T, Gillinov AM, et al: Percutaneous mitral valve repair for chronic ischemic mitral regurgitation: A real-time three-dimensional echocardiographic study in an ovine model. Circulation 2005;111:2183-2189.

Dang NC, Aboodi MS, Sakaguchi T, et al: Surgical revision after percutaneous mitral valve repair with a clip: Initial multicenter experience. Ann Thorac Surg 2005;80:2338-2342.

Feldman T: Proceedings of TCT: Current status of catheter-based mitral valve repair therapies. J Interv Cardiol 2006;19:396-400.

Feldman T: Percutaneous mitral annuloplasty: Not always a cinch. Catheter Cardiovasc Interv 2007;69:1062-1063.

Feldman T, Wasserman HS, Herrmann HC, et al: Percutaneous mitral valve repair using the edge-to-edge technique: Six-month results of the EVEREST phase I clinical trial. J Am Coll Cardiol 2005;46:2134-2140.

Liddicoat JR, Mac Neill BD, Gillinov AM, et al: Percutaneous mitral valve repair: A feasibility study in an ovine model of acute ischemic mitral regurgitation. Catheter Cardiovasc Interv 2003;60:410-416.

Silvestry FE, Rodriguez LL, Herrmann HC, et al: Echocardiographic guidance and assessment of percutaneous repair for mitral regurgitation with the Evalve MitraClip: Lessons learned from EVEREST I. J Am Soc Echocardiogr 2007;20:1131-1140.

Vassiliades TA Jr, Block PC, Cohn LH, et al: The clinical development of percutaneous heart valve technology: A position statement of the Society of Thoracic Surgeons (STS), the American Association for Thoracic Surgery (AATS), and the Society for Cardiovascular Angiography and Interventions (SCAI) Endorsed by the American College of Cardiology Foundation (ACCF) and the American Heart Association (AHA). J Am Coll Cardiol 2005;45:1554-1560.

Webb JG, Harnek J, Munt BI, et al: Percutaneous transvenous mitral annuloplasty: Initial human experience with device implantation in the coronary sinus. Circulation 2006;113:851-855.

CHAPTER 18

Tricuspid Valve Operations

Alexander Kulik and Thierry G. Mesana

Step 1. Surgical Anatomy

- The tricuspid valve is composed of three leaflets: the anterior, posterior, and septal. Compared with the mitral valve, the leaflets and chordae tendineae of the tricuspid valve are thinner, the tricuspid orifice is larger and more triangular, and the tricuspid annulus is thinner and more difficult to identify.
- The anterior leaflet is the largest of the three leaflets. Its chordae attach to the anterior and septal papillary muscles. The posterior leaflet is the smallest leaflet, and its chordae originate from the posterior and anterior papillary muscles. The septal leaflet is larger than the posterior leaflet, and its chordae attach to the posterior and septal papillary muscles.
- Structures surrounding the tricuspid valve that are of major surgical significance include the coronary sinus, the atrioventricular (AV) node, the membranous septum, the bundle of His, and the right coronary artery (Fig. 18-1).
- The conduction system is near the septal leaflet and its anterior-septal commissure. The AV node lies in the atrial septum bordering the septal leaflet, superior and anterior to the coronary sinus. Its exact location can be approximated at the apex of the triangle of Koch, an isosceles triangle composed of the septal annulus and the tendon of Todaro as its sides and the coronary sinus orifice as its base. The membranous septum usually lies beneath the septal leaflet inferior to the anterior-septal commissure. Extending from the AV node is the bundle of His, which penetrates the right trigone under the interventricular component of the membranous septum (approximately 5 mm inferior to the anterior-septal commissure) and runs along the crest of the muscular septum.
- The right coronary artery runs anterior to the anterior leaflet annulus and may be injured by deep sutures in the annulus.

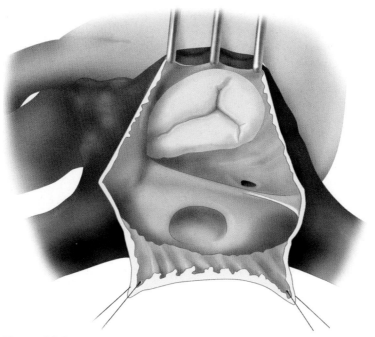

Figure 18-1

Step 2. Preoperative Considerations

- Tricuspid stenosis is most commonly rheumatic in origin. On rare occasions, infective endocarditis, congenital abnormalities, or carcinoid disease may be implicated. Rheumatic tricuspid involvement usually results in both tricuspid stenosis and regurgitation, and it typically coexists with mitral or aortic rheumatic disease. The hallmark features of rheumatic tricuspid stenosis are commissural fusion and leaflet thickening, but calcification is usually absent. Carcinoid syndrome leads to either focal or diffuse deposits of fibrous tissue on the endocardium of valve leaflets and the cardiac chambers. The tricuspid valve in carcinoid syndrome is thickened with retracted leaflets fixed in a semiopen position, resulting in both tricuspid stenosis and regurgitation.
- Tricuspid valve regurgitation (TR) can occur with abnormal or normal valve leaflets. Causes of TR associated with abnormalities of the tricuspid leaflets include rheumatic valve disease, endocarditis, carcinoid syndrome, radiation therapy, trauma, Marfan syndrome, papillary muscle dysfunction, and congenital disorders such as Ebstein anomaly.
- Regurgitation develops with normal tricuspid valve leaflets as a result of right ventricular (RV) dysfunction and tricuspid annular dilation (functional regurgitation), usually in the context of left-sided valvular disease. Pulmonary hypertension or RV dysfunction leads to elevations of RV systolic and diastolic pressures, RV cavity enlargement, and tricuspid annular dilation. The circumference of the tricuspid annulus lengthens primarily along the attachments of the anterior and posterior leaflets. The septal leaflet portion, on the other hand, is fixed between the right and left trigones and the atrial and ventricular septa, preventing its lengthening (Fig. 18-2). As annular and ventricular dilatation progress, the cordal–papillary muscle complex becomes functionally shortened, although it remains normal in appearance. This combination of RV enlargement and tricuspid annular dilation prevents leaflet coaptation and leads to valvular incompetence.
- Previously, it was believed that functional TR decreases or even disappears after surgical correction of left-sided valve disease. This concept influenced cardiac surgery practice for many years. More experience, however, has led to better appreciation of the potential for progression of functional TR and tricuspid annular dilation after left-sided surgery. This effect may occur in spite of the complete correction of the mitral and aortic disease and the resolution of pulmonary hypertension after surgery. Tricuspid annular dilation is the strongest and most consistent risk factor for the development of late TR after left-sided valve surgery.
- Severe TR and its resultant RV dysfunction and venous congestion contribute to an increase in both early and late morbidity and mortality after left-sided valve surgery. Moreover, reoperation to correct worsening postoperative TR is associated with a high operative mortality rate and disappointing long-term results. Therefore, a proactive strategy of repairing a dilated tricuspid annulus at the time of the initial left-sided valve surgery, regardless of the degree of TR, is being advocated as a strategy to help reduce the incidence of late TR and RV failure.

1. Indications for Tricuspid Valve Intervention

- The 2006 American College of Cardiology/American Heart Association valve guidelines recommend tricuspid valve repair for patients with severe functional TR who are undergoing concurrent surgery for mitral valve disease. This provides symptomatic improvement and may improve long-term survival. Tricuspid valve repair or replacement is also recommended for severe primary TR in symptomatic patients. When the tricuspid valve leaflets are too diseased and not amenable to repair, tricuspid valve replacement is believed to be reasonable for patients with severe TR.

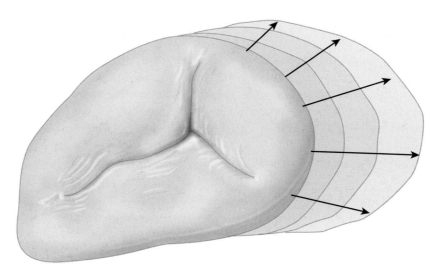

Figure 18-2

- Tricuspid valve repair may also be considered for less-than-severe TR in patients undergoing mitral valve surgery when there is pulmonary hypertension or tricuspid annular dilation. Several cardiac surgery centers currently advocate for the routine repair of the dilated tricuspid annulus at the time of left-sided heart surgery, regardless of the degree of TR. A tricuspid annular diameter (measured between the anterior-septal and posterior-septal commissures) of 70 mm has been suggested as an indication for the repair of tricuspid annular dilation. At our center, we repair a tricuspid annulus if the diameter is 50 mm or more even if there is no associated TR. This repair is believed to reduce the risk of RV dysfunction, both in the perioperative period and in the long term, as well as the need for a second operation.
- American College of Cardiology/American Heart Association practice guidelines recommend against tricuspid surgery for patients with only mild primary TR. Tricuspid surgery is also not indicated in those patients with some degree of TR who are asymptomatic, when there is no concurrent left-sided valve disease, or when severe pulmonary hypertension is absent.

2. Choice of Repair Technique

- Previously, it was believed that the type of tricuspid valve repair performed was of little importance, as long as the size of the tricuspid annulus was secured to avoid progressive dilation. For patients with functional TR secondary to left-sided valve disease, the De Vega annuloplasty was thought to be the most appropriate procedure to reduce the size of the tricuspid annulus. However, recent data demonstrate poor long-term results with the use of the De Vega technique. Although it is a safe and simple procedure, 30% or more of patients may develop recurrent moderate to severe TR after a De Vega repair, with progressive annular dilation and recurrence of symptoms.
- Long-term studies have also illustrated poor long-term durability and high rates of recurrent TR with the use of flexible rings and bands (Duran, Cosgrove-Edwards, Peri-Guard). Only rigid rings have yielded good long-term results, with the bulk of evidence favoring the semirigid Carpentier-Edwards ring as the most durable after tricuspid valve repair.
- At our center, we perform tricuspid valve repairs using rigid annuloplasty bands for all patients with tricuspid annular dilation of greater than 50 mm, regardless of the presence of TR, at the time of concurrent left-sided valve surgery. We also use annuloplasty bands in patients with annular dilations less than 50 mm but severe TR (more than 2+). The De Vega repair is reserved for patients undergoing left-sided valve surgery who have 2+ TR or less and tricuspid annular dimensions of less than 50 mm. In patients with a large annulus and severe TR, we perform annuloplasty and edge-to-edge techniques.

3. Choice of Prosthetic Valve Type

- Repair of the tricuspid valve is superior to valve replacement because it is associated with lower hospital mortality rates, better long-term survival, better preservation of ventricular function, fewer thromboembolic complications, and a reduced risk of endocarditis. However, in the context of organic tricuspid disease with severe leaflet thickening and cordal retraction, tricuspid valve replacement is the preferred surgical intervention.
- The choice of prosthesis type in the tricuspid position has been debated in the cardiac surgery community for many years. A recent meta-analysis summarized the published literature by comparing outcomes reported for contemporary mechanical and bioprosthetic tricuspid valves. A total of 11 studies, with 646 mechanical and 514 biologic tricuspid prostheses and 6046

follow-up years, were analyzed. Studies that reported prosthetic models from before 1970 were excluded. Overall, the pooled survival and reoperation data did not favor either prosthesis type. Furthermore, the incidence of mechanical valve thrombosis was comparable with the incidence of bioprosthetic valve deterioration. Therefore, the type of prosthetic valve is not a risk factor for adverse outcomes after tricuspid valve replacement, and there is no evidence favoring one prosthetic type or the other.

♦ As in other valve positions, there is no gold standard prosthetic valve available for tricuspid valve replacement. We believe that the choice between a mechanical or a bioprosthetic valve in the tricuspid position should be individualized according to the surgeon's clinical judgment, patient characteristics, anticoagulation considerations, likelihood of pregnancy, socioeconomic status, and lifestyle issues. A patient with drug addiction and a history of endocarditis, who may have difficulty with anticoagulation compliance, should have a bioprosthesis implanted.

4. Prosthesis and Ring Size

♦ Although it is not supported by good evidence, it is currently popular to implant undersized rings to improve coaptation during the repair of mitral regurgitation. This strategy may also apply to the repair of functional TR. However, there are no data to support the practice of implanting undersized rings in the tricuspid position. Long-term data from the Cleveland Clinic demonstrated that the use of a small tricuspid ring for the repair of functional TR did not protect against the development of recurrent late TR. We generally implant a tricuspid prosthesis (band or valve) identical in size to the mitral prosthesis used during concurrent mitral repair or replacement.

♦ When replacing the tricuspid valve, it is almost always possible to place large bioprosthetic or mechanical valves. Prostheses with an internal diameter greater than 27 mm do not have clinically significant gradients, and thus hemodynamic performance is rarely an issue in tricuspid valve replacement.

5. Tricuspid Valve Endocarditis

♦ In tricuspid endocarditis, the tricuspid valve may be infected in isolation or in the context of other infected valves. Isolated tricuspid bacterial endocarditis is usually seen in the presence of intravenous drug use or long-standing central venous catheters. The most common etiologic organisms include *Pseudomonas aeruginosa*, *Staphylococcus aureus*, gram-negative bacilli, and, rarely, *Candida albicans*.

♦ If at all possible, tricuspid valve repair with partial valve excision and reconstruction should be considered in less severe cases of tricuspid endocarditis. For complete destruction of the valve, however, tricuspid valve excision or replacement may be offered.

♦ In patients with ongoing intravenous drug addictions, valve excision may prove to be a useful approach that avoids the subsequent risk of prosthetic valve endocarditis. However, the resultant severe TR after valve excision compromises postoperative cardiac function, and a delayed reoperation for prosthesis implantation may prove to be technically difficult. Therefore, primary bioprosthetic valve replacement is usually preferred over total valve excision.

Step 3. Operative Steps

1. Surgical Exposure

- Tricuspid valve surgery may be performed through a full sternotomy or a right anterior thoracotomy. We prefer the median sternotomy approach to give full access to the mitral, aortic, and tricuspid valves. In a redo operation in a patient with a dilated RV, we perform femoral cannulation to decompress the heart before the redo sternotomy. Bicaval cannulation with snares is essential to isolate the right atrium and avoid an air lock in the cardiopulmonary bypass circuit. The inferior vena cava cannula is placed in the right atrial appendage and turned inferiorly, whereas the superior vena cava (SVC) cannula is inserted into body of the right atrium and turned superiorly. This strategy of crossing the cannulas permits them to be retracted easily out of the operative field during mitral and tricuspid surgery (Fig. 18-3).
- The operation is performed under cardiopulmonary bypass and mild hypothermia, with or without the use of aortic cross-clamping. During isolated tricuspid surgery, we may avoid cross-clamping the aorta. Not cross-clamping avoids cardiac ischemia and enables the evaluation of tricuspid valve motion and the consequences of each suture placement (conduction tissue). A sump sucker is placed in the coronary sinus to improve exposure.
- During multivalve surgery, aortic cross-clamping is essential, and we use antegrade cold blood cardioplegia supplemented with retrograde cardioplegia. We repair the tricuspid valve at the end of the operation (after the left-sided lesions have been addressed) while the patient is being rewarmed. Some centers advocate removing the cross-clamp at this point, but we keep it in place because it improves surgical exposure and puts less stress on the heart, while adding just a few minutes to the total aortic cross-clamp time.
- The tricuspid valve is exposed through a conventional oblique right atriotomy, starting from the atrial appendage and passing approximately 2 cm posterior to and parallel with the atrioventricular groove. The atriotomy edges are retracted with sutures or a retraction device.

2. De Vega Technique

- De Vega annuloplasty is a simple and inexpensive procedure that does not interfere with the conduction or leaflet tissue while effectively reducing the tricuspid annulus size. Because of its simplicity, it requires little additional cross-clamp time and can be performed concomitantly with aortic and mitral surgery.
- The De Vega technique is most applicable to those patients with TR as a result of mild annular dilation (<50 mm) in whom it is anticipated that good long-term function does not depend on the integrity of the repair. In these situations, the De Vega annuloplasty provides a competent tricuspid valve during the early postoperative course while the heart remodels after surgical treatment of the left-sided valvular lesions. This may diminish the risk of immediate postoperative RV dysfunction.
- We use the De Vega repair in patients undergoing left-sided valve surgery who have 2+ TR or less and a tricuspid annular dimension less than 50 mm. If there is more than 2+ TR or annular dilation greater than 50 mm, an annuloplasty band is implanted.
- We use a modification of the De Vega technique that involves the use of two double-armed, pledgeted 3-0 polytetrafluoroethylene sutures (Fig. 18-4 [follow arrows 1, 2, 3]). The first suture is passed as a circular stitch in a counterclockwise direction from the posterior-septal commissure to the middle of the anterior leaflet. Deep bites are taken every 5 to 6 mm into the endocardium and the fibrous ring at the junction of the tricuspid annulus and the RV free wall. The

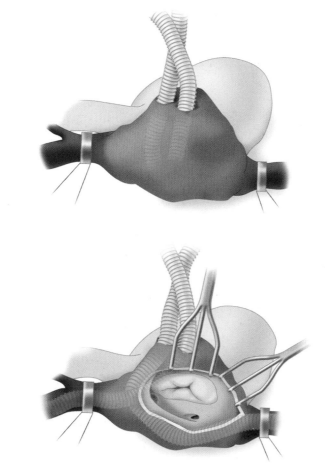

Figure 18-3

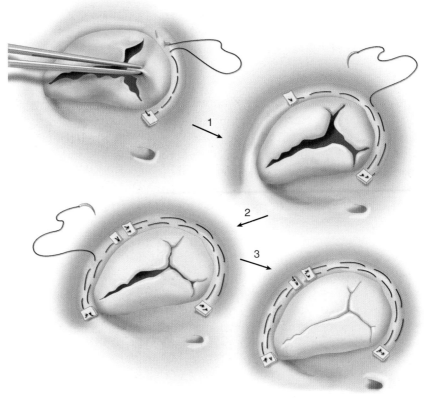

Figure 18-4

second limb of the first suture is run parallel and 1 to 2 mm outside the previous suture in the same counterclockwise direction. At the middle of the anterior leaflet, both sutures are placed through a second pledget. Another double-armed, pledgeted 3-0 Gore-Tex suture is passed as a circular stitch in the same manner in a clockwise direction starting from the anterior-septal commissure to the middle of the anterior leaflet. The two sutures are then tightened and tied, producing a pursestring effect to reduce the length of the anterior and posterior sections of the annulus and provide adequate leaflet coaptation. The orifice should be able to admit 2.5 to 3 fingerbreadths snugly through the valve, or a Hagar sizer (24 to 30 mm) may be used.

3. Bicuspidization

♦ Bicuspidization of the tricuspid valve is a simple technique to repair TR and may achieve good long-term results. Essentially, this procedure converts the tricuspid valve into a bicuspid valve. Interrupted 4-0 polypropylene sutures can be placed between the anterior and posterior leaflets, or between the posterior and septal leaflets, to create a bicuspid valve (Fig. 18-5). This process is always combined with an annuloplasty band and occasionally with an edge-to-edge repair. Concurrently, the posterior annulus may be plicated with a 2-0 or 3-0 polyester suture (with or without pledgets). This usually yields excellent leaflet coaptation while ensuring an adequate orifice for flow.

4. Annuloplasty Band Insertion

♦ To produce a reduction of the tricuspid annulus with the best long-term durability, an annuloplasty ring or band should be used. The options include the use of a rigid ring (Carpentier-Edwards; Edwards Lifesciences, LLC, Irvine, Calif), a flexible ring (Duran; Medtronic Inc., Minneapolis, Minn), or a flexible band (Cosgrove annuloplasty system; Edwards Lifesciences, LLC). The area of the anterior leaflet or the length of the base of the septal leaflet (intertrigonal distance) may be used to determine the appropriate size. Alternatively, we prefer to implant a tricuspid band identical in size to the mitral band used during the left-sided valve repair. These ring and band devices are designed to restore the valve to its normal configuration and, importantly, to avoid suture placement in the region of the AV node.
♦ Gentle tension is applied to the tricuspid leaflets during placement of the annulus sutures to identify the exact location of the thin tricuspid annulus. Mattress sutures are placed circumferentially, with wider bites (7 to 8 mm) on the annulus and smaller corresponding bites (4 to 5 mm) through the fabric of the ring or band (Fig. 18-6). We use a finer suture and needle, typically 4-0 polypropylene, with strong bites passing into the deeper part of the annulus to avoid sutures' tearing through the fragile annular tissue.

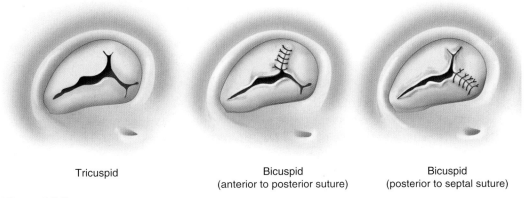

Tricuspid

Bicuspid
(anterior to posterior suture)

Bicuspid
(posterior to septal suture)

Figure 18-5

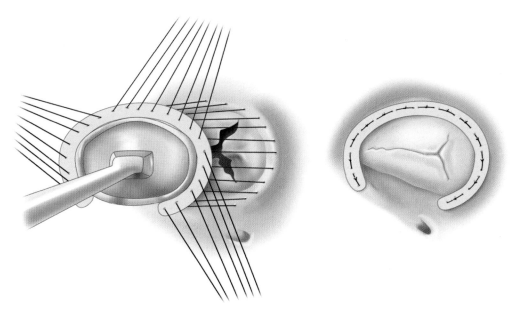

Figure 18-6

5. Edge-to-Edge Repair

- In the setting of complex lesions and severe residual TR, an edge-to-edge tricuspid valve repair may be used as an effective adjuvant procedure to annuloplasty repair. The edge-to-edge technique was originally described by Alfieri for the purpose of mitral valve repair and may be applied to the tricuspid valve in a similar fashion. One technique of edge-to-edge repair involves the use of a stay suture attaching the free edges of each of the three leaflets at the site of the regurgitation. A 4-0 or 5-0 polytetrafluoroethylene suture reinforced with a small pericardial pledget is passed through the middle point of the free edge of each of the leaflets, just at the level where the leaflet turns down to attach to the primary chordae. This effectively creates a triple-orifice tricuspid valve (Fig. 18-7A). A second suture is always used to reinforce the repair.
- Alternatively, a double-orifice technique may be employed. This is achieved first by bicuspidization of the tricuspid valve with a plication suture along the posterior leaflet annulus. Subsequently, the edge-to-edge repair approximates the septal and anterior leaflets using a 4-0 or 5-0 Gore-Tex "U" stitch at the midpoint of these two leaflets. This achieves a double-orifice edge-to-edge repair in a manner similar to the Alfieri mitral repair. A second suture is used to reinforce the repair, and the two orifices are measured with sizers to ensure that each is at least 14 mm in diameter (Fig. 18-7B).

6. Assessment of Tricuspid Valve Repair

- Assessment of tricuspid valve competence after repair is achieved by filling the RV with cold saline and applying pressure on the main pulmonary artery to observe leaflet apposition. Residual leakage or distortion mandates additional repair maneuvers to achieve coaptation. Although open assessment of the tricuspid valve is important, the most accurate evaluation of the adequacy of tricuspid repair is performed using transesophageal echocardiography after the patient has been weaned from cardiopulmonary bypass. If the result appears inadequate, further repair should be performed; alternatively, replacement may be necessary.
- TR function and RV function need to be assessed at the same time, particularly for functional TR repair.

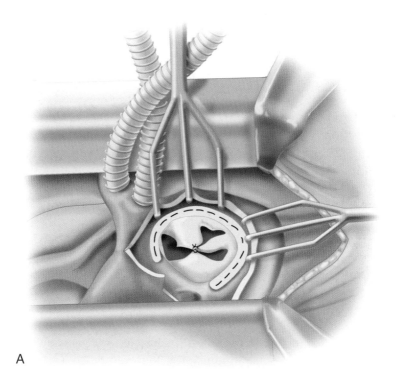

A

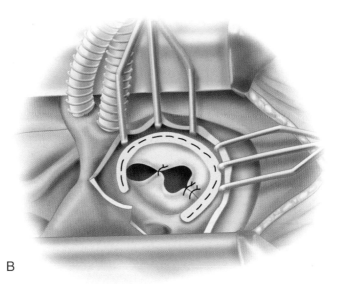

B

Figure 18-7

7. Tricuspid Valve Replacement

◆ When the severity of valvular distortion prevents a satisfactory repair procedure, valve replacement becomes mandatory. Ideally, the subvalvular apparatus should be retained to optimize postoperative RV function, with the leaflet tissues incorporated into the suturing of the prosthesis to the annulus. If the subvalvular apparatus and the leaflet tissues are diseased to the point that they will interfere with prosthesis insertion or function, their resection is necessary, but a 2- to 3-mm fringe of leaflet tissue is left on the annulus. The cordal attachments are divided deep in the RV.

◆ As in mitral valve replacement, the prosthesis size is selected based on the diameter of the AV ring sizing the anterior leaflet. Interrupted pledgeted mattress sutures (2-0 or 3-0 polyester) are passed through the annulus using an intra-annular everting technique (Fig. 18-8-1). Along the area occupied by the septal leaflet, the sutures are placed in the fringe of leaflet tissue to avoid damaging the AV node and bundle of His. The sutures are then passed through the sewing ring of the prosthesis (Fig. 18-8-2a), and the prosthesis is slipped down into its bed. Subsequently, the sutures are tied and cut (Fig. 18-8-3a). Care is taken to avoid injury to the RV endocardium as the prosthesis is passed into the decompressed ventricle. Alternatively, pledgeted mattress sutures may be placed along the septal annulus only, followed by continuous running sutures along the anterior and posterior sections of the annulus (Figs. 18-8-2b and 18-8-3b).

8. Tricuspid Valve Endocarditis Repair

◆ There is a growing interest in applying Carpentier repair techniques in patients with tricuspid valve endocarditis. Pericardial patching of perforations and ring annuloplasty are standard techniques to produce competent valves and avoid replacement. Moreover, limited resection of a diseased anterior or septal leaflet may be performed. The affected portion is excised in a trapezoidal fashion, and a 2-0 polyester suture is used to locally plicate that specific annulus segment. Subsequently, the resected leaflet edges are reapproximated with interrupted 5-0 or 6-0 polypropylene sutures. A permanent pacemaker may be necessary in patients who require septal leaflet resection and repair (patients with complete heart block). If the posterior leaflet is involved, the diseased tissue is removed, and bicuspidization of the tricuspid valve usually results in a competent valve.

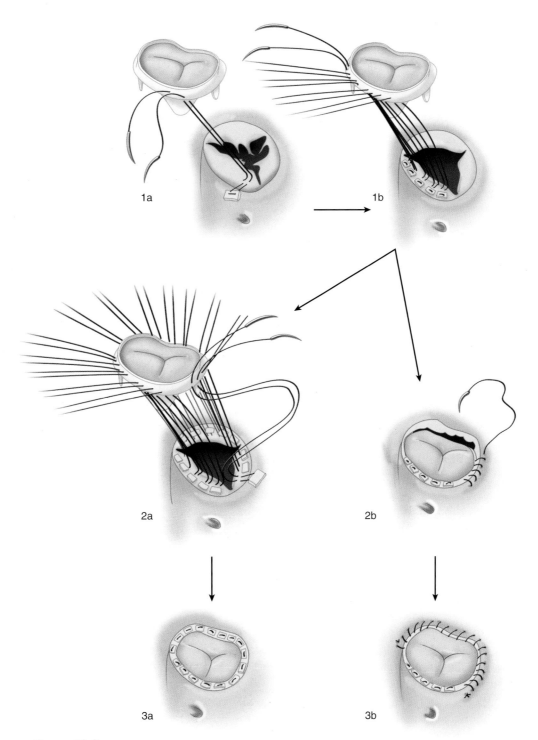

Figure 18-8

9. Tricuspid Valve Endocarditis Resection

◆ There is an inherent risk involved with valve replacement in patients with ongoing intravenous drug addiction. With active tricuspid valve endocarditis in the setting of drug addiction, the three leaflets and their chordae can simply be excised. A 2- to 3-mm fringe of leaflet tissue is left on the annulus to enable late prosthesis insertion during a reoperation when the addiction is under better control.

Step 4. Postoperative Care

◆ Weaning from cardiopulmonary bypass and early postoperative care may be particularly challenging in patients with severe preoperative pulmonary hypertension (i.e., mitral stenosis) and RV dysfunction. RV preload should be optimized with volume infusions to improve contractility. However, a right atrial pressure higher than 18 mm Hg may lead to overdilation of the RV. Transesophageal echocardiography may be helpful in titrating the patient's volume status. Inotropic support with intravenous milrinone or dobutamine is usually necessary to allow weaning from cardiopulmonary bypass. In severe cases of pulmonary hypertension, however, pulmonary vasodilators (e.g., inhaled nitric oxide, intravenous prostaglandins) may be required to reduce RV afterload in the early postoperative period. Later in the postoperative period, when patients are off inotropic support and recovering on the ward, diuretic agents are aggressively used to treat the characteristic fluid retention in these patients.

◆ Complete heart block can occur after surgery owing to damage to the conduction system during tricuspid valve procedures (1% to 2%). Ideally, the anchoring sutures for the tricuspid prosthesis should be placed well away from the conduction tissue. After concurrent tricuspid and mitral valve replacement, complete heart block is fairly common. The presence of two rigid prosthetic sewing rings is thought to produce ongoing trauma and eventually lead to AV node dysfunction, either in the immediate postoperative period or months to years after surgery. Approximately 10% of patients receiving double-valve replacement require insertion of a pacemaker in the postoperative period, and the prevalence is 25% up to 10 years after surgery. Because of this risk of complete heart block during the initial hospital stay, electrocardiographic monitoring should be continued until discharge. Consideration should also be given to placing permanent epicardial pacemaker leads at the time of surgery.

◆ Long-term anticoagulation is necessary when mechanical prostheses have been inserted in any of the valve positions. Warfarin administration is started on the evening of postoperative day 1 or 2. Occasionally, intravenous heparin is used until the international normalized ratio is therapeutic, particularly in the context of two or more mechanical prostheses and atrial fibrillation. However, there does not appear to be any evidence to support the practice of intravenous heparin therapy early in the postoperative course in a patient with a single mechanical prosthesis. Long-term anticoagulation is controversial if a bioprosthesis is used in the tricuspid position when bioprostheses have been used for other valve replacements. Regardless, a large number of patients with tricuspid bioprostheses eventually develop other indications (such as atrial fibrillation) for long-term anticoagulant treatment.

Step 5. Pearls and Pitfalls

- In patients requiring redo operations for tricuspid valve surgery, the RV is often dilated and adherent to the posterior sternum. Great care should be exercised during the redo sternotomy. We use a combination of sharp dissection, oscillating saw, and sternal elevation to perform the redo sternotomy. Blunt digital dissection should be avoided because of the risk of injury to the often friable RV free wall.
- Bicaval cannulation is necessary during tricuspid operations. The SVC cannula may be placed in the body of the right atrium and steered superiorly, or it may be placed directly in the SVC itself. The sinoatrial (SA) node rests at the anteromedial junction of the right atrium and SVC. Therefore, the cannulation site should be 2 cm superior or inferior to this region to avoid SA node injury. The atrial incision should be well away from the SA node, and the superior extension of the incision should be limited to 1 to 2 cm from the superior margin of the right atrium.
- One of the major challenges of tricuspid surgery lies in the placement of sutures. The depths of the suture bites in the annulus must be substantial to avoid tearing through the tissues. However, the sutures should be placed well away from the conduction tissue, the coronary sinus, and the right coronary artery to avoid iatrogenic injury.
- Long-term surgical follow-up studies have demonstrated that 2+ TR or more and severe tricuspid annular dilation predict the development of late severe TR and the need for tricuspid reoperation. Therefore, ensuring the adequacy of tricuspid repair during the initial operation is critically important.
- Special care should be taken to assess the foramen ovale for patency in all tricuspid operations. These lesions can easily be closed with sutures to reduce the possibility of systemic desaturation from right-to-left shunting, especially in the context of pulmonary hypertension, and to reduce the risk of paradoxical embolization.
- Consideration should be given to placing permanent epicardial ventricular pacing leads in patients undergoing tricuspid valve surgery, especially during combined mitral and tricuspid valve replacement (up to 25% postoperative complete heart block). Epicardial pacemaker leads can be placed with ease at the time of surgery, and they can be buried in a pocket anterior to the posterior rectus sheath in the left upper quadrant for later permanent pacemaker implantation, if required.

Bibliography

Arbulu A, Holmes RJ, Asfaw I: Surgical treatment of intractable right-sided infective endocarditis in drug addicts: 25 years experience. J Heart Valve Dis 1993;2:129-137; discussion 138-139.

Bonow RO, Carabello BA, Kanu C, et al: ACC/AHA 2006 guidelines for the management of patients with valvular heart disease: A report of the American College of Cardiology/American Heart Association Task Force on Practice Guidelines (writing committee to revise the 1998 Guidelines for the Management of Patients With Valvular Heart Disease). Developed in collaboration with the Society of Cardiovascular Anesthesiologists, Endorsed by the Society for Cardiovascular Angiography and Interventions and the Society of Thoracic Surgeons. Circulation 2006;114:e84-e231.

Carpentier A, Deloche A, Hanania G, et al: Surgical management of acquired tricuspid valve disease. J Thorac Cardiovasc Surg 1974;67:53-65.

Cohn LH: Tricuspid regurgitation secondary to mitral valve disease: When and how to repair. J Cardiac Surg 1994;9:237-241.

Cohn LH, Edmunds LH Jr (eds): Cardiac Surgery in the Adult, 2nd ed. New York, McGraw-Hill, 2003.

De Vega NG: Selective, adjustable and permanent annuloplasty: An original technic for the treatment of tricuspid insufficiency [in Spanish]. Rev Esp Cardiol 1972;25:555-556.

Dreyfus GD, Corbi PJ, Chan KM, Bahrami T: Secondary tricuspid regurgitation or dilatation: Which should be the criteria for surgical repair? Ann Thorac Surg 2005;79:127-132.

Khonsari S, Sintek CF: Cardiac Surgery: Safeguards and Pitfalls in Operative Technique, 3rd ed. New York, Lippincott Williams & Wilkins, 2003.

Kouchoukos NT, Karp RB, Blackstone EH, et al (eds): Kirklin/Barratt-Boyes Cardiac Surgery, 3rd ed. New York, Churchill Livingstone, 2003.

Kulik A, Rubens FD, Wells PS, et al: Early postoperative anticoagulation after mechanical valve replacement: A systematic review. Ann Thorac Surg 2006;81:770-781.

Lai YQ, Meng X, Bai T, et al: Edge-to-edge tricuspid valve repair: An adjuvant technique for residual tricuspid regurgitation. Ann Thorac Surg 2006;81:2179-2182.

McCarthy PM, Bhudia SK, Rajeswaran J, et al: Tricuspid valve repair: Durability and risk factors for failure. J Thorac Cardiovasc Surg 2004;127:674-685.

Rivera R, Duran E, Ajuria M: Carpentier's flexible ring versus De Vega's annuloplasty: A prospective randomized study. J Thorac Cardiovasc Surg 1985;89:196-203.

Rizzoli G, Vendramin I, Nesseris G, et al: Biological or mechanical prostheses in tricuspid position? A meta-analysis of intra-institutional results. Ann Thorac Surg 2004;77:1607-1614.

Sarraj A, Duarte J: Adjustable segmental tricuspid annuloplasty: A new modified technique. Ann Thorac Surg 2007;83:698-699.

Tang GH, David TE, Singh SK, et al: Tricuspid valve repair with an annuloplasty ring results in improved long-term outcomes. Circulation 2006;114:1577-1581.

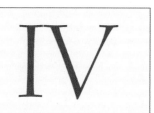

Operations for Aortic Disease

CHAPTER 19

TYPE A AORTIC DISSECTIONS

Michael A. Coady and Thomas G. Gleason

Step 1. Surgical Anatomy

- A comprehensive understanding of the anatomy of the aortic root and ascending aorta as well as the pathologic process involved in type A dissections is critical for undertaking surgical reconstructive procedures.
- A type A aortic dissection begins with a primary intimal tear in the ascending aorta. Tears usually occur along points of fixation where the wall tension is more pronounced (i.e., the sinotubular junction).[1] The tear creates an intimal flap, which divides the aortic wall into true and false lumens.
- The intimal tear in type A dissections is typically transverse, and the dissection progresses rapidly along the thinner, outermost third of the aortic media. This is precisely why rupture often occurs into the pericardial or pleural spaces through this outer wall (rather than reentry occurring into the true lumen distally).[2] In ascending aortic dissections, the false lumen typically occupies the right anterior portion of the aorta, and the medial half of the aorta remains intact.

◆ Figure 19-1 demonstrates a type A dissection viewed through a median sternotomy and pericardiotomy. The ascending aorta is dilated and thinned from blood coursing through the false lumen; the right coronary artery is distorted. Note the subadventitial hematoma and extension into the brachiocephalic arteries.

◆ Figure 19-2 displays the two primary anatomic segments of the ascending aorta: the aortic root or sinus portion, and the tubular portion.

▲ The *aortic root*, which begins at the base of the heart and the left ventricle, is the portion of the ventricular outflow tract that supports the cusps of the aortic valve; it consists of the sinuses of Valsalva, the valvular leaflets, the interleaflet triangles or subcommissural triangles, and the right and left coronary ostia. The noncoronary leaflet is slightly larger than the right or left. The aortic annulus or aortoventricular junction attaches the aortic root to the left ventricle; it is not physically a ring, but rather is defined by the semilunar attachment of each cusp to the aortic wall at the distalmost point of the left ventricular outflow tract. The normal annulus does not exceed a diameter of 25 to 27 mm in adults.

▲ The *sinotubular junction* (STJ) or ridge is a circular structure that defines the junction of the sinuses of Valsalva and the tubular ascending aorta. The STJ separates the aortic root from the tubular ascending aorta. The STJ is usually 10% to 15% smaller than the diameter of the aortic annulus in young people, but becomes equal to or slightly larger than the annular diameter in the elderly.

▲ The *tubular ascending aorta* extends from the STJ to just proximal to the innominate artery.

◆ These anatomic distinctions (aortic root and tubular ascending aorta) are important because they add clarity to a description of the ascending aortic pathologic process characterizing type A aortic dissections. Operations involving the aortic root (sinus portion) of the ascending aorta are technically more challenging because they can involve repair or replacement of the aortic valve or reimplantation of the coronary arteries into a graft.

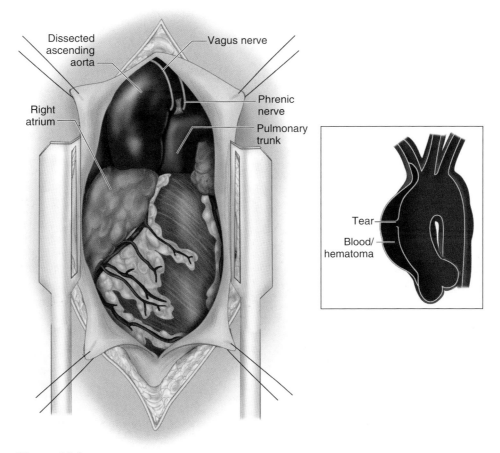

Figure 19-1

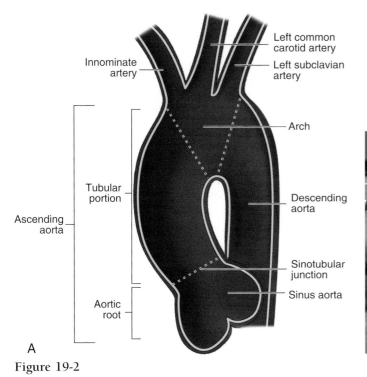

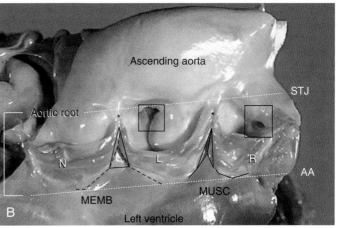

A

Figure 19-2

Step 2. Preoperative Considerations

- Untreated Stanford type A dissections are associated with a mortality rate approximating 1% to 2% per hour during the first 24 to 48 hours. Immediate operative repair is indicated in the majority of these patients unless there is deemed to be a prohibitively high operative risk.[3]
- Advanced age, malperfusion syndromes, or preoperative paraplegia predict a poorer outcome but are not considered absolute contraindications to surgery. However, patients who present neurologically devastated from an associated stroke almost uniformly do poorly. In this rare group of patients, expectant care is often justified.[4]
- Aggressive medical (anti-impulse and antihypertensive) therapy should be initiated at the first clinical suspicion of an aortic dissection in order to control heart rate, blood pressure, and the rate of rise of the arterial pulse (dP/dt). This should begin on presentation and should continue throughout the initial work-up.
- All patients should have appropriate monitoring, including an indwelling arterial catheter, central venous access, and a Foley catheter. Optimal pain control and management of the patient's blood pressure are paramount.
- Cardiac-specific β_1-selective blocking agents are first-line interventions. Esmolol (loading dose 0.5 mg/kg over 5 minutes, followed by an infusion of 0.1 to 0.2 mg/kg/min) is added to keep the heart rate at 60 to 80 bpm. Other agents may be added if the blood pressure is not adequately controlled, to further reduce the afterload and the strain on the aortic wall. Vasodilating agents such as labetalol (2 to 10 mg/min), nicardipine (5 to 10 mg/hr), or sodium nitroprusside (initial dose 0.25 μg/kg/min) should be used, keeping the mean arterial pressure from 60 to 80 mm Hg. Labetalol has both β_1 and α blocking activity, and its use typically precludes the need for esmolol.
- The electrocardiogram, pulse oximetry, radial or femoral arterial pressure, central venous pressure, and bladder and tympanic membrane temperatures are monitored throughout the operation.
- Transesophageal echocardiography (TEE) should be used in all patients to assess the dissected aorta, interrogate valve competency and left ventricular function, and demonstrate flow in the dissected lumens.
- Antifibrinolytic therapies have been shown to limit blood transfusion requirements during emergent cardiac surgery. α-Aminocaproic acid (Amicar), tranexamic acid, and aprotinin have all been used safely for type A aortic dissection operations with and without the use of deep hypothermia and circulatory arrest. We recommend the use of an antifibrinolytic for all cases of type A aortic dissection repair.
- As the operative steps are described in the following, the five tenets of acute type A dissection repair to keep in mind are (1) myocardial protection, (2) neurocerebral protection, (3) restoration of a competent aortic valve, (4) excision of the intimal tear site, and (5) elimination of false lumen blood flow with maintenance of true lumen blood flow.

Step 3. Operative Steps

1. Arterial Cannulation

- Right axillary (or subclavian) artery cannulation is our preferred method in the repair of an acute type A dissection to facilitate antegrade true lumen blood flow and selective antegrade cerebral blood flow during periods of deep hypothermia and circulatory arrest. Right axillary artery cannulation is particularly useful when atherosclerotic disease is prominent in the aortic arch. Local wound complications are rarer with axillary arterial cannulation than with femoral arterial cannulation. After arterial inflow cannulation at any site in cases of aortic dissection, antegrade blood flow should be confirmed in both carotid arteries and the true lumen of the descending thoracic aorta. This can be achieved using a combination of TEE and cervical transcutaneous echocardiography by the anesthesia team.
- Alternatively, the use of femoral cannulation (see Chapter 2) may be the quickest method of arterial access for patients who present in extremis, and it has been used safely and reliably for type A dissection repair. Femoral arterial perfusion, however, has the potential for causing malperfusion to the brain or other organs on institution of retrograde aortic blood flow with cardiopulmonary bypass (CPB) because of changes in flow patterns related either to the dissection flap or to the embolization of thrombus. Despite these risks, several studies have demonstrated relatively low rates of operative mortality, malperfusion, and stroke.[5-7] Although many surgeons advocate cannulation of the femoral artery with the strongest pulse, confirmation of true-lumen entry using a guidewire advanced into the aortic true lumen with TEE guidance is more reliable.
- Alternative modes of arterial cannulation include innominate artery cannulation or direct cannulation of the aortic true lumen using a guidewire technique under echocardiographic guidance. As in any mode of arterial perfusion, the surgeon needs to prevent inadvertent false lumen pressurization, cerebral embolization, and systemic malperfusion by securing cannulation of the true lumen.

2. Axillary Arterial Cannulation

- If the right subclavian–axillary artery is not dissected, the axillary artery may be used for arterial cannulation. The surgical dissection of the subclavian–axillary artery should be done before performing a median sternotomy.
- The right axillary artery is exposed through a right infraclavicular incision approximately one to two fingerbreadths below and parallel to the clavicle, exposing the pectoralis major fascia (Fig. 19-3A). This fascia is divided, and the muscle is spread in the direction of its fibers. The clavipectoral fascia is divided beneath the pectoralis major muscle, and the pectoralis minor muscle is then exposed. The pectoralis minor can be encircled with a sweeping motion of the surgeon's index finger (Fig. 19-3B) and divided near its insertion onto the coracoid process. Alternatively, the right subclavian vein that is visible in the fat plane medial to the pectoralis minor can be retracted caudad to expose the right subclavian artery without dividing the pectoralis minor.
- The axillary or subclavian artery lies posterior and cephalic to the vein. The axillary artery is controlled with Silastic vessel loops. A partial occlusion clamp is placed on the artery after administration of 5000 U of intravenous heparin sulfate. An elliptical arteriotomy is created and an 8- to 10-mm knitted or woven Dacron vascular graft is then sewn end-to-side to the anterosuperior surface of the axillary artery with 5-0 polypropylene suture (Fig. 19-3C).
- The graft is trimmed and, after adequate heparinization for CPB, is cannulated directly near the skin incision with a 20F aortic cannula. The cannula is secured in the graft with a heavy mesentery suture (Fig. 19-3D). The arterial cannula is then de-aired and connected to the arterial portion of the CPB system. This final connection is typically performed after sternal entry and mediastinal dissection to avoid the need for full heparinization before sternal entry.

3. Incision, Venous Cannulation, and Preparation for Bypass

- A midline sternotomy incision is used for repair of a type A dissection. The pericardium is carefully opened and the aorta is not manipulated until cannulation is complete and CPB has been instituted.
- A single double-stage cannula is placed in the right atrium. Alternatively, two separate venous cannulae can be used, inserted into the superior and inferior venae cavae, respectively.
- A CO_2 line secured to the skin edge used throughout the procedure at 5 to 10 L/min can minimize air entrapment in the left ventricle. A balloon-tipped retrograde catheter is placed through the right atrium into the coronary sinus and is used for retrograde cardioplegia during the procedure.
- As mentioned later, upon aortic cross-clamping and proximal aortic transection, direct ostial antegrade cardioplegia is administered for cardioplegic induction. A myocardial temperature probe is placed in the septum and is useful in guiding the amount of cardioplegia to be given during the operation. A strategy of continuous retrograde cardioplegia or intermittent antegrade or retrograde cardioplegia is effective. Maintenance of a myocardial temperature of 7°C to 10°C is optimal.
- A venting catheter is inserted through the right superior pulmonary vein and advanced into the left ventricle if aortic regurgitation is present. A left ventricular vent is also helpful to maintain a bloodless field during aortic root reconstruction.

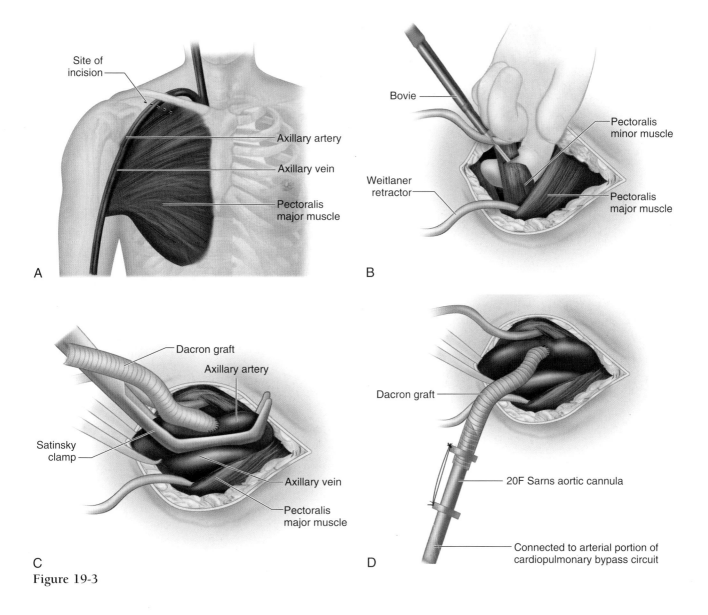

Site of incision

Axillary artery

Axillary vein

Pectoralis major muscle

A

Bovie

Pectoralis minor muscle

Weitlaner retractor

Pectoralis major muscle

B

Dacron graft

Axillary artery

Satinsky clamp

Axillary vein

Pectoralis major muscle

C

Dacron graft

20F Sarns aortic cannula

Connected to arterial portion of cardiopulmonary bypass circuit

D

Figure 19-3

4. Initiation of Cardiopulmonary Bypass

- Once systemic heparinization is completed and the activated clotting time is adequate, CPB is established slowly with continuous TEE monitoring of the flow pattern in the ascending and descending aortas to detect any evidence of malperfusion (i.e., the true lumen shrinks or is obliterated).[8]
- As the patient begins to be systemically cooled on CPB, the ascending aorta is carefully dissected.
- The ascending aorta is carefully separated from the pulmonary trunk and right pulmonary artery posteriorly.
- Dexamethasone (8 to 12 mg) or methylprednisolone (1 g) and thiopental (7 to 15 mg/kg) are administered during cooling to provide additional cerebral and spinal cord protection during deep hypothermia and circulatory arrest.[9] Alternatively, continuous electroencephalography (EEG) can be used to monitor neurocerebral function; when the EEG is isoelectric, indicating electrocerebral silence, circulatory arrest may be safely commenced. The use of barbiturates, however, interferes with EEG monitoring by inducing pharmacologic slowing of cerebral electrical activity, or even isoelectricity, thus obviating the utility of EEG monitoring in determining the extent of protection with cooling or the return of function with rewarming.
- Once the heart begins to fibrillate, the aorta is cross-clamped, the ascending aorta is transected, and a full dose of direct ostial antegrade or retrograde cold blood cardioplegia is administered. Cardioplegia is administered every 20 minutes throughout the procedure. Although retrograde cardioplegia provides excellent left ventricular protection, intermittent boluses of ostial right coronary artery antegrade cardioplegia provide additional protection for the right ventricle. If antegrade cardioplegia is used, great care should be exercised in placing ostial catheters in the area of aortic dissection to prevent arterial injury.
- The aortic cross-clamp should be placed several centimeters proximal to the takeoff of the innominate artery to avoid injury to the fragile aortic tissue.

5. Location of the Primary Intimal Tear

- Once the aortic cross-clamp is applied, the ascending aorta is opened proximal to the cross-clamp to locate the primary intimal tear (Fig. 19-4A).
- The initial incision is into the false lumen. Any clot that is present is removed from the false lumen, exposing the primary intimal tear (Fig. 19-4B).
- The aorta is trimmed circumferentially approximately 2 to 5 mm distal to the peaks of the aortic valve commissures (Fig. 19-4C).
- The aortic valve and coronary ostia are carefully inspected. If the coronary artery ostia are not compromised by the dissection, hand-held cardioplegic catheters may also be used to deliver cardioplegia.

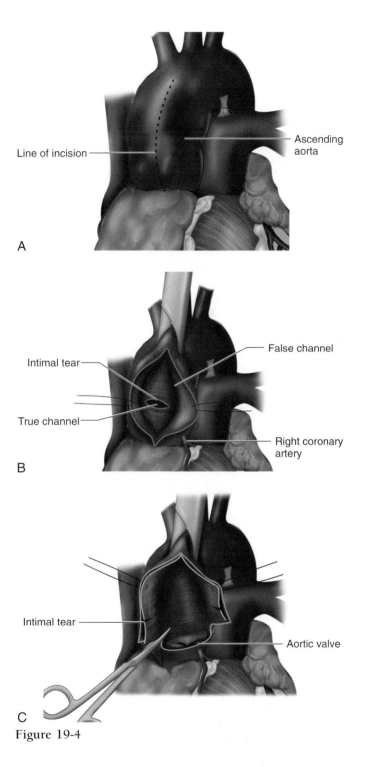

Figure 19-4

6. Management of the Aortic Root

- If the dissection flap has detached one or more commissures, they may be resuspended by using a pledgeted, double-armed polypropylene suture placed across each detached commissure and through the outer layer of the aorta. After drying the layers of the disrupted aortic wall with a peanut sponge, a layer of Teflon felt may be placed in the dissected plane for neomedial integrity, or a biologic glue can be used to obliterate the false channel (Fig. 19-5A). The aortic wall may be further reinforced using Teflon strips[10,11] (Fig. 19-5B).
- If the aortic valve is structurally abnormal, resuspension of the aortic valve is inadequate, or salvage of the valve seems unlikely, aortic root replacement is necessary.
- In patients with Marfan syndrome or pre-existing ascending aortic aneurysm, root replacement with a valved conduit or bioprosthetic root is optimal, depending on the patient's age. Some patients, particularly younger ones, are candidates for a valve-sparing root replacement, and a valve reimplantation strategy appears to have the best durability in the setting of dissection.
- Each coronary artery ostium is examined, and if dissection extends to one or both coronary arteries but the artery remains intact, the separated aortic wall layers may be repaired by adjoining the dissected layers with or without felt reinforcement. With circumferential coronary ostial dissection, it is often better to make slightly larger buttons (5 mm of aortic cuff) to allow for reconstitution of the dissected ostium. The Cabrol modification for coronary reattachment is rarely necessary but may be required if an adequately sized button for orthotopic transfer cannot be fashioned.
- A woven Dacron graft is selected for aortic replacement. Because the STJ is optimally 10% to 15% smaller than the aortic annulus, the graft size selected is typically one size smaller than the aortic annulus in order to promote central coaptation of the aortic cusps.

7. Circulatory Arrest and Open Distal Anastomosis

- By the time the aortic root has been inspected and aortic lesion addressed proximally, the patient has been cooled to a nasopharyngeal and bladder temperature of 18°C or, if an EEG-based strategy is being used, has displayed electrocerebral silence for greater than 4 minutes.
- Mannitol (0.3 to 0.4 g/kg) is given before circulatory arrest to induce an osmotic diuresis and help preserve renal function.
- The operating table is placed in Trendelenburg position. CPB is interrupted and the aortic cross-clamp is removed.
- We often use selective antegrade cerebral perfusion (SACP) for neurocerebral protection during circulatory arrest, especially when circulatory arrest times exceed 20 minutes. SACP strategies improve neurologic outcome because perfusion is provided to the entire brain through an intact and redundant circle of Willis. SACP is begun by clamping the innominate artery. CPB flow is resumed slowly through the axillary cannula to a rate of 5 mL/kg/min. Back-bleeding is typically seen down the left common carotid and left subclavian arteries during SACP. When a total aortic arch replacement is required, primarily because of the presence of an intimal tear in the arch that involves and extends beyond the brachiocephalic ostia, the left common carotid artery is also selectively cannulated endoluminally with a balloon-tipped catheter and perfused in concert with the right carotid through the axillary artery cannulation. Antegrade cerebral perfusion is initiated, the left subclavian is clamped to prevent steal, and the cerebral perfusion pressure is maintained at 50 mm Hg during hypothermic arrest.
- Retrograde cerebral perfusion can be used to flush out debris, de-air the brain, and effectively maintain deep hypothermic cerebral temperatures for up to 45 minutes.

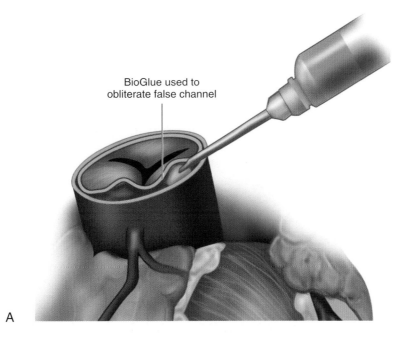

BioGlue used to
obliterate false channel

A

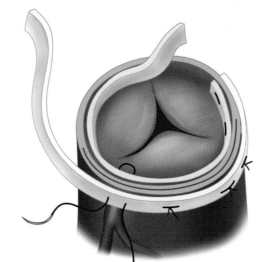

B

Figure 19-5

- In the majority of type A aortic dissections, only a hemiarch reconstruction is necessary to restore antegrade true-lumen flow and eliminate false-lumen flow. For hemiarch replacement, the aortic arch is trimmed circumferentially in an oblique fashion from the ostium of the innominate artery proximally to the distalmost aspect of the lesser curve of the arch opposite the left subclavian artery (Fig. 19-6).
- Similar to reconstruction of the proximal aortic layers, reapproximation of the distal ascending dissected aortic wall can be accomplished with biologic glue between dissected layers or by placement of neomedial felt to promote adherence of the layers and add integrity to the dissected wall. An outer layer of Teflon felt can also be used to reinforce the layers if the other measures are inadequate.
- There are two strategies of hemiarch reconstruction with respect to graft orientation. The Mount Sinai (Griepp) approach rotates the beveled end of the graft 180 degrees such that the toe of the graft apposes the greater curve of the arch near the innominate artery. In some cases this enables redirection of the proximal graft toward the root to prevent kinking of the graft if a single graft is desired for the entire reconstruction (Fig. 19-7). Alternatively, placing the toe of the bevel at the distal lesser curve can create a more natural lesser curve that extends toward the superior vena cava; however, to recreate normal angulation of the entire lesser curve from the root, a separate root graft should be used so that both the distal end of the root graft and the proximal end of the arch graft can subsequently be beveled and anastomosed to avoid any graft kinking.
- The hemiarch anastomosis is completed in an end-to-end manner using 4-0 Sh-1 polypropylene suture (Fig. 19-8).
- SACP is interrupted, the patient is placed in the Trendelenburg position, and the innominate clamp is removed. The arch and great vessels are de-aired by elevating the graft, massaging it to evacuate air. Once de-aired, the graft is clamped and CPB is resumed in an antegrade fashion and increased to full flow (Fig. 19-9). We often cannulate the distal graft for antegrade flow after arch reconstruction to provide more uniformly distributed inflow to the reconstructed arch and descending thoracic aorta. Flow again is checked by TEE.

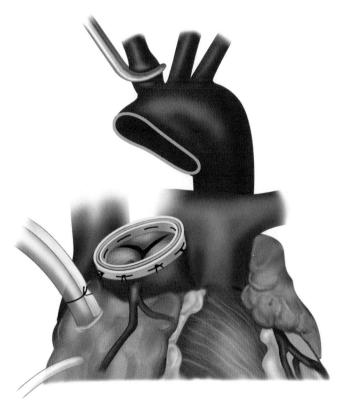

Figure 19-6

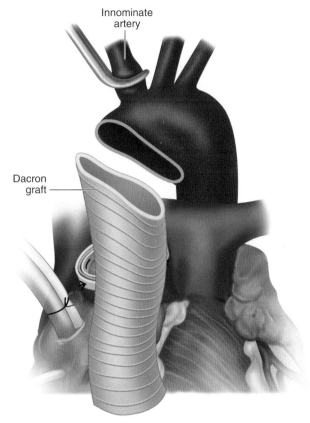

Innominate
artery

Dacron
graft

Figure 19-7

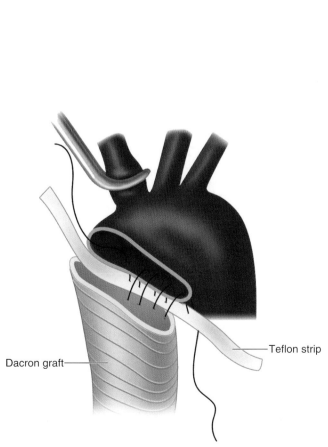

Dacron graft

Teflon strip

Figure 19-8

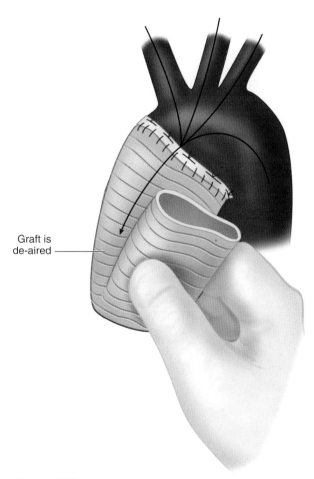

Graft is
de-aired

Figure 19-9

8. Proximal Anastomosis

- Once CPB is resumed, the patient is gradually rewarmed to 36°C to 37°C.
- The graft is then gently stretched to approximate the appropriate length necessary to complete the proximal anastomosis (in the Mt. Sinai technique). The graft is anastomosed to the reconstructed proximal aortic cuff in an end-to-end fashion using 4-0 Sh-1 polypropylene suture (Fig. 19-10). Alternatively, a separate graft is anastomosed proximally, then both the distal end of this graft and the proximal end of the arch graft are beveled, with the heel of each bevel at the lesser curve and the toe of each graft at the greater curve. The two grafts are then anastomosed with polypropylene suture.
- A root vent is placed into the graft for de-airing. Normothermic nutrient-enriched blood is delivered just before termination of CPB to facilitate earlier postcardiotomy myocardial recovery. Lidocaine (1 to 2 mg/kg) and magnesium sulfate (2 g) are placed into the pump, the patient is again placed in steep Trendelenburg position, and the cross-clamp is released.
- TEE is used to confirm aortic valve competence. All anastomoses are carefully inspected for adequate hemostasis. The completed procedure is shown in Figure 19-11.
- CPB is discontinued in the standard manner and protamine sulfate is administered once all anastomoses are found to be satisfactory.

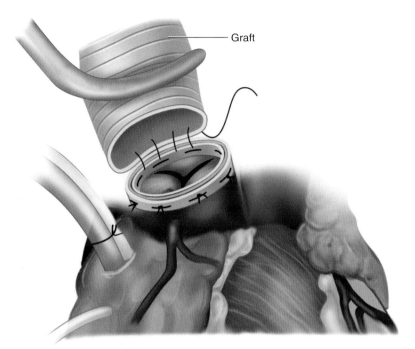

Figure 19-10

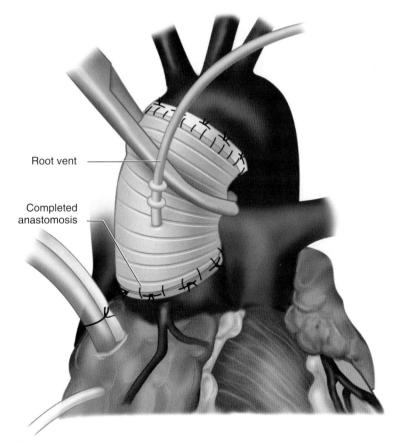

Figure 19-11

Step 4. Postoperative Care

- Control of hypertension is particularly important because this predisposes to excessive bleeding from suture lines and possible redissection or rupture of the false lumen in the early postoperative period.
- Peripheral pulses and organ function are carefully monitored after surgery because malperfusion of major aortic branches may occur or become apparent.
- Strict control of blood pressure is also necessary over the long term. Long-term follow-up surveillance with computed tomographic angiography is imperative to monitor signs of aneurysmal dilation and false channel enlargement.

Step 5. Pearls and Pitfalls

- An open distal anastomosis should always be used to avoid intimal damage by the aortic cross-clamp and to allow for careful inspection of the aortic arch.
- If severe aortic regurgitation is present, a sump vent is inserted into the left ventricle through the right superior pulmonary vein to prevent distention.
- Malperfusion can occur and may be observed on TEE. In malperfusion, the true lumen becomes progressively smaller or obliterated. If this occurs, true-lumen cannulation must be carried out immediately. Options include direct cannulation of the true lumen in the aortic arch using TEE guidance with a guidewire; passing a long arterial cannula through the left ventricular apex and across the aortic valve into the true lumen; and conversion to femoral arterial cannulation.
- The arterial perfusion tubing is always branched (Y-branch configuration) to enable immediate cannulation of an alternative site should arterial perfusion prove to be problematic during the case. Some surgeons do not like to perfuse the body solely through the axillary artery. For this reason, once the distal anastomosis is completed, the graft itself may be cannulated through the branched connection. This enables dual arterial perfusion in an antegrade manner.
- The five tenets of acute type A dissection repair are (1) myocardial protection, (2) neurocerebral protection, (3) restoration of a competent aortic valve, (4) excision of the intimal tear site, and (5) elimination of false-lumen blood flow with maintenance of true-lumen blood flow.

References

1. Sorenson HR, Olsen H: Rupture and dissecting aneurysms of the aorta: Incidence and prospects of surgery. Acta Chic Scand 1961;128:644.
2. Roberts WC: The aorta: Its acquired diseases and their consequences as viewed from a morphologic perspective. In Lindsay J Jr, Hurst JW (eds): The Aorta. New York, Grune and Stratton, 1979.
3. Elefteriades JA, Griepp R: Surgical procedures: A primer. In Elefteriades JA (ed): Acute Aortic Disease. New York, Informa Healthcare USA, 2007, pp 251-267.
4. Szeto WY, Gleason TG: Operative management of ascending aortic dissections. Semin Thorac Cardiovasc Surg 2005;17:247-255.
5. Svensson LG, Blackstone EH, Rajeswaran J, et al: Does the arterial cannulation site for circulatory arrest influence stroke risk? Ann Thorac Surg 2004;78:1274-1284.
6. Bavaria JE, Pochettino A, Brinster DR, et al: New paradigms and improved results for the surgical treatment of acute type A dissection. Ann Surg 2001;234:336-342.
7. Fusco DS, Shaw RK, Tranquilli M, et al: Femoral cannulation is safe for type A dissection repair. Ann Thorac Surg 2004;78:1285-1289.
8. Kyo S, Takamoto S, Omoto R, et al: Intraoperative echocardiography for diagnosis and treatment of aortic dissection: Utility of color flow mapping for surgical decision making in acute stage. Herz 1992;17:377-389.
9. Demers P, Miller DC: Surgery of the aortic arch, descending thoracic and thoracoabdominal surgery, and aortic dissection. In Sellke FW, Swanson S, del Nido P (eds): Sabiston & Spencer Surgery of the Chest, 7th ed, vol 2. Philadelphia, Elsevier, 2005, pp 1195-1220.
10. Yun KL, Miller DC: Technique of aortic valve preservation in acute type A aortic dissection. Oper Tech Cardiol Thorac Surg 1996;1:68.
11. Stone C, Borst H: Dissecting aortic aneurysms. In Edmunds LJ Jr (ed): Cardiac Surgery in the Adult. New York, McGraw-Hill, 1997, p 1124.

CHAPTER 20

TYPE B AORTIC DISSECTIONS

Michael P. Fischbein, Kapil Sharma, and R. Scott Mitchell

Step 1. Surgical Anatomy

- The ascending aorta begins at the sinotubular junction. The transverse arch begins at the superior attachment of the pericardial reflection, just proximal to the innominate artery. The most common transverse arch branching pattern includes three individual arteries: the innominate artery, the left common carotid artery, and the left subclavian artery. The second most common branching pattern has a common origin for the innominate artery and the left common carotid artery, referred to as a *bovine arch*.[1] The descending aorta begins distal to the transverse arch and continues to the diaphragmatic crura.
- Dissection of the aorta is characterized by the separation of the aortic media from the adventitia, creating a false lumen in the aortic wall that parallels the true lumen. A primary intimal tear (PIT) initiates the dissection and allows communication between the true and false lumens.
- Stanford type A dissections involve the ascending aorta. Stanford type B dissections involve the descending thoracic aorta or arch[2] (Fig. 20-1).

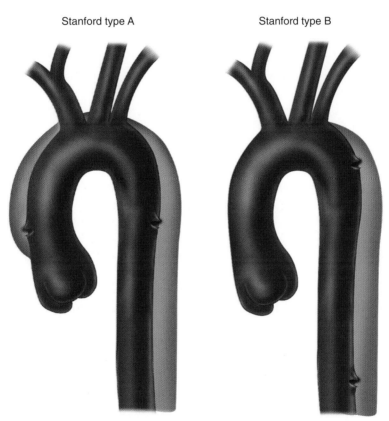

Figure 20-1

◆ Intramural hematomas (IMH) and penetrating aortic ulcers (PAU) are pathologic variants of the classic aortic dissection. Importantly, in contrast to the dissection, neither IMH nor PAU has blood flow down a false lumen. IMH likely results after aortic vasa vasorum rupture, causing hemorrhage into the aortic media.[3] PAU originates from an intimal lesion (ruptured atherosclerotic plaque) that penetrates into the aortic media and results in a variable amount of IMH[4] (Fig. 20-2A through C).

◆ The left phrenic and vagus nerves course over the anterolateral aspect of the distal arch. The left recurrent laryngeal nerve originates from the vagus nerve, runs inferiorly around the ligamentum arteriosum, and ascends on the posteromedial aspect of the arch.

◆ The anterior spinal artery perfuses the anterior two thirds of the spinal cord (location of motor neural fibers). Two posterior spinal arteries supply the posterior one third of the cord. Blood flow to the anterior spinal artery usually arises from intercostal arteries T7 to L1. Frequently, a dominant arterial branch can be identified, called the *artery of Adamkiewicz*.

Step 2. Preoperative Considerations

◆ Because there is no difference in early outcome between patients with acute type B dissection treated medically and those treated surgically, most surgeons favor a complication-specific surgical approach.[5-9] For patients with uncomplicated acute type B dissections, medical treatment has evolved as the therapy of choice. Medical treatment includes reduction of mean, peak, and rate of rise of arterial pressure (dP/dt) with both an intravenous beta blocker (e.g., esmolol) and a vasodilator (e.g., nitroprusside).

◆ Surgical or radiologic intervention has been reserved for complications, including aortic rupture or impending rupture, sudden increase in aortic size, intractable pain, or malperfusion syndromes.

◆ After determining that an intervention is required, the surgeon must decide between an open or an endovascular approach. At Stanford University, we consider an endovascular stent graft in patients who are older, are poor operative risks (e.g., in renal failure, have chronic obstructive pulmonary disease, have poor cardiac function, are acidotic from malperfusion), and have favorable anatomy. Younger patients, good surgical candidates, patients with connective tissue diseases, and patients with unfavorable endovascular stent graft anatomy receive a central aortic operation.

◆ Management of IMH and PAU is similar to that of uncomplicated type B dissection treated medically. Early surgical intervention should be considered in patients with persistent pain or an increasing pleural effusion (indicative of disease progression or impending rupture). Repeat diagnostic imaging should be performed after 24 hours and 5 to 7 days to monitor the lesion and confirm absence of progression.

◆ Diagnostic procedure options include computed tomographic (CT) angiographic scanning, transesophageal echocardiography, and magnetic resonance angiography. Study interpretation should include (1) dissection classification; (2) extent of the lesion; (3) PIT location; (4) presence or absence of organ malperfusion; (5) size of true and false lumens; and (6) dimension of the descending aorta, arch branch vessel anatomy, potential landing zones, and femoral/iliac dimensions for possible endovascular stent graft insertion.

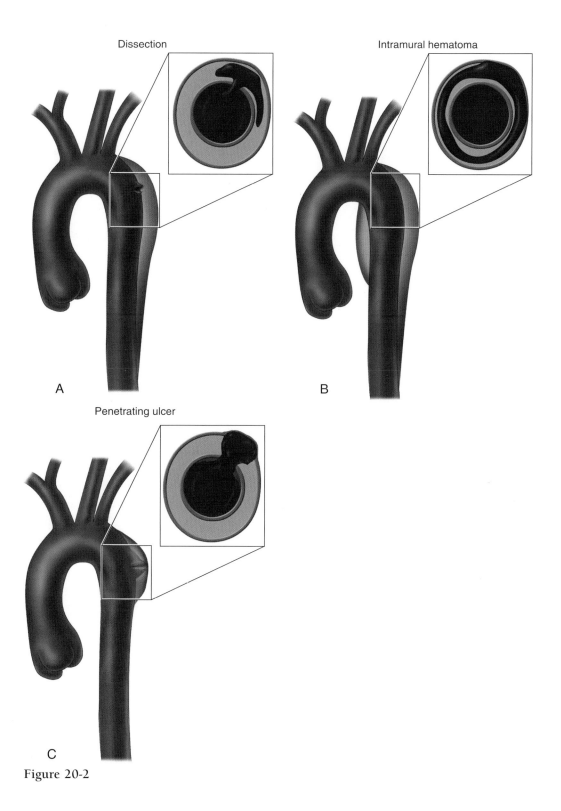

A

B

C

Figure 20-2

◆ Malperfusion results when a dissection compromises blood flow to end organs (abdominal viscera or lower extremities). Williams and colleagues described two pathophysiologic mechanisms of malperfusion—dynamic branch compromise and static branch compromise.[10] *Dynamic branch compromise* occurs when the true lumen is narrowed or compressed because the majority of flow is through the false lumen (Fig. 20-3A). *Static branch compromise* occurs when the dissection flap or intimal tears extend into a branch vessel ostium, leading to mechanical obstruction of flow from the intimal intussusception (Fig. 20-3B). False-lumen reentry tears may occur into the arterial true lumen beyond the obstruction, thereby reconstituting blood flow to the involved organ (Fig. 20-3C).

Step 3. Operative Steps

1. Open Surgical Repair

Incision

◆ The patient should be intubated with a double-lumen endotracheal tube for selective right lung ventilation. We recommend placement of an epidural catheter for pain control and a lumbar drain for cerebrospinal fluid (CSF) drainage (improves perioperative spinal cord perfusion and potentially reduces the incidence of postoperative paraplegia). Monitoring lines include central venous access and arterial pressure lines. Core body and cerebral temperatures are monitored by bladder and tympanic probes, respectively. Neurologic monitoring by noninvasive near-infrared spectroscopy cerebral oxygenation monitoring may be used.

◆ The patient is positioned in the right lateral decubitus position for a left posterolateral thoracotomy. The hips are rotated back to the left for bilateral femoral vessel access. Skin preparation should include access to the left carotid, right axillary, and bilateral femoral arteries. The left thorax is entered through the fourth intercostal space, providing access to the transverse arch and proximal descending aorta. The fifth rib may need to be divided posteriorly to obtain access to the distal thoracic aorta. Alternatively, a second entry point into the seventh intercostal space may provide access to the distal thoracic aorta (Fig. 20-4A and B).

◆ Full cardiopulmonary bypass with antegrade perfusion is preferred. Arterial cannulation strategies include perfusion into the arch, left subclavian artery, left common carotid artery, right subclavian artery, left ventricular apex and across the aortic valve, or femoral artery (perfusing the true lumen). Venous return can be accomplished with central venous cannulation through the femoral vein or retrograde cannulation through the main pulmonary artery.

◆ Hypothermic circulatory arrest is used to perform an open proximal anastomosis. Clamping between the left common carotid and left subclavian arteries may be used, but it frequently results in insufficient length for a proximal anastomosis. If left ventricular distention occurs during systemic cooling and subsequent ventricular fibrillation, the left heart may need to be decompressed with a vent through the left superior pulmonary vein or left ventricular apex. In the setting of good ventricular function and short hypothermic circulatory arrest times, systemic hypothermia alone is usually sufficient for myocardial protection. If the patient has poor ventricular function or the surgeon anticipates a long or complex open proximal anastomosis, myocardial protection strategies include more aggressive systemic cooling (18°C to 20°C) or administration of cardioplegia through an occlusion/infusion catheter positioned in the ascending aorta.[11]

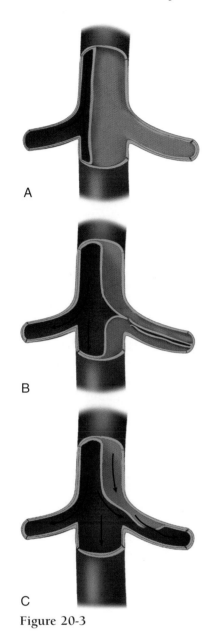

A

B

C

Figure 20-3

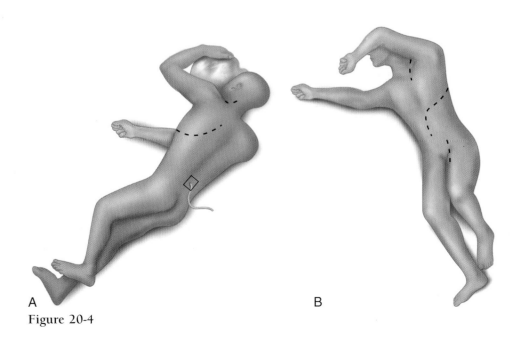

A   B

Figure 20-4

Dissection and Repair

- The phrenic and vagus nerves are identified and dissected free from the transverse arch.
- The transverse arch, proximal and middle descending thoracic aorta, and left subclavian artery are circumferentially dissected. Division of the ligamentum arteriosum helps mobilize the distal transverse arch and exposes the recurrent laryngeal nerve.
- The surgeon mobilizes and dissects circumferentially around the descending aorta for the distal anastomotic site. The primary goal is to replace only a short segment of aorta to redirect flow into the true lumen. This strategy allows one to stay above T7 and therefore prevents having to reimplant intercostal arteries.
- When the goal hypothermic temperature is achieved (18°C to 22°C core temperature), the pump is turned off and the proximal descending aorta opened. CO_2 may be infused into the operative field. The proximal aorta and distal aorta are completely transected to ensure circumferential inclusion of the intima and adventitia within the suture line (Fig. 20-5A). An appropriately sized woven Dacron graft is selected and sewn proximally to undissected aorta with an open technique (the entire PIT is excised; Fig. 20-5B). If the dissection extends into the arch, both the aortic intima and the adventitia are incorporated while performing the anastomosis to obliterate the false lumen. The left subclavian artery may need to be individually reimplanted if the PIT is very close or proximal to the left subclavian artery. The recurrent laryngeal nerve along the proximal aortic neck must be carefully identified, especially while transecting the aorta along the posterior wall; this is a common site of nerve injury while performing the proximal anatomosis.
- An arterial perfusion cannula is inserted into the proximal graft, and the patient is placed in the Trendelenburg position. After the transverse arch and graft have been de-aired, cardiopulmonary bypass is resumed to the head, heart, and upper extremities by placing a cross-clamp on the graft (Fig. 20-6). The anastomosis is checked for hemostasis. Systemic rewarming is commenced approximately 10 minutes after reperfusion to allow oxygen debt reversal.
- Proximal intercostal arteries are oversewn (above T7) to eliminate steal of blood from the spinal cord.
- Attention is now focused on the distal anastomosis, which is also performed with an open technique. Distally, intima and adventitia are occasionally reapproximated with a Teflon felt medial or adventitial bolster. The distal anastomosis is reconstructed, redirecting flow into the reconstructed true lumen (Fig. 20-7A).
- The proximal cross-clamp is released, air is evacuated both proximally and distally before tying the sutures, and both anastomoses are checked for hemostasis.
- The patient is resuscitated and rewarmed to 35°C to 36°C, with cardiopulmonary bypass subsequently discontinued. Transesophageal echocardiography should be used to ensure perfusion of the true lumen at the level of the diaphragm.
- Postoperative visceral malperfusion should be monitored with urine output and serial serum lactate levels and arterial blood gases. If visceral malperfusion persists (very unusual in our experience), it may be treated percutaneously with balloon septal fenestration and uncovered stenting in collaboration with the interventional radiologist.
- Surgical intervention for chronic type B dissections may be considered for both symptomatic patients (e.g., pain, mesenteric ischemia) and asymptomatic patients (e.g., rapidly expanding or large 5- to 6-cm aortic dissections). The techniques used are identical to those for an acute type B dissection, although the extent of resection is usually greater in that all of the enlarged aorta is removed. Before performing the distal anastomosis, a "tongue" of chronic dissection flap is excised from the aorta, allowing blood flow into both true and false lumens distally (the visceral or iliac arteries may originate from either the true or false lumen; Fig. 20-7B through D). Surgical resections distal to T7 may require reimplantation of large intercostal arteries to avoid spinal cord ischemia.

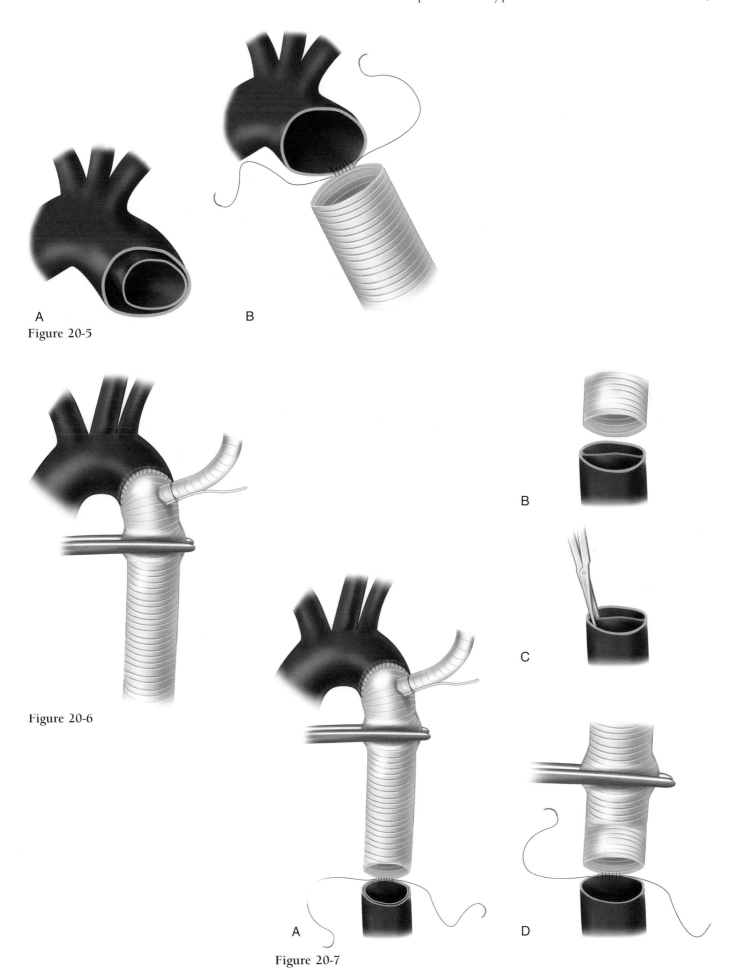

A

B

Figure 20-5

Figure 20-6

A

Figure 20-7

B

C

D

Closure

◆ The native aorta is closed over the Dacron graft. Chest tubes are placed in the left thorax. The left lung is reinflated under direct vision. The thoracotomy is closed in the usual fashion.

2. Endovascular Stent Grafts

Anatomic Requirements

◆ Contrast-enhanced CT of the chest/abdomen/pelvis (including femoral vessels) is the primary diagnostic tool to determine candidacy for endovascular stent graft placement.
◆ Endovascular stent grafts are oversized by approximately 7% to 18% based on CT cross-sectional intraluminal diameter to obtain sufficient radial force and create an adequate endoseal. Although it is currently approved only for the treatment of descending thoracic aortic aneurysms, we have used the Gore TAG Thoracic Endoprosthesis (W. L. Gore & Associates, Inc., Flagstaff, Ariz) to treat acute type B dissections under a PSIDE (Physician-Sponsored Investigational Device Exemption). Most devices require 2-cm landing zones (proximal and distal) to ensure adequate fixation. Balloon dilation is avoided.
◆ Endovascular stent grafts require introducer sheath access into the abdominal aorta. Introducer sheath size is determined by the stent graft size selected and varies from 20F to 24F outside diameter. The common femoral and iliac arteries must measure 8 to 10 mm. Vessel tortuosity and severe calcification are contraindications to the procedure.
◆ The endovascular stent graft only needs to cover the PIT. The PIT is measured and the endovascular stent graft length selected. Placement proximal to T6-T8 minimizes the risk for postprocedure paraplegia.
◆ To obtain an adequate proximal landing zone length for fixation and sealing, the left subclavian artery may need to be covered. If this strategy is used, a left carotid–subclavian bypass may be indicated if any of the following is present: (1) a large vertebral artery off the left subclavian artery, (2) a patent left internal mammary artery graft, or (3) an incomplete circle of Willis.

Incision

◆ The patient is placed in the supine position. Arterial access is obtained through the common femoral artery with an open technique (Fig. 20-8). Alternatively, if the common femoral artery size is not adequate, the external or common iliac artery may be used after obtaining exposure with a retroperitoneal technique. Frequently, a 10-mm Dacron graft is anastomosed to the common iliac artery for vascular access (Fig. 20-9).

Deployment

◆ The patient is administered intravenous heparin. An introducer sheath (20F to 24F) is introduced over a super-stiff guidewire under fluoroscopic guidance. The device is subsequently advanced over the guidewire and the endovascular stent graft carefully positioned with regard to previously determined landmarks (i.e., left subclavian artery). The stent graft is then deployed. We have never balloon-dilated the endovascular stent graft in the setting of an acute dissection.
◆ Accurate endovascular stent graft deployment, as well as redirection of aortic blood flow, may be confirmed by aortography (Figs. 20-10 and 20-11).

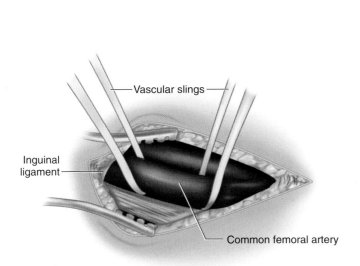

Figure 20-8

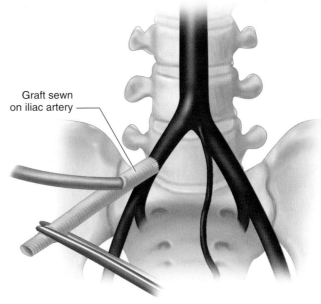

Figure 20-9

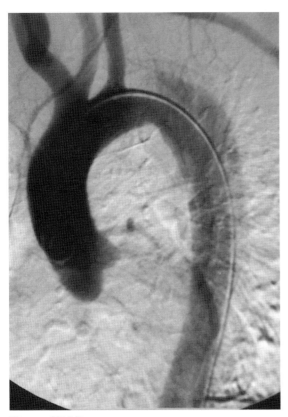

Figure 20-10

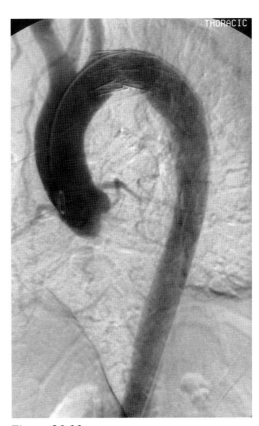

Figure 20-11

- Endovascular stent graft coverage of the primary intimal tear redirects flow into the true lumen (Fig. 20-12B), reversing malperfusion secondary to true lumen collapse, or *dynamic malperfusion* (Fig. 20-12A). Note the increased size of the true lumen with increased flow in the celiac artery (see Fig. 20-12B). Endovascular stenting (uncovered) of the individual branch vessel orifice alone or in combination with fenestration of the dissection septum may be required for *static malperfusion* of end organs. The patient in Figure 20-13 required right renal artery angioplasty and stenting into the true lumen (see Fig. 20-13A). Figure 20-13B is the poststent angiogram.

Closure

- Proximal and distal arterial control is obtained before removing the introducer sheath. We recommend leaving a guidewire in place during the sheath removal. If a catastrophic vascular injury is identified, a balloon catheter may be placed over the guidewire to obtain vascular control until open surgical or endovascular repair. After removing the guidewire, the artery is repaired.
- The groin dissection or retroperitoneal exposure is closed in the usual fashion.

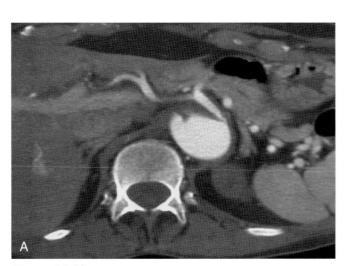

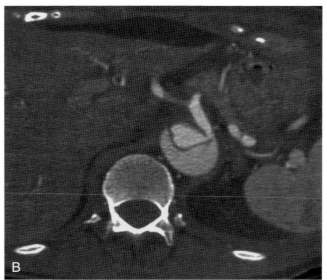

Figure 20-12

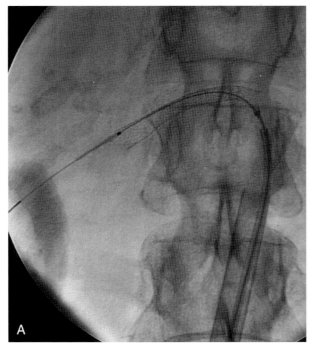

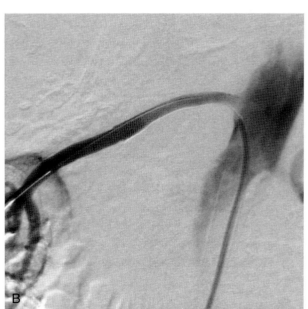

Figure 20-13

Step 4. Postoperative Care

- If safe to do so, the double-lumen endotracheal tube should be changed to a single-lumen tube before leaving the operating room.
- Postoperative care in the intensive care unit includes blood pressure control with mean arterial pressures of 70 to 80 mm Hg. Patients should have serial abdominal, neurologic, and pulse examinations.
- CSF is drained continuously to maintain CSF pressures less than 10 mm Hg. The CSF drain is usually removed after 3 days if there are no neurologic complications.
- Follow-up CT scans of the chest/abdomen/pelvis should be obtained before discharge. The patient should also have annual CT scans to monitor the size of the residual aortic dissection.

Step 5. Pearls and Pitfalls

- The standard treatment for end-organ malperfusion remains proximal repair of the dissection with either open or endovascular stent graft surgery, as described, covering or excising the proximal intimal tear. If intra-abdominal visceral malperfusion persists after repair, and percutaneous intervention is not available, open surgical fenestration of the descending thoracic or suprarenal aorta can be performed (midline laparotomy). Alternatively, extra-anatomic bypass may be used. Similarly, persistent malperfusion of the lower extremities can be treated with percutaneous interventional techniques, surgical fenestration, or bypass grafting (femoral–femoral bypass for unilateral lower extremity malperfusion, or axillary–femoral/femoral–femoral bypass for bilateral malperfusion).
- In the setting of postoperative paraplegia, mean arterial pressures should be augmented (goal ≥90 mm Hg), the CSF lumbar drain continued or placed (goal CSF pressure ≤10 mm Hg), and the patient's body temperature allowed to remain cool.

References

1. Layton KF, Kallmes DF, Cloft HJ, et al: Bovine aortic arch variant in humans: Clarification of a common misnomer. AJNR Am J Neuroradiol 2006;27:1541-1542.
2. Daily PO, Trueblood HW, Stinson EB, et al: Management of acute aortic dissections. Ann Thorac Surg 1970;10:237-247.
3. Robbins RC, McManus RP, Mitchell RS, et al: Management of patients with intramural hematoma of the thoracic aorta. Circulation 1993;88(5 Pt 2):II1-II10.
4. Stanson AW, Kazmier FJ, Hollier LH, et al: Penetrating atherosclerotic ulcers of the thoracic aorta: Natural history and clinicopathologic correlations. Ann Vasc Surg 1986;1:15-23.
5. Crawford ES: The diagnosis and management of aortic dissection. JAMA 1990;264:2537-2541.
6. Doroghazi RM, Slater EE, DeSanctis RW, et al: Long-term survival of patients with treated aortic dissection. J Am Coll Cardiol 1984;3:1026-1034.
7. DeSanctis RW, Doroghazi RM, Austen WG, Buckley MJ: Aortic dissection. N Engl J Med 1987;317:1060-1067.
8. Glower DD, Fann JI, Speier RH, et al: Comparison of medical and surgical therapy for uncomplicated descending aortic dissection. Circulation 1990;82(5 Suppl):IV39-IV46.
9. Umana JP, Lai DT, Mitchell RS, et al: Is medical therapy still the optimal treatment strategy for patients with acute type B aortic dissections? J Thorac Cardiovasc Surg 2002;124:896-910.
10. Williams DM, Lee DY, Hamilton BH, et al: The dissected aorta: Part III. Anatomy and radiologic diagnosis of branch-vessel compromise. Radiology 1997;203:37-44.
11. Melissano G, Maisano F, Civilini E, et al: Direct cerebral perfusion and myocardial protection with moderate systemic hypothermic arrest for high descending aortic aneurysm. J Thorac Cardiovasc Surg 2004;127:1530-1531.

CHAPTER 21

AORTIC ARCH ANEURYSMS

John S. Ikonomidis

Step 1. Surgical Anatomy

- Academic anatomists refer to the aortic arch as that part of the aorta that begins and ends with a line drawn in cross-section across the aorta at a level corresponding to the lesser curvature of the aortic arch. This therefore implies that the arch of the aorta starts at approximately the level of the superior reflection of the pericardial cavity. However, surgical anatomists and surgeons alike tend to consider the aortic arch as that portion of the aorta that begins with a line drawn cross-sectionally across the aorta at the level of the proximal origin of the ostium of the innominate artery and ending at the distal margin of the ostium of the left subclavian artery.

- The aortic arch tapers somewhat from anterior to posterior owing to the takeoff of the three large arterial branches—the innominate artery, the left common carotid artery, and the left subclavian artery. In approximately 5% of patients, this anatomic configuration consists of a double ostium or *bovine aortic arch*, where the innominate artery and left common carotid artery arise from a somewhat larger, but single aortic ostium (Fig. 21-1).

- Other anatomic structures of importance during aortic arch surgery include the left recurrent laryngeal nerve, the left phrenic nerve, and the right recurrent laryngeal nerve; these become important when considering separate replacement of the branch vessels in conjunction with aortic arch surgery.

- Aortic arch aneurysms seldom occur as isolated structures, but rather occur in conjunction with aneurysmal dilation of the proximal ascending aorta or the distal aorta. Aneurysmal dilation often causes the aortic arch aneurysm to shift anteriorly and laterally to the right. Because most cases of aortic arch aneurysm surgery are performed through a median sternotomy, this anatomic change brings critical structures more anteriorly and may facilitate the repair (Fig. 21-2).

Normal   Bovine

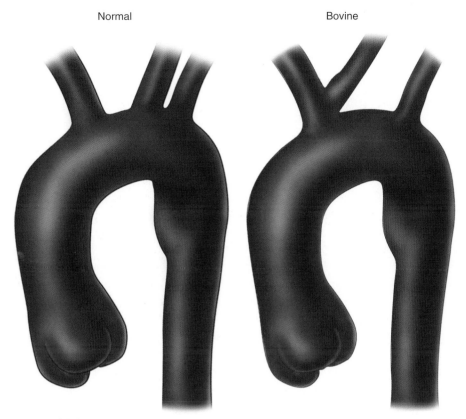

Figure 21-1

Normal   Aneurysm

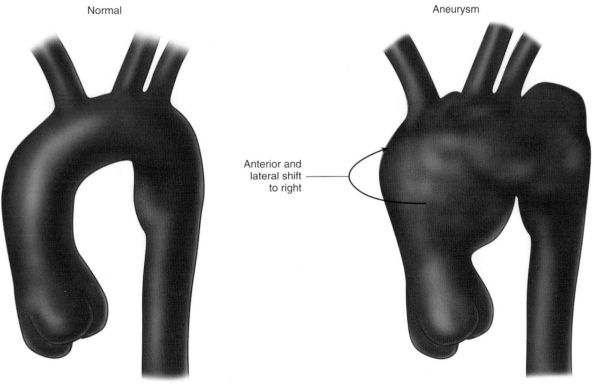

Anterior and
lateral shift
to right

Figure 21-2

Step 2. Preoperative Considerations

◆ Assessment of the patient's fitness for aortic arch replacement has multiple facets. Most importantly, the patient needs to be of an age and physical condition that would withstand a major operation such as this. A careful consideration of noncardiovascular comorbidity such as respiratory and renal disease should be undertaken because these are significant independent predictors of poor outcome.

◆ From a cardiovascular point of view, left ventricular function and the presence or absence of significant valvular disease are important variables to consider. The presence of coronary disease does not preclude operation, but it would mandate additional coronary artery bypass procedures that would add to the length of the surgical procedure.

◆ The presence of significant peripheral vascular disease in the carotid arteries, subclavian arteries, or femoral arteries is an important consideration in terms of determining cannulation and perfusion strategies during circulatory arrest. Similar anatomic considerations apply to the configuration of the aortic arch anatomy as far as the great vessels are concerned. A history of previous stroke or transient ischemic attacks may indicate the presence of significant cerebrovascular disease, and this must be investigated thoroughly with thin-slice computed tomography scans, magnetic resonance imaging, or cerebral angiography. A recommended standard preoperative work-up for patients undergoing aortic arch replacement is shown in Table 21-1.

TABLE 21-1.   **Preoperative Assessment for Aortic Arch Replacement**

History and Physical Examination

Family history of aneurysm disease or connective tissue disorders

Cardiovascular risk factors

History of cerebrovascular events

History of renal or pulmonary disease

Previous operations on the vascular system

Previous cardiac surgery through sternotomy

Cardiac murmurs on auscultation

Palpable peripheral pulses

Investigations

Peripheral vascular studies
   Carotid arteries
   Lower extremity arteries

Pulmonary function testing

Transthoracic echocardiogram

Coronary arteriogram

Thin-slice computed tomographic angiogram of chest/abdomen/pelvis

Step 3. Operative Steps

1. Pharmacologic Adjuncts

- An important consideration with aortic arch replacement is cerebral preservation. Circulatory arrest in some form is required for aortic arch replacement, so a strategy should be undertaken to minimize the period and extent of cerebral hypoperfusion. A standard premedication strategy includes methylprednisone 500 mg to 1 g intravenously, mannitol 0.5 g/kg to maintain diuresis, and sodium pentobarbital approximately 10 to 15 mg/kg to reduce brain injury. To maximize the effect of the sodium pentobarbital, I administer this approximately 5 minutes before the start of hypothermic circulatory arrest. The patient's head should also be packed in ice.

2. Cannulation Site and Adjunct Perfusion Strategy

- Selection of cannulation site is important. In general, for circulatory arrest times anticipated to be less than 30 minutes, current literature suggests that direct cannulation of the aneurysm distally, cooling the patient down to 18°C to 20°C, and discontinuation of the pump with no perfusion adjuncts for 10 to 15 minutes is safe. I have typically used this strategy for a proximal hemiarch replacement with good results.
- If it is anticipated that a longer time on circulatory arrest will be required, such as for full arch replacement, a strategy should be used to maintain some form of cerebral perfusion at this temperature. This strategy should provide the best cerebral perfusion while minimizing the clutter in the operative field. Between the currently available techniques of retrograde cerebral perfusion, direct perfusion of the great vessels with separate cannulae, and selective perfusion through the right axillary artery, I recommend selective perfusion, especially if the patient has a bovine aortic arch. I believe this is the best strategy because (1) the vast majority of patients have an intact circle of Willis, and therefore selective antegrade cerebral perfusion is usually appropriate for most cases of arch replacement; (2) retrograde cerebral perfusion has been associated with development of brain edema and perhaps some neurologic dysfunction, and detailed studies indicate that very little blood flow given this way actually reaches the cerebral cortex; and (3) insertion of antegrade catheters into the ostia of the arch vessels is cumbersome, complicates the operative field, and may dislodge plaques if the arch is involved with atherosclerosis, possibly contributing to postoperative neurologic sequelae.
- The arterial side of the pump should be split to provide perfusion for this cannula and a separate cannula to be inserted into the aortic arch graft.

3. Right Axillary Artery Cannulation

- The right axillary artery is accessed through a right infraclavicular incision approximately 2 to 3 cm below the clavicle inferiorly along the lateral aspect of the clavicle just before the deltopectoral groove (Fig. 21-3). This incision is approximately 5 to 7 cm long, depending on the patient's habitus, through which a portion of the pectoralis major and usually most, if not all, of the pectoralis minor is divided. The axillary artery sits in the brachial plexus and is easily palpable. Electrocautery is not advised during this portion of the dissection to expose the axillary artery because of risk of thermal injury to the brachial plexus. It is usually straightforward to identify and encircle the axillary artery over a distance of 3 to 4 cm.
- Cannulation strategies for the axillary artery can include direct cannulation or placement of a side graft. I prefer a 10-mm Dacron side graft because this maintains perfusion to the right arm. There also is evidence in the literature that a side graft strategy for cannulation of the axillary artery may be more beneficial in reducing neurologic injury than direct cannulation. In addition, because the axillary artery is such a friable vessel, once the graft is inserted, it is not necessary to repair this artery when the cannula is removed; rather, the graft can be tied off at the end of the procedure with maintenance of excellent arterial patency.
- The patient must be heparinized to avoid clotting of the graft during sternotomy and preparation for bypass. Also, a right radial artery arterial catheter should be placed beforehand to monitor arterial pressure during the circulatory arrest period.

4. Establishment of Cardiopulmonary Bypass and Systemic Cooling

- A standard median sternotomy is performed and the heart is supported in a standard pericardial cradle. Extensive dissection is undertaken around the aneurysm and extending as far into the arch as is thought comfortable before institution of cardiopulmonary bypass. Double-stage venous cannulation is performed, an antegrade cardioplegia cannula is placed in the aneurysm, and a coronary sinus catheter is placed in preparation for cardioplegia administration (Fig. 21-4).
- After systemic heparinization and confirmation of an activated clotting time of 400 seconds, cardiopulmonary bypass is instituted. Systemic cooling with alpha-stat acid-base management strategy is immediately begun, and systemic temperature is monitored by both nasopharyngeal and bladder probes. As much of the aortic arch dissection is completed as possible to eliminate its necessity during the circulatory arrest period. It is usually possible to mobilize the arch aneurysm to the level of the left subclavian artery, bearing in mind that this is the region of the left recurrent laryngeal nerve, which should be identified and preserved if feasible. The innominate vein should be widely mobilized for easy cephalad or caudad retraction.

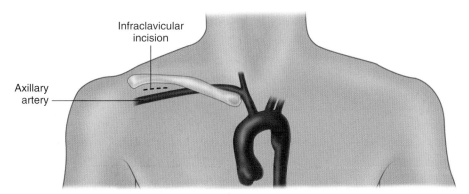

Figure 21-3

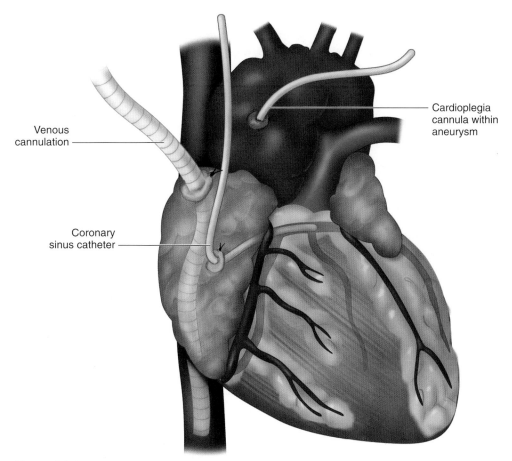

Figure 21-4

◆ Ventricular fibrillation usually occurs at a blood temperature around 26°C to 28°C, but this can be prevented to some extent with a 100- to 200-mg intravenous bolus of lidocaine. If the heart fibrillates, care must be taken to ensure that the left ventricle does not distend. If this happens, the options include cross-clamping and cardioplegic arrest or insertion of a left ventricular vent through the right superior pulmonary vein or the left ventricular apex (my preference). To arrest the heart, the cross-clamp is applied across the aneurysm with the pump flows decreased to minimize tension on the dilated aortic wall. Pump flows are then brought back up and the heart is arrested with cold blood cardioplegia given first antegrade to bring about a satisfactory cardiac arrest, then switching to retrograde coronary sinus administration. The heart is further protected with a myocardial cooling jacket, and I usually place a cold laparotomy sponge on the right ventricle to further preserve the right ventricle. Cardioplegic infusions of 250 to 500 mL are given every 20 minutes throughout the surgical procedure. I use a myocardial temperature probe placed in the interventricular septum under the left anterior descending coronary artery to maintain the myocardial temperature between 10°C and 15°C throughout the operation.

◆ For patients in whom proximal ascending and aortic root operations are necessary, this cooling period is the time to resect the ascending aneurysm or perform as much of the root replacement as possible. However, once desired cooling is achieved, the proximal operation should not continue but should be deferred for reconstruction of the aortic arch. This avoids unnecessary time on cardiopulmonary bypass; in addition, sufficient time will be available to complete the operation as rewarming is performed after the arch replacement is completed.

5. Circulatory Arrest and Preparation for Aortic Arch Replacement

◆ When the bladder temperature reaches 18°C to 20°C, the pump is discontinued but the patient is not exsanguinated. A small clamp is placed on the innominate artery proximally, and flow is initiated to maintain a normal arterial infusion pressure (mean radial artery pressure around 60 mm Hg). The main cross-clamp is removed, and blood is cleared from the field with cardiotomy bypass suction.

◆ Once selective antegrade cerebral perfusion is begun, back-bleeding from the remainder of the great vessel ostia sometimes necessitates placement of small clamps across these vessels. Once this is achieved, dissection is undertaken whereby the arch vessels are prepared for implantation and a distal anastomotic site is prepared (Fig. 21-5). In the patient with no connective tissue disorder and good tissue in the aortic arch, it is appropriate to replace the aortic arch with the great vessels as a single Carrel island; however, in patients with known connective tissue disease, the aortic arch should be completely replaced, excluding all aortic tissue to prevent late aneurysm formation at the island site. For this procedure, special branched grafts are available for separate implantation of the great vessels.

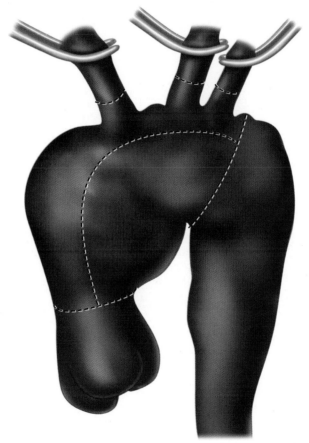

Figure 21-5

6. Aortic Arch Replacement

- Once the distal anastomotic site in the descending thoracic aorta is prepared, a four-branch graft is brought into the field and invaginated into itself. This is inserted into the distal descending thoracic aorta, and an anastomosis is performed between the aorta and the cuff, usually with 3-0 polypropylene suture (Fig. 21-6A). I do not use felt material for this anastomosis.
- Once the anastomosis is completed, the inside of the graft is evaginated and a small amount of surgical adhesive is laid down around the anastomotic site to seal any needle holes. The side branch of the graft is then cannulated and perfusion to the body is resumed, during which time the graft is de-aired; a cross-clamp is then placed just proximal to the branch to allow distal cold perfusion (Fig. 21-6B).
- Anastomoses then proceed with the left subclavian, left common carotid, and innominate arteries, with sequential moving of the clamp proximally with completion of each anastomosis to maximize cerebral flow. After completion of all of the anastomoses, the clamp is then moved proximal to the innominate artery graft, thus restoring complete perfusion to the head (Fig. 21-6C). At this point, the pump flow is increased as appropriate, and rewarming is begun.

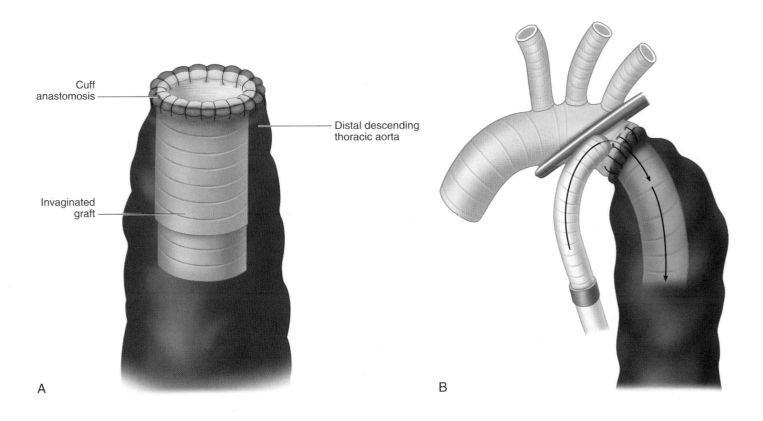

Cuff anastomosis

Distal descending thoracic aorta

Invaginated graft

A

B

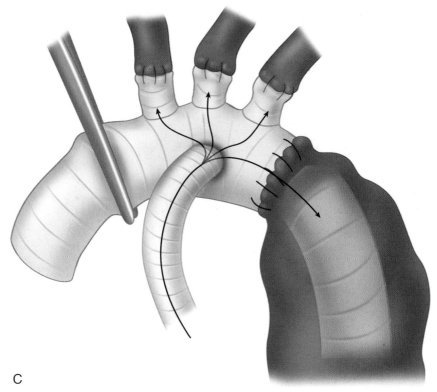

C

Figure 21-6

7. **Closure**

- During the rewarming procedure, the ascending aorta–to–graft anastomosis is performed, or proximal aortic work or valve replacement or root replacement can be completed, after which a graft-to-graft anastomosis is performed. An ascending aortic vent is inserted, and after appropriate de-airing maneuvers, the cross-clamp is removed and myocardial perfusion begun (Fig. 21-7). Atrial and ventricular pacemaker wires are inserted, the heart is allowed to recover on cardiopulmonary bypass, and ventilation is begun with continued de-airing. All suture lines are inspected for bleeding requiring surgical repair, and the axillary artery graft is tied off and divided.
- When the bladder temperature has reached at least 36.5°C, de-airing has been completed, normal sinus rhythm is restored, and blood gas and laboratory values have normalized, the patient is weaned from cardiopulmonary bypass. The venous cannula is removed, and protamine is administered through the inflow limb of the arch graft, after which the limb is ligated and divided close to the arch graft (Fig. 21-8). After confirmation of complete hemostasis, drains are inserted, usually a flexible drain posteriorly and one anterior chest tube. The sternum is closed with stainless steel wires followed by opposition of soft tissues in layers with absorbable sutures.

Step 4. Postoperative Care

- Patients who undergo aortic arch replacement are critically ill. Important postoperative considerations are maintenance of appropriate hemodynamics and urine output and careful monitoring for bleeding. Hypertension swings are not uncommon in these patients, and a single hypertension swing may trigger bleeding from one of the many suture lines used in this operation.
- Careful vigilance regarding the patient's filling pressures is mandatory to identify any problems with cardiac tamponade from bleeding. The clinical examination of the patient going into tamponade shows cold and mottled extremities and an abrupt decline in urine output. Early reexploration in these patients is mandatory and lifesaving. After an appropriate period of stability, the patient is weaned from anesthetic and is allowed to awaken. Extubation then proceeds by standard criteria predicated on the patient's appropriate neurologic recovery.

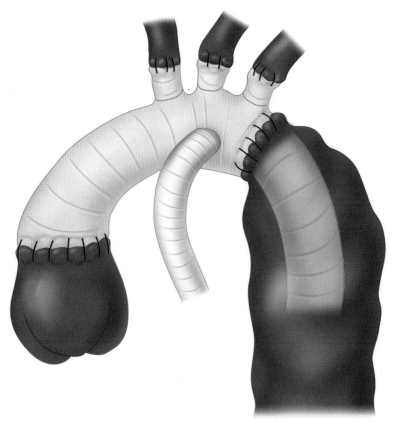

Figure 21-7

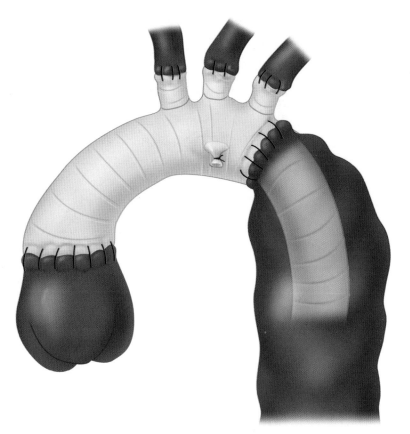

Figure 21-8

Step 5. Pearls and Pitfalls

- It is important, especially when a branch replacement of the arch is used, to identify and preserve the recurrent laryngeal nerves. There is a possibility with this operation that both nerves can be destroyed, which is irreparably debilitating for the patient.
- Orientation of the branch graft is important. When the graft is invaginated, it is advisable to mark the graft cuff with a marking pencil on the side where the branches will be oriented to allow appropriate orientation of the cuff in the descending thoracic aorta. This is performed under circulatory arrest; having to revise this anastomosis because of improper orientation can have dire consequences.
- Another important consideration is suture technique. The vessels being sewn are usually histologically abnormal (especially if involved with connective tissue disease), and great care must be taken with each pass of the needle to avoid microtears that may translate into troublesome bleeding problems later.
- Bleeding can seem unstoppable at times with this operation. The best way to deal with this is, first, to visually ensure that there are no sites of bleeding that require direct surgical repair while on bypass. Second, make sure that the patient is completely rewarmed (i.e., at least 36.5°C bladder temperature) before weaning from bypass. Third, reverse anticoagulation with protamine given slowly, pack all surgical sites, and wait 5 minutes. Have platelets and fresh frozen plasma hanging and dripping in during this time. After this period, most needle holes will seal and the bleeding will either cease or decrease to the point where sites that need further attention can be easily identified. From here, if the patient remains coagulopathic, keep the patient as warm as possible and correct all coagulation abnormalities with blood products and extra protamine. If bleeding is still troublesome, consider administration of activated recombinant factor VIIa concentrate.

Bibliography

Hagl C, Khaladj N, Karck M, et al: Hypothermic circulatory arrest during ascending and aortic arch surgery: The theoretical impact of different cerebral perfusion techniques and other methods of cerebral protection. Eur J Cardiothorac Surg 2003;24:371-378.

Kamiya H, Klima U, Hagl C, et al: Short moderate hypothermic circulatory arrest without any adjunctive cerebral protection for surgical repair of the ascending aorta extending into the proximal aortic arch: Is it safe? Heart Surg Forum 2006;9:E759-E761.

Reich DL, Uysal S, Ergin MA, Griepp RB: Retrograde cerebral protection as a method of neuroprotection during thoracic aortic surgery. Ann Thorac Surg 2001;72:1774-1782.

Spielvogel D, Lansman SL, Griepp RB: Aortic arch replacement/selective antegrade cerebral perfusion. Op Tech Thorac Cardiovasc Surg 2005;10:23-44.

Svensson LG, Blackstone EH, Rajeswaran J, et al: Does the arterial cannulation site for circulatory arrest influence stroke risk? Ann Thorac Surg 2004;78:1274-1284.

CHAPTER 22

THORACOABDOMINAL ANEURYSMS

Peter I. Tsai, Scott A. LeMaire, and Joseph S. Coselli

Step 1. Surgical Anatomy

- Thoracoabdominal aortic aneurysms (TAAAs) are characterized by dilation of the aorta (to at least 1.5 times its normal diameter) at the diaphragmatic hiatus—the boundary that separates the descending thoracic and abdominal aortic segments—with varying degrees of extension into the chest and abdomen.
- The normal diameter of the aorta varies by anatomic location and by the patient's sex, age, and body size. Average normal aortic diameters for men and women, respectively, are 28 mm and 26 mm at the level of mid-descending thoracic aorta, 23 mm and 20 mm at the celiac axis, and 19.5 mm and 16.5 mm at the infrarenal aorta. Body surface area is a better predictor of aortic size than is height or weight, particularly in patients younger than 50 years of age.
- The Crawford classification of TAAA repairs (Fig. 22-1) enables appropriate risk stratification and selection of specific perioperative treatment modalities based on the extent of the aortic replacement. Extent I aneurysms involve most or all of the descending thoracic aorta and the upper abdominal aorta. Extent II aneurysms involve most or all of the descending thoracic aorta and extend into the infrarenal abdominal aorta. Extent III aneurysms involve the distal half or less of the descending thoracic aorta and varying portions of the abdominal aorta. Extent IV aneurysms involve most or all of the abdominal aorta.
- Understanding the anatomy of the spinal cord circulation is necessary to prevent spinal cord ischemia. The arteria radicularis magna (artery of Adamkiewicz) is the largest of the radicular medullary arteries supplying the anterior spinal artery and is therefore often targeted for reimplantation during TAAA repair. This artery has a variable origin; it arises from a lower intercostal artery (T9-T12) in 60% of persons, from a lumbar artery (L1-L4) in approximately 25%, and from an upper intercostal artery (T5-T8) in about 15%.

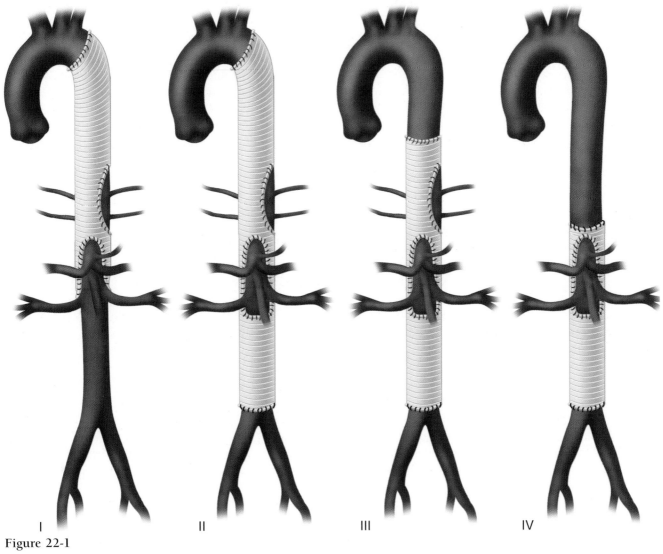

Figure 22-1

I   II   III   IV

Step 2. Preoperative Considerations

- Nonoperative management—which consists of strict blood pressure control, cessation of smoking, and at least yearly surveillance with imaging studies—is appropriate for asymptomatic patients who have small aneurysms.
- Indications for operation in asymptomatic patients include an aortic diameter exceeding 5 to 6 cm or a rate of dilation greater than 1 cm per year. In patients with Marfan syndrome or related connective tissue disorders, the threshold for operation is lower for both absolute size and rate of growth. In the case of TAAAs that cause symptoms—especially pain—or that are complicated by superimposed acute dissection, the risk of impending rupture warrants expeditious evaluation and urgent aneurysm repair, even when the aforementioned threshold diameters have not been reached.
- With the exception of patients who require emergency operation, all patients undergo a thorough preoperative evaluation, with emphasis on cardiac, pulmonary, and renal function. Patients who have asymptomatic aneurysms and severe coronary artery occlusive disease undergo myocardial revascularization before aneurysm repair. If clamping proximal to the left subclavian artery is anticipated in patients in whom the left internal thoracic artery has been used as a coronary artery bypass graft, a left common carotid–to–subclavian artery bypass is performed to prevent cardiac ischemia when the aortic clamp is applied.
- Preoperative renal insufficiency has been a major risk factor for early mortality throughout the history of TAAA repair. Strategies to reduce the risk of contrast-induced nephropathy from preoperative imaging studies include periprocedural administration of acetylcysteine and intravenous hydration. Ideally, surgery is delayed for 24 hours or longer after contrast administration. If renal insufficiency occurs or worsens after a patient receives contrast, the surgical procedure is postponed until renal function recovers or is satisfactorily stabilized.
- Pulmonary complications are the most common form of postoperative morbidity in patients undergoing TAAA repairs. Patients with a forced expiratory volume at 1 second (FEV_1) greater than 1 L and a Pco_2 less than 45 mm Hg are considered satisfactory surgical candidates. In suitable patients, borderline pulmonary function frequently is improved by smoking cessation, treatment of bronchitis, weight loss, and a general exercise program that the patient follows for a period of 1 to 3 months before operation.
- An evolving aspect of selecting appropriate treatment in patients with TAAAs is the choice between performing a traditional open graft replacement and using an endovascular approach. Purely endovascular TAAA repairs require the use of fenestrated or branched stent grafts, and these repairs are currently considered experimental. Hybrid repairs, during which open visceral bypass grafting is performed to secure organ perfusion before the entire aneurysm is covered with a stent graft, appear well suited for patients with limited physiologic reserve and are becoming increasingly popular.

Step 3. Operative Steps

1. **Intraoperative Management Strategy**

♦ Shortly after the induction of anesthesia, 25 to 50 g of mannitol is given intravenously to promote vigorous diuresis. To prevent acidosis, sodium bicarbonate solution is administered by continuous infusion at a rate of 2 to 3 mEq/kg/hr while the aorta is clamped. A cell-saving device is used throughout the procedure to salvage shed blood from the operative field. The patient's temperature is allowed to drift down to a nasopharyngeal temperature of 32°C to 33°C.

♦ Left heart bypass (LHB) and cerebrospinal fluid (CSF) drainage are used to optimize organ protection in patients undergoing Crawford extent I and II TAAA repairs and in patients who are undergoing extent III or IV TAAA repair after previous descending thoracic aortic replacement. In addition, in patients with poor cardiac function, LHB is used to reduce cardiac strain, thus improving the patients' ability to tolerate aortic clamping. Enough CSF is drained to keep CSF pressure between 8 and 10 mm Hg during the operation.

♦ Motor-evoked potential monitoring can provide information about spinal cord function and thereby anterior spinal perfusion during aortic repair. This method of spinal cord monitoring, which precludes complete neuromuscular blockade, requires special anesthetic techniques.

2. Incisions and Aortic Exposure

• The patient is turned to a right lateral decubitus position with the shoulders placed at 60 to 80 degrees and the hips flexed to 30 to 40 degrees from horizontal and stabilized with a beanbag (Fig. 22-2). For TAAAs that extend into the superior aspect of the thorax (i.e., extents I and II; Fig. 22-3), the upper portion of the thoracoabdominal incision is generally made through the sixth intercostal space (see Fig. 22-2A); the sixth or seventh ribs may be divided posteriorly to achieve additional proximal or distal exposure, respectively, as needed. With extent III aneurysms, a similar incision is made but the pleural space is entered through the seventh or eighth intercostal space, depending on the desired level of exposure. The incision is gently curved as it crosses the costal margin to reduce the risk of tissue necrosis at the apex of the lower portion of the musculoskeletal tissue flap. In contrast, to approach extent IV aneurysms, a straight oblique incision through the 9th or 10th interspace is used (see Fig. 22-2B). In most cases, the distal extent of the incision is at the level of the umbilicus. The incision is extended toward the pubis if iliac aneurysms are to be repaired.

• Fixed metal retractors attached to the operating table provide consistent static exposure. The diaphragm is divided in a circular fashion to protect the phrenic nerve and to preserve a 3- to 4-cm rim of diaphragmatic tissue posterolaterally to facilitate closure when the operation is complete. The abdominal aortic segment is exposed by a transperitoneal approach; the retroperitoneum is entered lateral to the left colon, where the spleen, the left kidney, and the ureter are retracted anteriorly and to the right. The crus of the diaphragm is divided, and the left renal artery is identified but not circumferentially dissected or encircled with a tape. An open abdominal approach permits direct inspection of the bowel, abdominal viscera, and visceral blood supply after aortic reconstruction is completed.

• When the aneurysm encroaches on the left subclavian artery, the distal aortic arch is mobilized gently by dividing the remnant of the ductus arteriosus. The vagus and recurrent laryngeal nerves are identified. Occasionally, the vagus nerve is divided below the recurrent nerve to provide additional mobility, thereby protecting the recurrent nerve from injury. If clamping proximal to the left subclavian artery is anticipated, this artery is separately and circumferentially mobilized to enable placement of a bulldog clamp. After adequate exposure of the aorta is achieved, heparin (1 mg/kg) is administered before aortic clamping or the start of LHB.

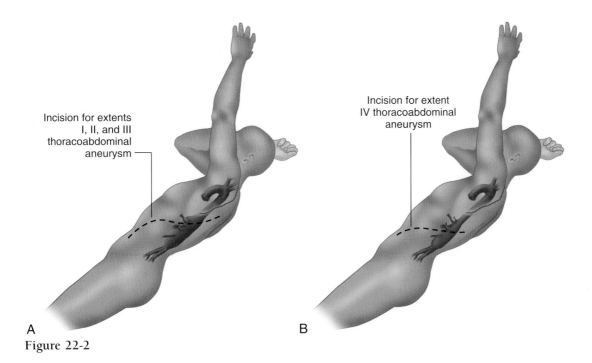

Incision for extents
I, II, and III
thoracoabdominal
aneurysm

Incision for extent
IV thoracoabdominal
aneurysm

A

B

Figure 22-2

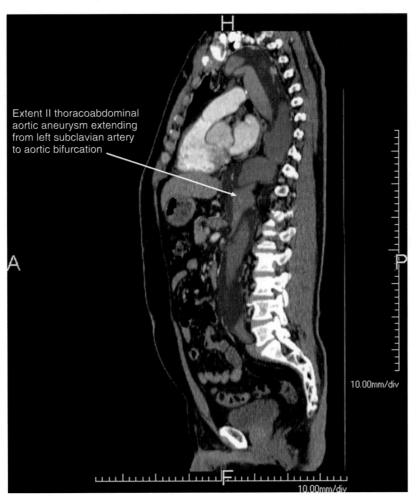

Extent II thoracoabdominal
aortic aneurysm extending
from left subclavian artery
to aortic bifurcation

10.00mm/div

10.00mm/div

Figure 22-3

3. Graft Replacement of the Aorta

+ Patients with extensive TAAAs (extents I and II) are at greatest risk for development of postoperative paraplegia or paraparesis, and LHB is used to provide distal aortic perfusion during the proximal portion of the aortic repair. This is achieved by using temporary bypass from the left atrium (through a cannula inserted through the inferior pulmonary vein) to either the femoral artery (most commonly the left) or the distal descending thoracic aorta with a closed-circuit, in-line centrifugal pump (Fig. 22-4). Carefully examining computed tomography scans or magnetic resonance images helps the surgeon to select an appropriate site for direct aortic cannulation. Areas with intraluminal thrombus are avoided because cannulating them can lead to distal embolization (Fig. 22-5).
+ A clamp is applied to the distal transverse arch (between the left common carotid and left subclavian arteries) or the proximal descending thoracic aorta. When LHB is used, a distal aortic clamp is placed between T4 and T7 (see Fig. 22-4). Bypass flows are adjusted to maintain normal proximal arterial and venous filling pressures. Flows between 1500 and 2500 mL/min are generally required. The aorta is opened, transected 2 to 3 cm beyond the proximal clamp, and dissected from the esophagus. Patent upper intercostal arteries are oversewn.
+ The proximal anastomosis is performed between the aorta and a 22- or 24-mm Dacron graft with continuous 3-0 polypropylene suture. In patients with fragile aortic tissues (such as those with acute aortic dissection or Marfan syndrome), 4-0 polypropylene is often used. Interrupted polypropylene mattress sutures with felt pledgets are used to reinforce selected portions of the anastomoses. Surgical adhesives are avoided in these operations.

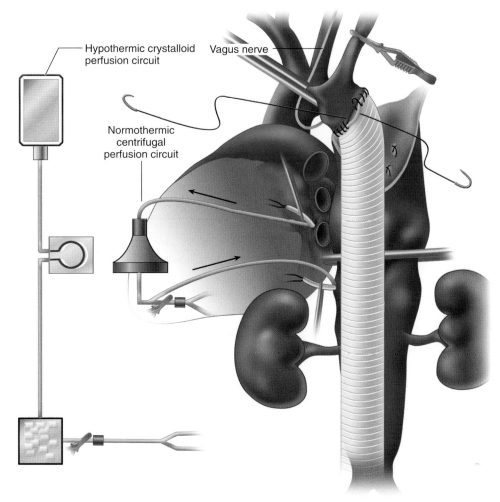

Hypothermic crystalloid perfusion circuit

Vagus nerve

Normothermic centrifugal perfusion circuit

Figure 22-4

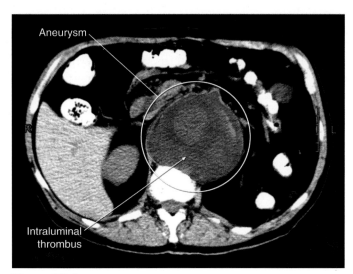

Aneurysm

Intraluminal thrombus

Figure 22-5

- After the proximal anastomosis is completed, LHB is stopped, the aortic cannula is removed, and the entire remaining aneurysm is opened longitudinally. The origins of the visceral and renal branches are identified, and cold (4°C) lactated Ringer solution is intermittently delivered to the renal arteries by using balloon catheters (Fig. 22-6). In patients receiving LHB, balloon catheters are also placed in the celiac and superior mesenteric arteries so that selective visceral perfusion can be delivered from the pump circuit.
- For most extent I and II repairs, patent lower intercostal arteries are selected and reattached to an opening cut in the side of the graft (see Fig. 22-6); large arteries with little or no back-bleeding are considered particularly important. When none of these arteries is patent, endarterectomy of that aortic wall and removal of calcified intimal disease should be considered as a means of identifying arteries suitable for reattachment. After this anastomosis is complete, the proximal clamp is often moved down the graft to restore intercostal perfusion (Fig. 22-7).
- In extent I repairs, the reattachment of the visceral arteries is often incorporated into a beveled distal anastomosis. In extent II and III repairs, the visceral artery origins (where 25% of patients have stenosis and require endarterectomy, stenting, or interposition bypass grafting) are reattached to one or more oval openings in the graft (see Fig. 22-7). The left renal artery requires attachment to a separate opening in the graft in 30% to 40% of cases (see Fig. 22-7, *inset*).
- When the aneurysm extends below the renal arteries, a distal anastomosis is performed near the aortic bifurcation (Fig. 22-8). In patients with iliac artery aneurysms, a bifurcation graft is sewn onto the end of the straight graft, and routine distal bypass anastomoses are performed. Care is taken to preserve circulation to at least one of the internal iliac arteries.

4. Closure

- After protamine sulfate is administered, meticulous hemostasis is achieved; the renal, visceral, and peripheral circulations are assessed; and the body is rewarmed with warm-water irrigation of the operative field. The aneurysm wall is then loosely wrapped around the aortic graft. Two posteriorly located thoracic drainage tubes and a closed-suction retroperitoneal drain are placed before closure. The diaphragm is closed with continuous heavy polypropylene suture, and the thoracotomy is closed with braided polyester sutures and reinforced with figure-of-eight steel wires.

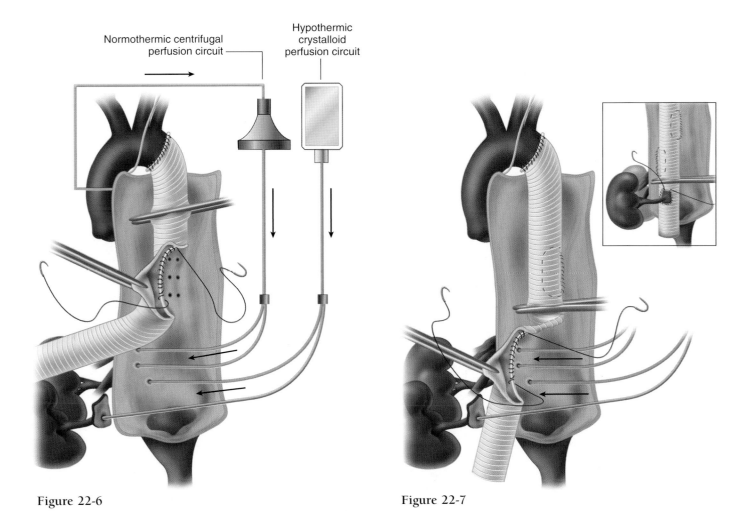

Figure 22-6

Figure 22-7

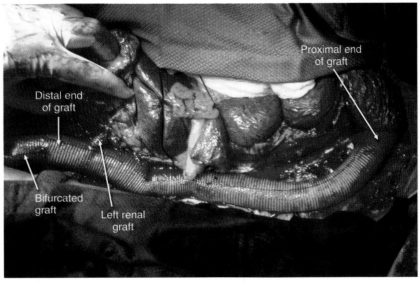

Figure 22-8

5. Alternative Techniques

Reversed Elephant Trunk Technique

♦ The reversed elephant trunk technique is performed as an initial operation in patients with extensive aneurysmal disease involving the ascending aorta, transverse aortic arch, and thoracoabdominal aorta who present with a TAAA that is causing symptoms (back pain), has ruptured, or is considerably larger than the ascending aorta (Fig. 22-9). The TAAA is replaced during the first stage of aortic repair (Fig. 22-10); a portion of the proximal end of the aortic graft is invaginated into the graft lumen, and the folded graft edge is used for the proximal anastomosis. During the second-stage operation, the suspended section of graft is retrieved (Fig. 22-11A) and used to replace the ascending and transverse aortic arch (Fig. 22-11B).

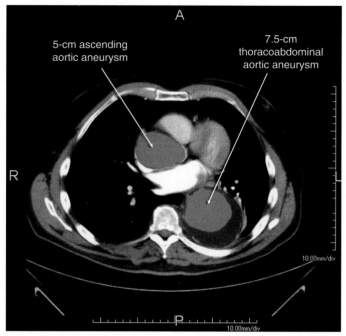

Figure 22-9

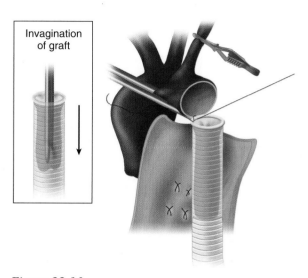

Figure 22-10

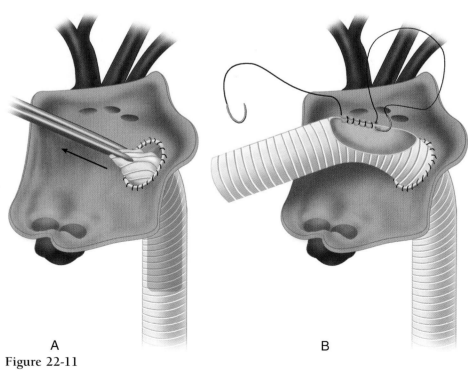

A

B

Figure 22-11

Hypothermic Circulatory Arrest

- Hypothermic circulatory arrest is selectively used in cases in which the distal aortic arch cannot be safely clamped because it is too large (Fig. 22-12) or because the aneurysm has ruptured. Arterial and venous cannulae are placed through the left femoral vessels. A second venous cannula is placed in the left atrium through the inferior pulmonary vein to enhance venous drainage and prevent cardiac distention. After the patient has been cooled to electrocerebral silence and circulatory arrest has been initiated, the aneurysm is opened and a proximal anastomosis to the distal aortic arch is performed, after which a Y-limb from the arterial line is connected to a side-branch of the graft. The graft is then de-aired and clamped, pump flow to the upper body is resumed, and the remainder of the aortic repair is completed.

Step 4. Postoperative Care

1. Early Postoperative Management

- Complications that are commonly associated with an increased risk of death include paraplegia, renal failure, respiratory failure, cardiac events, and bleeding.
- Meticulous blood pressure control is maintained during the first 24 to 48 hours by using nitroprusside and intravenous β-adrenergic antagonists to maintain the mean arterial blood pressure at 80 to 90 mm Hg. In patients with particularly fragile aortic tissue (i.e., patients with Marfan syndrome or acute dissection), a target range of 70 to 80 mm Hg is used to help maintain hemostasis. Hypertensive episodes are controlled to prevent suture line disruption, which can cause severe bleeding or pseudoaneurysm formation. Hypotensive episodes must also be avoided because they can precipitate ischemic complications, including paraplegia and renal failure.
- Drainage of CSF is usually continued for 2 days after surgery. Fluid is drained with a closed collection system as needed to keep CSF pressure between 10 and 12 mm Hg during the early postoperative period and between 12 and 15 mm Hg after patients have confirmed that they are able to move their legs.
- Patients in whom paraplegia or paraparesis develops are treated aggressively in an attempt to reverse the deficit. Treatment includes draining CSF, administering steroids and osmotic diuretics, optimizing hemodynamics, correcting anemia, and preventing fever.
- Vocal cord paralysis can contribute to respiratory complications and should be suspected in patients with postoperative hoarseness and confirmed by direct examination. Effective treatment can be provided by direct cord medialization or, in higher risk patients, by polytetrafluoroethylene injection.
- Infection of a TAAA graft is often fatal; thus, intravenous antibiotics are continued until all drains, chest tubes, and central venous lines have been removed.

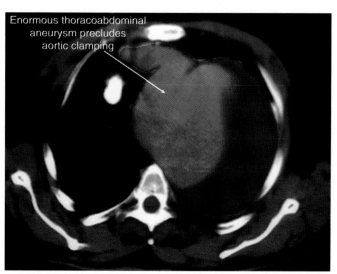

Figure 22-12

2. Long-term Surveillance

◆ Patients who have undergone TAAA repair remain at risk for development of new aneurysms in other aortic segments or in reattachment patches. Life-long surveillance with annual computed tomography or magnetic resonance imaging of the chest and abdomen is important, especially in patients with connective tissue disorders. Subsequent aortic repairs can be performed with surprisingly low mortality and morbidity rates, particularly when done electively.

Step 5. Pearls and Pitfalls

◆ Beware of the potential presence of a retroaortic left renal vein, which can be injured during TAAA exposure. When this vein is encountered, it is occasionally possible to mobilize the intact vessel and work underneath it. More commonly, however, the vein is temporarily ligated and divided, and after the aortic replacement is completed, the vein is repaired with either a direct end-to-end anastomosis or a short interposition graft.

◆ During extent I and II repairs, the aorta at the site of the proximal anastomosis is transected and carefully dissected off the esophagus. This enables placement of full-thickness aortic sutures while preventing esophageal injury. When the thoracic duct is encountered in this region, it should be ligated to prevent postoperative chylothorax.

◆ After the aorta is unclamped, intravenous indigo carmine is administered to confirm renal perfusion. Extravasation of dye into the retroperitoneal field indicates injury of the left ureter, which can then be repaired.

◆ It is not uncommon to encounter a tear in the splenic capsule during dissection, particularly during thoracoabdominal reoperations, when the surgeon may find that dense adhesions have fused the spleen and diaphragm. A very low threshold for performing splenectomy is necessary to prevent dangerous postoperative splenic bleeding and ischemic sequelae.

Acknowledgments

The authors thank Brook Wainwright, MS, and Scott A. Weldon, MA, CMI, for developing the medical illustrations, and Stephen N. Palmer, PhD, ELS, for providing editorial support.

Bibliography

Brockstein B, Johns L, Gewertz BL: Blood supply to the spinal cord: Anatomic and physiologic correlations. Ann Vasc Surg 1994;8:394-399.

Coselli JS, Bozinovski J, LeMaire SA: Open surgical repair of 2286 thoracoabdominal aortic aneurysms. Ann Thorac Surg 2007;83:S862-S864.

Coselli JS, LeMaire SA: Left heart bypass reduces paraplegia rates after thoracoabdominal aortic aneurysm repair. Ann Thorac Surg 1999;67:1931-1934.

Coselli JS, LeMaire SA: Descending and thoracoabdominal aneurysms. In Cohn LH (ed): Cardiac Surgery in the Adult, 3rd ed. New York, McGraw-Hill, 2008, pp 1277-1298.

Coselli JS, LeMaire SA, Carter SA, Conklin LD: The reversed elephant trunk technique used for treatment of complex aneurysms of the entire thoracic aorta. Ann Thorac Surg 2005;80:2166-2172.

Coselli JS, LeMaire SA, Köksoy C, et al: Cerebrospinal fluid drainage reduces paraplegia after thoracoabdominal aortic aneurysm repair: Results of a randomized clinical trial. J Vasc Surg 2002;35:631-639.

Huh J, LeMaire SA, Bozinovski J, Coselli JS: Perfusion for thoracic aortic surgery. In Gravlee GP, Davis RE, Stammers AH, Ungerleider RM (eds): Cardiopulmonary Bypass: Principles and Practice, 3rd ed. Philadelphia, Lippincott Williams & Wilkins, 2008, pp 647-661.

Jacobs MJ, Elenbaas TW, Schurink GW, et al: Assessment of spinal cord integrity during thoracoabdominal aortic aneurysm repair. Ann Thorac Surg 2002;74:S1864-S1866.

Köksoy C, LeMaire SA, Curling PE, et al: Renal perfusion during thoracoabdominal aortic operations: Cold crystalloid is superior to normothermic blood. Ann Thorac Surg 2002;73:730-738.

Kouchoukos NT, Masetti P, Murphy SF: Hypothermic cardiopulmonary bypass and circulatory arrest in the management of extensive thoracic and thoracoabdominal aortic aneurysms. Semin Thorac Cardiovasc Surg 2003;15:333-339.

LeMaire SA, Jamison AL, Carter SA, et al: Deployment of balloon expandable stents during open repair of thoracoabdominal aortic aneurysms: A new strategy for managing renal and mesenteric artery lesions. Eur J Cardiothorac Surg 2004;26:599-607.

MacArthur RG, Carter SA, Coselli JS, LeMaire SA: Organ protection during thoracoabdominal aortic surgery: Rationale for a multimodality approach. Semin Cardiothorac Vasc Anesth 2005;9:143-149.

Roselli EE, Greenberg RK, Pfaff K, et al: Endovascular treatment of thoracoabdominal aortic aneurysms. J Thorac Cardiovasc Surg 2007;133:1474-1482.

van Dongen EP, Schepens MA, Morshuis WJ, et al: Thoracic and thoracoabdominal aortic aneurysm repair: Use of evoked potential monitoring in 118 patients. J Vasc Surg 2001;34:1035-1040.

Wong DR, Coselli JS, Amerman K, et al: Delayed spinal cord deficits after thoracoabdominal aortic aneurysm repair. Ann Thorac Surg 2007;83:1345-1355.

THORACIC ENDOVASCULAR AORTIC REPAIR FOR DESCENDING THORACIC AORTIC AND AORTIC ARCH ANEURYSMS

Wilson Y. Szeto, William T. Brinkman, and Joseph E. Bavaria

- Thoracic endovascular aortic repair (TEVAR) has become an effective treatment for various descending thoracic aortic pathologic processes, including aortic aneurysm and dissection. Although long-term outcome data for this therapy are not available, the short-term and intermediate results have been promising.
- Multiple devices have been investigated in multicenter trials. Three devices are currently approved for the treatment of descending thoracic aortic aneurysms: the Gore TAG (W. L. Gore & Associates, Inc., Flagstaff, Ariz), Medtronic's Talent (Medtronic, Inc., Minneapolis, Minn), and the Cook Zenith TX2 (Cook Medical Inc., Bloomington, Ind).
- At present, device and anatomic limitations have restricted the applicability of TEVAR to the descending thoracic aorta. However, with improvement in device design and surgical technique, endovascular therapy for aortic disease will likely widen its applicability to disease located in the ascending aorta, the aortic arch, and the thoracoabdominal aorta.

Step 1. Surgical Anatomy

- Beginning distal to the left subclavian artery, the descending thoracic aorta is the continuation of the aortic arch. As it descends through the posterior mediastinum, the descending thoracic aorta lies to the left of the vertebral bodies and gradually approaches the midline. At the level of the 12th vertebra, it passes through the aortic hiatus in the diaphragm and becomes the abdominal aorta (Fig. 23-1).
- Anterior branches of the descending thoracic aorta include bronchial and esophageal arteries. These branches continue as segmental arterial supply to their respective structures.
- Intercostal arteries are posterior branches along the length of the descending thoracic aorta and provide segmental arterial blood supply to the spinal cord.
- In most patients, a dominant anterior medullary artery, the artery of Adamkiewicz, arises between levels T7 and L1 and provides the majority of the blood supply to the anterior spinal artery, perfusing the anterior two thirds of the spinal cord. Anteriorly, the intercostal arteries continue along the inferior margins of the ribs and form collaterals with the internal thoracic arteries located at the anterior chest wall.

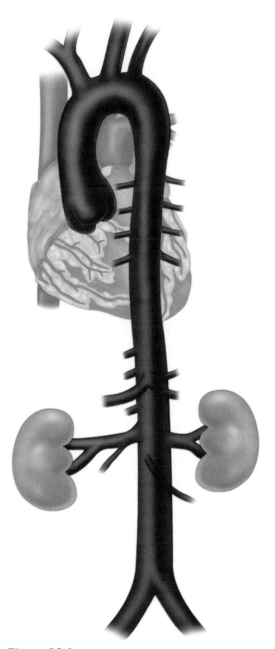

Figure 23-1

♦ There are no major arterial branches in the descending thoracic aorta, enabling the treatment of the entire descending thoracic aorta with TEVAR. The first major branch is the celiac artery, which arises in the abdominal aorta to supply the upper gastrointestinal tract. However, complete coverage of the entire descending thoracic aorta, including the left subclavian artery, is associated with an increased risk of stroke and spinal cord ischemia.

Step 2. Preoperative Considerations

♦ Extensive preoperative planning with appropriate imaging is essential with TEVAR. Preoperative assessment must address two important issues: anatomic requirements and vascular access. The gold standard is computed tomographic angiography of the thorax, abdomen, and pelvis, with distal arterial runoffs. Thin-slice helical computed tomography scanning with 3-mm slices is ideal to create three-dimensional reconstructions of the aorta. In patients with contraindications to intravenous contrast, magnetic resonance angiography is an acceptable alternative.

1. Anatomic Requirements

♦ Anatomic requirements center on the suitability of the proximal and distal landing zones. TEVAR involves the deployment of an intraluminal endoprosthesis resulting in the exclusion of the thoracic aneurysm. Therefore, the essential requirement is suitable proximal and distal landing zones to achieve adequate seal and prevent endoleaks.
♦ The evaluation for the suitability of the landing zones involves two major criteria: the length of the zone and the aortic diameter. Although device specific, the length of the landing zone must be sufficient to achieve adequate exclusion. For most devices, the requirement is 2 cm of aorta without significant tapering. The aortic diameter must safely accommodate a self-expanding endovascular device. For aneurysmal disease, the device should be upsized (compared with the diameter of the landing zone) by 10% to 20% to achieve adequate exclusion. Available devices allow safe treatment for aortic diameters between 19 and 43 mm.
♦ For nonaneurysmal disease such as dissections or traumatic transection, less aggressive upsizing (<10%) is generally recommended.
♦ Additional factors to consider in the evaluation of the landing zones include the presence of thrombus, rapid tapering, calcification, tortuosity, and angulation (Fig. 23-2A).
♦ Circumferential thrombus and extensive calcification at a landing zone may not allow adequate seal, resulting in endoleaks.
♦ Minimal tapering of the aortic diameter over the length of the landing zone (<15%) with minimal tortuosity and angulation are also desirable to ensure adequate exclusion.
♦ Angulation is often a proximal landing zone issue at the level of the distal arch. Severe angulation may result in "bird-beaking" of the endograft. These and other factors may require extension of the proximal and distal landing zones. If coverage of branch vessels is necessary at the proximal or distal landing zone, extra-anatomic bypasses such as carotid–subclavian bypass or mesenteric–visceral bypass, respectively, may be necessary.

2. Vascular Access

♦ TEVAR cannot be performed with inadequate vascular access (Fig. 23-2B).
♦ Vascular complication is a major component of the morbidity and mortality associated with TEVAR. All current devices require a large-caliber delivery system, ranging from 20F to 24F outer diameter.

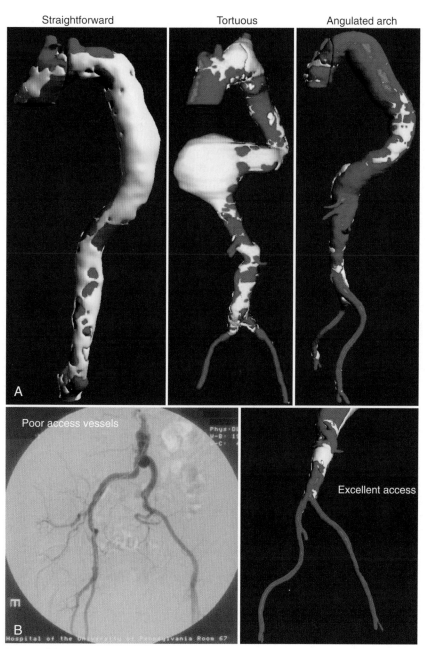

Figure 23-2

- Preoperative imaging must include assessment of the iliofemoral vasculature. In addition to diameter, factors such as excessive calcification, tortuosity, history of peripheral vascular disease, and previous aortoiliac surgery may prevent safe delivery of the endograft.
- If severe peripheral occlusive disease is prohibitive to safe delivery of the endograft, endovascular balloon angioplasty may be performed either preoperatively or concomitantly during TEVAR before introduction of the delivery devices.
- In the event that femoral arterial access is inadequate, aortoiliac exposure through a retroperitoneal approach may be required.

3. Intraoperative Neuromonitoring

- Patients undergoing TEVAR are at risk for neurologic complications, including stroke and spinal cord ischemia. Intraoperative neuromonitoring using electroencephalography and somatosensory-evoked potentials should be routinely used for patients undergoing TEVAR.
- Stroke is associated with wire manipulation in the severely atherosclerotic aortic arch.
- Spinal cord ischemia may result in permanent lower extremity paraplegia. Factors such as the length of aortic coverage, previous abdominal aortic aneurysm repair, occlusive aortoiliac disease, and coverage of the left subclavian artery may affect collateral arterial supply to the spinal cord and increase the risk of paraplegia.
- Intraoperative neuromonitoring may detect early evidence of spinal cord ischemia before a reliable neurologic examination can be obtained. Maneuvers such as volume expansion and lumbar drainage should be used to prevent permanent paraplegia if intraoperative neuromonitoring suggests spinal cord ischemia.
- In patients with preoperative risk factors for spinal cord ischemia (i.e., previous abdominal aortic aneurysm repair, occlusive aortoiliac disease, or total coverage of descending thoracic aorta), preemptive lumbar drainage should be considered.

Step 3. Operative Steps

1. Imaging

- The primary modality of intraoperative imaging for TEVAR is fluoroscopy. Using either a fixed or portable C-arm, fluoroscopy provides real-time imaging.
- Additional helpful features include digital subtraction angiography and road mapping.
- Digital subtraction angiography allows subtraction and removal of background images such as bony structures to enhance visualization of the object injected with contrast (i.e., descending thoracic aorta).
- Road mapping involves the transfer of a reference image superimposed onto a live image for guidance during deployment of the device (Fig. 23-3A).
- Intravascular ultrasonography (IVUS) is an option for patients with renal insufficiency or any other contraindication to intravenous contrast. Introduced from the femoral artery, IVUS provides the advantage of direct intraluminal imaging, particularly in cases of dissection, where the true and false lumens must be identified. Furthermore, intraoperative evaluation of the aorta, particularly the landing zones, can be performed.
- Information regarding the characteristics of the landing zones, such as diameter and the presence of thrombus, may be obtained and verified with preoperative imaging (Fig. 23-3B).

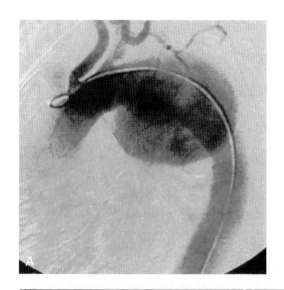

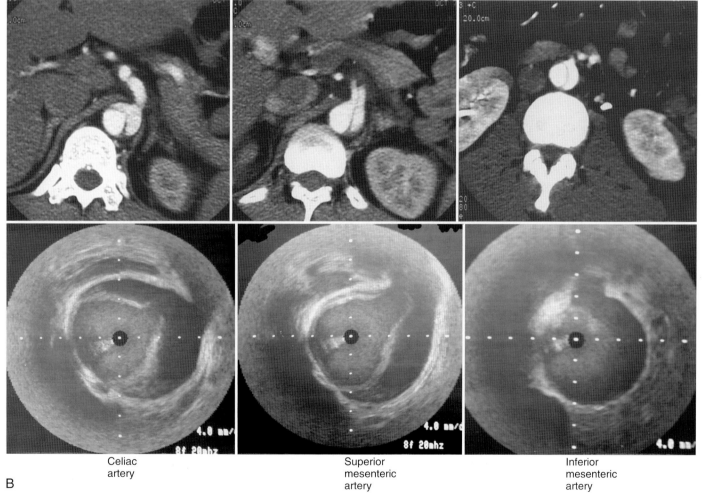

Celiac
artery

Superior
mesenteric
artery

Inferior
mesenteric
artery

B

Figure 23-3

2. Access

- For most patients, the femoral artery provides adequate vascular access for deployment of the endograft (Fig. 23-4A and B). A transverse incision is made at the level of the inguinal ligament. The femoral artery is exposed and proximal control is obtained. An 18-gauge needle is used for direct puncture of the femoral artery, and a flexible guidewire (0.035-inch Bentson wire; Boston Scientific Corporation, Natick, Mass) is introduced retrograde to the aortic arch using the Seldinger technique under fluoroscopy.
- Because of the angulation and tortuosity of the aortic arch, it is often difficult to deliver the endograft with a flexible guidewire, and a super-stiff guidewire (0.035-inch Lunderquist wire; Cook Medical, Bloomington, Ind) is often required. A super-stiff guidewire should never be introduced into the arch without a guide catheter because of risk of rupture or dissection. Therefore, a wire exchange maneuver is needed.
- Under fluoroscopy, a long guide catheter (100-cm MPA [multipurpose angle]; Cordis, Johnson & Johnson, Miami, Fla) is advanced to the arch over the flexible guidewire. Once in position, the MPA is secured, and the flexible guidewire is removed.
- The Lunderquist wire is then advanced within the MPA to the level of the aortic arch under fluoroscopy.
- The MPA is removed and the super-stiff guidewire is in position for the deployment of the endograft.
- If the femoral artery is suboptimal for access, the iliac artery may be exposed with a retroperitoneal approach (Fig. 23-4C). The iliac artery can be directly accessed using a technique similar to that described for the femoral artery. A double pursestring of 4-0 polypropylene sutures is used to secure the vessel and provide hemostasis with the application of two sets of tourniquets.
- Alternatively, a 10-mm Dacron graft can be sewn to the iliac artery as a conduit for the delivery of the endograft. The conduit may be brought through a separate counter-incision in the groin to allow for better angulation of the relatively long and stiff deployment device.
- A diagnostic catheter (5F pigtail; Cordis) with multiple side holes is placed percutaneously in the contralateral femoral artery. The standard percutaneous puncture with the Seldinger technique is used, and a 5F or 7F introducer sheath (Cordis) may be placed for access. The pigtail catheter is advanced to the aortic arch under fluoroscopy.
- Occasionally, brachial access is needed for coil embolization of the left subclavian artery to create an adequate proximal landing zone if a carotid–subclavian artery bypass was performed.
- In addition, precise deployment of the endograft at the left subclavian artery or the left common carotid artery can be facilitated with the placement of the pigtail catheter (through a left brachial artery access) at the respective origin in the arch.
- Brachial access can often be achieved percutaneously using the Seldinger technique with placement of a 5F introducer sheath. Systemic heparinization is recommended before any wire manipulation in the arch.

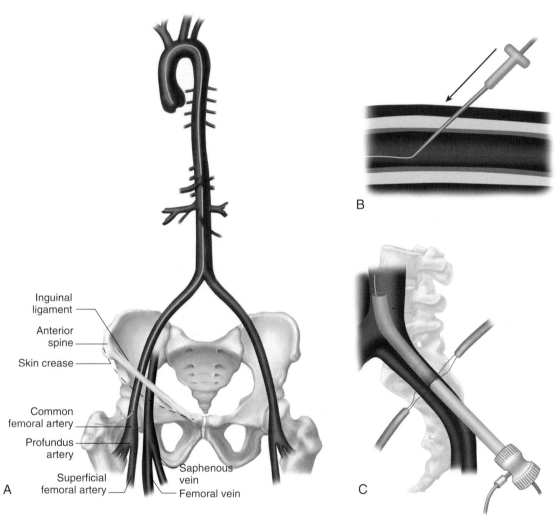

Inguinal ligament

Anterior spine

Skin crease

Common femoral artery

Profundus artery

Superficial femoral artery

Saphenous vein

Femoral vein

A

B

C

Figure 23-4

3. Deployment of the Endograft—Aneurysm

• Extensive preoperative planning will have determined the number, the size, and the sequence of deployment of the endografts.

• The total treatment length (coverage length) of the descending thoracic aorta determines the length and number of endografts.

• The diameter of the endografts is determined by the diameter of the aortic landing zones. Although there are device-specific variabilities, the endografts are generally deployed in a proximal-to-distal sequence. However, if the proximal endograft is larger than the distal device, or precise deployment is required at the celiac artery, it may be preferable to deploy the endografts in a distal-to-proximal sequence.

• Under fluoroscopic guidance, the endograft is delivered to the proximal landing zone using the Lunderquist guidewire (Figs. 23-5 and 23-6A through C).

• For the Gore TAG endoprosthesis, an introducer sheath is available to provide hemostasis during endograft exchanges if multiple devices are deployed.

• Other devices, such as the Medtronic Talent and Valiant endografts (Medtronic Vascular, Santa Clara, Calif) and the Zenith TX2 (Cook Medical), are deployed directly into the access artery without an introducer sheath.

• For optimal imaging of the arch and visualization of the brachiocephalic vessels, the C-arm is placed in a left anterior oblique position of 45 to 50 degrees. Once the endograft is in place, a diagnostic arteriogram is obtained to confirm the location of the aneurysm and position of the endograft in relation to the landing zone. If satisfactory, the pigtail catheter is withdrawn from behind the endograft and the device is deployed. The mechanism of deployment is device specific, each with its own advantages and disadvantages. Road mapping may be used to facilitate precise deployment of the endograft.

• To deploy a second endograft, it is exchanged with the first device over the Lunderquist guidewire (Fig. 23-7).

• If precise deployment at the celiac artery is necessary, the C-arm is placed in a full lateral position for optimal imaging and a second diagnostic angiogram is obtained.

• Similar to the proximal device, the distal endograft is advanced to the appropriate landing zone with the use of angiography and road mapping. Once satisfactory position is achieved, the endograft is deployed.

• Adequate overlap of the devices is necessary to prevent junctional, or type III, endoleaks. Although overlaps are device specific, a minimum overlap of 5 cm is recommended.

• Ballooning of the landing zones as well as the junction between endografts is device specific, but it is generally recommended that optimal apposition of the endografts be achieved to prevent endoleaks.

• Under fluoroscopic guidance, a compliant balloon is advanced to the appropriate location and inflated. Overly aggressive ballooning may result in aortic dissection or stent fractures.

• In general, the ballooning is performed in a proximal-to-distal sequence with final ballooning at the junctions.

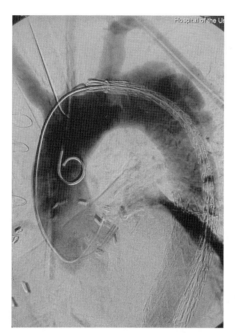

Figure 23-5

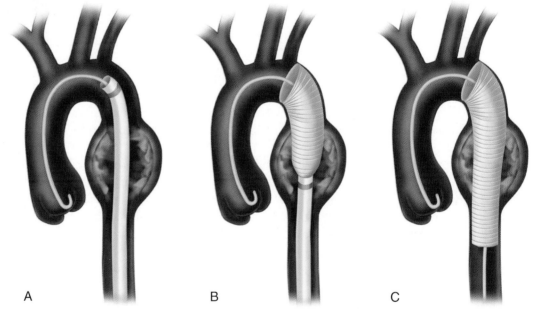

A   B   C

Figure 23-6

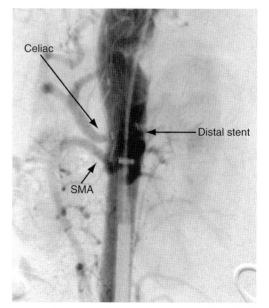

Figure 23-7

- Once all ballooning has been completed and the positions of the endografts are satisfactory, a completion angiography is performed (Fig. 23-8A and B).
- The previously withdrawn diagnostic pigtail catheter is advanced into the aortic arch under fluoroscopic guidance.
- The completion angiogram is performed to examine for endograft migration and endoleak. If endoleak is detected, treatments such as ballooning or placement of additional devices should be performed.
- If all is satisfactory, the delivery system is withdrawn from the access vessel. The Lunderquist guidewire is left in place in the event of vascular injury or avulsion. By retaining wire access, an occlusive balloon can be advanced over the Lunderquist wire to achieve proximal control if necessary. Once the surgeon is confident there is no vascular injury, the Lunderquist guidewire is removed and the access vessel repaired.
- If there is concern over iliac rupture or dissection, a retrograde aortoiliac angiogram should be obtained.
- If a subclavian–carotid bypass was previously performed, coil embolization of the proximal left subclavian artery can be performed.

4. Subclavian–Carotid Bypass

- The proximal aorta is divided into landing zones as illustrated in Figure 23-9. Landing zones Z0, Z1, and Z2 involve coverage of branch vessels and require extra-anatomic bypasses.
- Often, Z2 is required to ensure a suitable proximal landing zone, necessitating a left subclavian–carotid transposition or bypass before TEVAR.
- At our institution, the bypass is preferred because transposition requires a more proximal exposure of the subclavian artery. In the setting of thoracic aneurysm, the anatomy of the proximal left subclavian artery can be distorted. However, a left subclavian–carotid bypass requires a concomitant coil embolization of the proximal subclavian artery at the time of the thoracic endografting procedure to prevent the development of a type II endoleak. As described earlier, this can be accomplished through left brachial access at the time of TEVAR.
- The procedure is carried out through a supraclavicular approach to the left subclavian and common carotid arteries.
- An incision is made approximately 1 to 2 cm superior to the clavicle (Fig. 23-10A).
- Along with the sternocleidomastoid and the omohyoid muscles, the platysma is divided with electrocautery.
- The anterior scalene muscle is identified, with the phrenic nerve coursing across the muscle fibers.
- Along with the phrenic nerve, the thoracic duct should be identified, and care should be taken to avoid injury to both structures.
- The subclavian artery can be found deep to the anterior scalene muscle.
- The vertebral and internal mammary arteries are identified.
- Proximal and distal dissection is performed and vessel loops may be used for vascular control (Fig. 23-10B). With medial retraction of the internal jugular vein, the common carotid artery is exposed. Vessel loops may also be used for vascular control and to optimize exposure of the common carotid artery.
- Systemic heparinization should be achieved before occlusion of the vessels.
- With the clamps in place, arteriotomies are performed in both the common carotid and the left subclavian arteries (Fig. 23-10C).
- It is important to construct the synthetic graft (i.e., expanded polytetrafluoroethylene [ePTFE] or Dacron) with the correct length and configuration to avoid tension or kinking. The anastomoses are performed using running 5-0 or 6-0 polypropylene sutures.

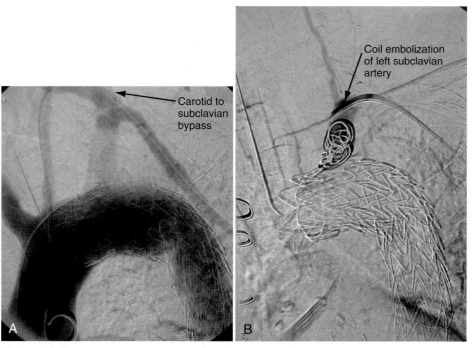

Carotid to subclavian bypass

Coil embolization of left subclavian artery

A

B

Figure 23-8

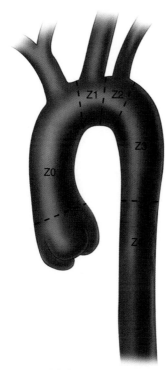

Figure 23-9

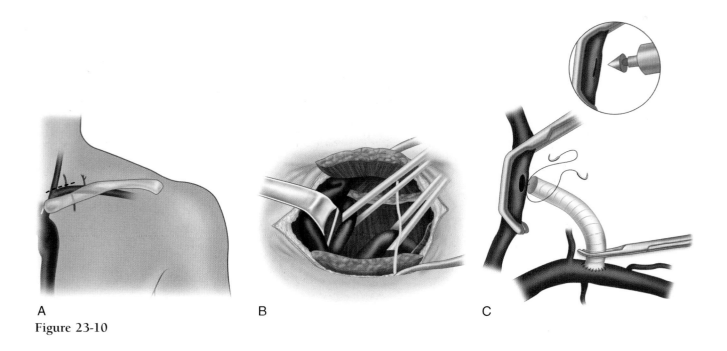

A

B

C

Figure 23-10

◆ Once completed, the clamps are removed and the anastomoses are examined for hemostasis. Once the surgeon is satisfied, the wound is closed in the correct anatomic layers.

5. Deployment of the Endograft—Aortic Dissection

◆ Conventional open repair of descending thoracic aortic aneurysm resulting from chronic type B aortic dissection remains a surgical challenge, with significant morbidity and mortality. The role of TEVAR in this population is currently unclear. Complete expansion of the endograft with exclusion of the thrombosed false lumen may be difficult to achieve.

◆ Furthermore, often neither proximal nor distal landing zones are ideal, with continuation of the dissection flap or false lumen into important branch vessels, precluding an endovascular repair (Fig. 23-11).

◆ However, TEVAR may potentially exert its biggest impact on acute aortic syndromes such as acute aortic dissection.

◆ Emergent open repair of acute type B dissection complicated by rupture or malperfusion has historically been associated with significant morbidity and mortality. Reports have suggested improved outcome in patients with complicated acute type B aortic dissection treated by TEVAR, compared with conventional open repair. However, the role of TEVAR in uncomplicated type B aortic dissection remains unclear and is under investigation.

◆ Endovascular treatment of acute aortic dissection in the descending thoracic aorta presents additional technical challenges. In contrast to nondissecting aneurysmal disease, the principal concept in the treatment of acute aortic dissection is the identification and coverage of the primary tear site. Particularly in cases of malperfusion, the goal is to obliterate the false lumen with reestablishment of blood flow and reexpansion of the true lumen (Fig. 23-12A and B).

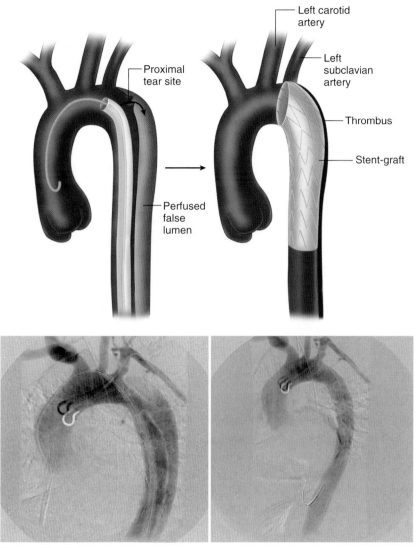

Figure 23-11

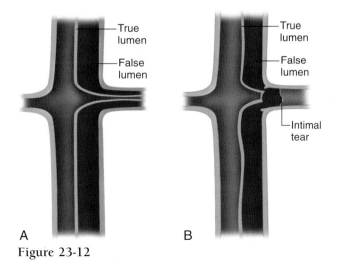

Figure 23-12

- Often, additional reentry sites and fenestrations are present in the distal aorta. Treatment with bare metal or uncovered stents may be necessary if important branches such as the renal, visceral, or lower extremity arteries continue to be malperfused after proximal therapy with TEVAR (Fig. 23-13).
- Access to the true lumen may be difficult to achieve and often requires alternative sites such as brachial or axillary arteries.
- Confirmation of wire access in the true lumen is mandatory before deployment of the device and may be aided by use of IVUS. Involvement of important side branches and compromise of their true lumens may also be evaluated with IVUS. In cases of renal malperfusion, the use of IVUS may also minimize the amount of contrast used.
- Finally, coverage of the left subclavian artery may be necessary to achieve adequate proximal seal because the primary tear site with type B aortic dissection is located at the level of the left subclavian artery in the majority of patients.
- For patients with previous coronary artery bypass (e.g., left internal mammary artery to left anterior descending coronary artery) or with subsequent neurovascular compromise associated with acute coverage of the left subclavian artery, a concomitant left subclavian–carotid artery bypass should be performed (Fig. 23-14).

6. Hybrid Total Arch Repair for Aortic Arch Aneurysms

- Surgical management of aortic arch aneurysms remains a challenge, requiring deep hypothermic circulatory arrest (DHCA) and a complex cerebral perfusion strategy.
- The success of endovascular technique in the treatment of descending thoracic aortic aneurysms has led to the development of hybrid procedures for aortic arch aneurysm repair. The hybrid total arch repair involves open brachiocephalic bypass (debranching procedure) with concomitant endovascular arch stent grafting.
- In contrast to traditional open total arch repair, these hybrid procedures have the advantages of avoiding DHCA and possible cardiopulmonary bypass (CPB).
- The hybrid arch repair has been reported in small series with encouraging early results.

Operative Technique
- Hybrid arch repairs can be performed as concomitant or staged procedures.
- The patient is placed in a supine position, and a median sternotomy provides adequate exposure to the arch.
- Neuromonitoring with continuous electroencephalography is used for detection of neurologic events throughout the operation, as per our standard arch protocol.
- Fluoroscopic imaging is provided by either a portable or a floor-mounted angiographic C-arm system.
- Based on exposure and the size of the arch aneurysms, CPB and aortic occlusion may be necessary to perform the proximal anastomosis of the brachiocephalic bypass.
- The goal is to create an adequate proximal landing zone in the ascending aorta for the concomitant arch stent graft deployment. This often requires the proximal anastomosis of the brachiocephalic bypass to be performed at the level of the sinotubular junction.
- Because of the limited length of the ascending aorta, the aortic and cardioplegia cannulae are placed in full recognition of the location of both the proximal anastomosis of the brachiocephalic bypass and the proximal landing zone of the arch stent graft. If adequate aortic length is present, a side-biting clamp can be placed at the level of the ascending aorta during the proximal anastomosis, and CPB may be avoided.

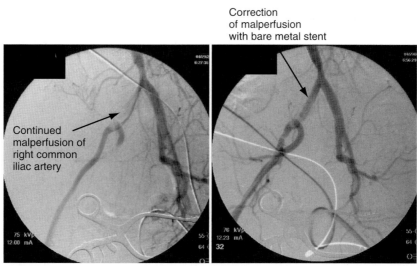

Correction
of malperfusion
with bare metal stent

Continued
malperfusion of
right common
iliac artery

Figure 23-13

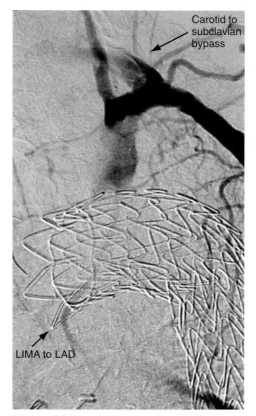

Carotid to
subclavian
bypass

LIMA to LAD

Figure 23-14

- A modified trifurcated Dacron graft with an additional fourth branch for stent graft deployment (Vascutek-Terumo, Ltd., Ann Arbor, Mich) is used for the brachiocephalic bypass to the great vessels.
- The proximal anastomosis to the ascending aorta is performed as proximal as possible, just distal to the sinotubular junction, to allow deployment of the stent graft in the ascending aorta without compromise to the proximal inflow anastomosis. (The average length of the ascending aorta from the sinotubular junction to the innominate artery is 6 to 7 cm, thus allowing an optimal 3- to 4-cm proximal landing zone.) The proximal reconstruction of the brachiocephalic bypass can be performed as an aortic patch or an interposition graft.
- Once the anastomosis is completed, the distal end-to-end anastomoses of the trifurcated grafts to the arch vessels are performed from left to right with sequential clamping: first the left subclavian, then the left common carotid, and finally the innominate artery anastomoses are performed. The proximal takeoff of each arch vessel is detached.
- A de-airing maneuver is performed for each anastomosis before release of the distal clamp.
- Intraoperative neuromonitoring is used to detect neurologic events during all manipulations of the arch.
- Deployment of the stent graft is achieved either antegrade through the fourth arm of the modified trifurcated graft or retrograde through the femoral artery. The technical aspects of deployment of the device are similar to those for TEVAR in the descending thoracic aorta, as described in the previous section. Fluoroscopic guidance is required for precise deployment of the aortic stent graft. The sequence of the operation is illustrated in Figure 23-15A through E.
- Although the short-term results are encouraging, the long-term durability of the hybrid approach to arch aneurysms remains to be determined.
- Furthermore, sternotomy is still required, with the associated potential complications and morbidity.
- The hybrid approach may be a bridging strategy while branched stent graft devices are being developed for arch aneurysms. Future development and improvement of total endovascular repair of arch aneurysms may mean performance of fewer hybrid arch procedures. However, until such total endovascular arch repair devices are developed, the hybrid arch procedures offer a surgical option for high-risk patients who are not candidates for the traditional open total arch repair.

Step 4. Postoperative Care

- Postoperative care of the patient undergoing TEVAR involves the standard resuscitation protocol used with any major cardiac operation.
- Hemodynamic monitoring is recommended in an intensive care unit setting. Because of the lack of an aortic suture line, higher blood pressure may be tolerated postoperatively to optimize spinal cord perfusion.
- Patients should also be allowed to emerge from anesthesia expeditiously for early neurologic assessment. If spinal cord ischemia is suspected, immediate salvage maneuvers, including spinal drainage, hypertension, and volume expansion, should be used.

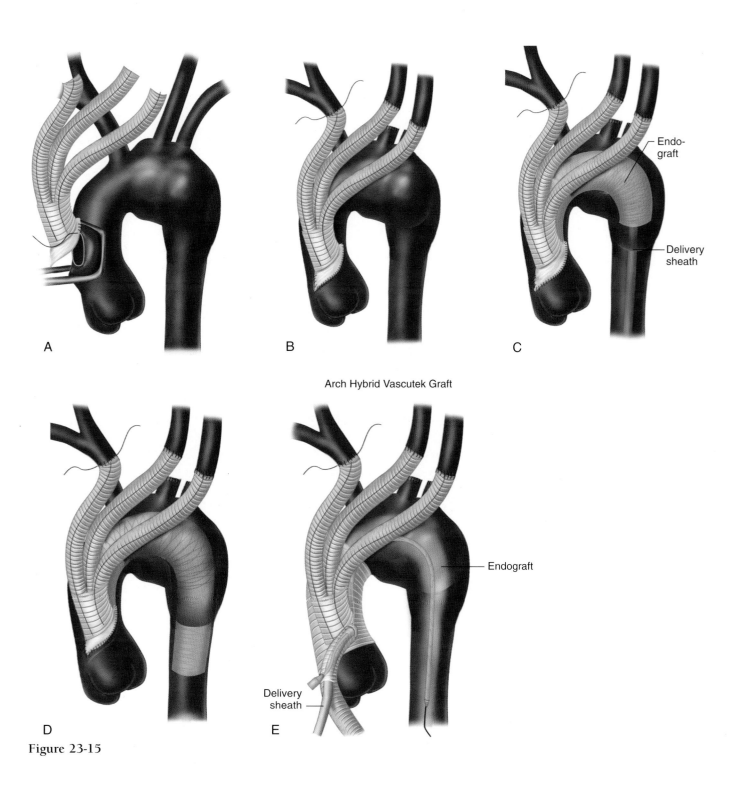

Arch Hybrid Vascutek Graft

Figure 23-15

Step 5. Pearls and Pitfalls

- ◆ Success with TEVAR requires extensive preoperative planning with regard not only to device selection, but to comprehensive evaluation of vascular access–related issues. Size, tortuosity, and calcification of the iliofemoral vasculature must be carefully examined.
- ◆ In the event of iliofemoral injury (Fig. 23-16A), the surgeon must be able to expeditiously address this potentially lethal complication. The importance of maintaining wire access until the integrity of the iliofemoral vasculature is ensured cannot be overemphasized.
- ◆ Device selection as well as the technical considerations of deployment must be carefully planned.
- ◆ Thorough evaluation of the proximal landing zone is required to prevent "bird-beaking" of the device (Fig. 23-16B).
- ◆ Also, incorrect sizing of the device can have catastrophic consequences. For aneurysms, the recommendation is upsizing of 10% to 20% based on the true diameter on cross-sectional examination of the aorta. Downsizing may result in inadequate exclusion, predisposing the patient to stent migration or endoleak (Fig. 23-16C). Aggressive upsizing should also be discouraged because device collapse is a potential complication (Fig. 23-17A and B).

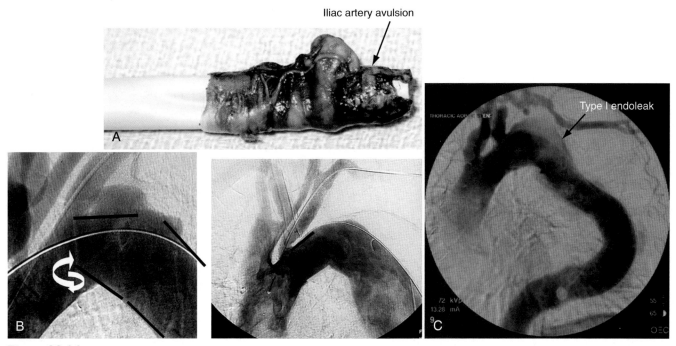

Figure 23-16

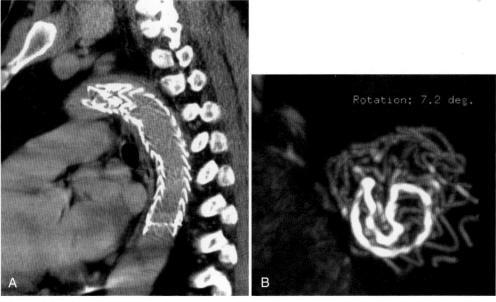

Figure 23-17

- ◆ Another possible complication is aortic dissection (Fig. 23-18A through C). Aggressive ballooning may result in the development of aortic dissection and should also be avoided.
- ◆ Finally, if multiple devices are deployed, it is crucial to allow adequate overlap to prevent development of junctional, or type III, endoleaks (Fig. 23-19).

Bibliography

Appoo JJ, Moser WG, Fairman RM, et al: Thoracic aortic stent grafting: Improving results with newer generation investigational devices. J Thorac Cardiovasc Surg 2006;131:1087-1094.

Bavaria JE, Appoo JJ, Makaroun MS, et al: Endovascular stent grafting versus open surgical repair of descending thoracic aortic aneurysms in low-risk patients: A multicenter comparative trial. J Thorac Cardiovasc Surg 2007;133:369-377.

Brinkman WT, Szeto WY, Bavaria JE: Stent graft treatment for transverse arch and descending thoracic aorta aneurysms. Curr Opin Cardiol 2007;22:510-516.

Cheung AT, Pochettino A, McGarvey ML, et al: Strategies to manage paraplegia risk after endovascular stent repair of descending thoracic aortic aneurysms. Ann Thorac Surg 2005;80:1280-1288; discussion 1288-1289.

Chuter TA, Buck DG, Schneider DB, et al: Development of a branched stent-graft for endovascular repair of aortic arch aneurysms. J Endovasc Ther 2003;10:940-945.

Eggebrecht H, Nienaber CA, Neuhauser M, et al: Endovascular stent-graft placement in aortic dissection: A meta-analysis. Eur Heart J 2006;27:489-498.

Fattori R, Nienaber CA, Rousseau H, et al: Results of endovascular repair of the thoracic aorta with the Talent Thoracic stent graft: The Talent Thoracic Retrospective Registry. J Thorac Cardiovasc Surg 2006;132:332-339.

Gutsche JT, Cheung AT, McGarvey ML, et al: Risk factors for perioperative stroke following thoracic endovascular aortic repair. Ann Thorac Surg 2007;84:1195-1200.

Mitchell RS, Miller DC, Dake MD, et al: Thoracic aortic aneurysm repair with an endovascular stent graft: The "first generation." Ann Thorac Surg 1999;67:1971-1974; discussion 1979-1980.

Suzuki T, Mehta RH, Ince H, et al: Clinical profiles and outcomes of acute type B aortic dissection in the current era: Lessons from the International Registry of Aortic Dissection (IRAD). Circulation 2003;108(Suppl 1):II312-II317.

Szeto WY, Bavaria JE, Bowen FW, et al: The hybrid total arch repair: Brachiocephalic bypass and concomitant endovascular aortic arch stent graft placement. J Card Surg 2007;22:97-102; discussion 103-104.

Wheatley GH 3rd, Gurbuz AT, Rodriguez-Lopez JA, et al: Midterm outcome in 158 consecutive Gore TAG thoracic endoprostheses: Single center experience. Ann Thorac Surg 2006;81:1570-1577; discussion 1577.

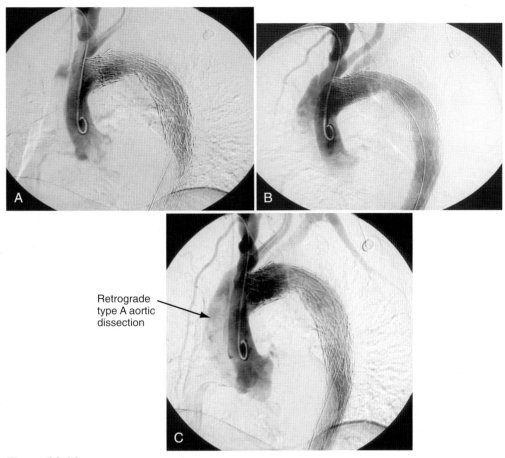

Retrograde
type A aortic
dissection

Figure 23-18

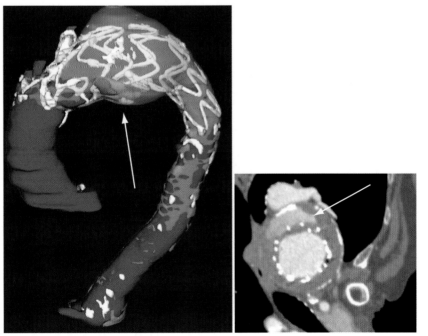

Figure 23-19

SECTION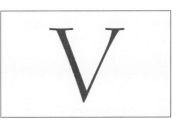

Miscellaneous Operations

24

SURGERY FOR ATRIAL FIBRILLATION

A. Marc Gillinov and Tomislav Mihaljevic

Step 1. Surgical Anatomy

- In most patients, atrial fibrillation is thought to arise from the left atrium, with the region around the pulmonary vein orifices and posterior left atrium representing the most important sites for the initiation and maintenance of atrial fibrillation.
- The right atrium is important in the pathogenesis of typical atrial flutter and, in some patients, contributes to the initiation and maintenance of atrial fibrillation.

Step 2. Preoperative Considerations

- The two settings in which cardiac surgeons encounter patients seeking ablation of atrial fibrillation are (1) atrial fibrillation in patients undergoing concomitant cardiac surgery and (2) atrial fibrillation alone as an indication for a stand-alone procedure.
  - ▲ In the concomitant setting, ablation is most commonly performed in patients with mitral valve disease and atrial fibrillation. Almost all such patients should have a combined procedure that includes correction of the mitral valve dysfunction and ablation of atrial fibrillation. An exception might be made in a very high-risk patient undergoing a complex and lengthy reoperative procedure; in that instance, it might be prudent to oversew the left atrial appendage but forgo ablation to save cross-clamp time.
  - ▲ Stand-alone surgical ablation is uncommon, and there are few data documenting long-term results of newer, less invasive procedures. Stand-alone surgical ablation is indicated in (1) patients who fail medical therapy and catheter ablation; (2) patients who fail medical therapy and have contraindications to catheter ablation (e.g., left atrial thrombus, discontinuous inferior vena cava, contraindication to warfarin); and (3) selected highly symptomatic individuals who desire the procedure with the highest probability of success. Surgical approaches in these patients include the Cox-Maze III or IV and a variety of less invasive procedures. Long-term results of the Cox-Maze III operation suggest 10-year success exceeding 90%. In patients with left atrial thrombus, the Cox-Maze III or IV procedure with cardiopulmonary bypass is indicated because less invasive, off-pump approaches may result in dislodgement of thrombus.

Step 3. Operative Steps

1. Cox-Maze III

- The heart is approached through a median sternotomy with a limited skin incision. Bicaval cannulation is used.
- After cardiac arrest, the pulmonary vein–encircling incision is started by performing a standard incision in the left atrium anterior to the right pulmonary veins. This incision is carried over to the left atrial appendage (Fig. 24-1). The left atrial appendage is excised (Fig. 24-2).

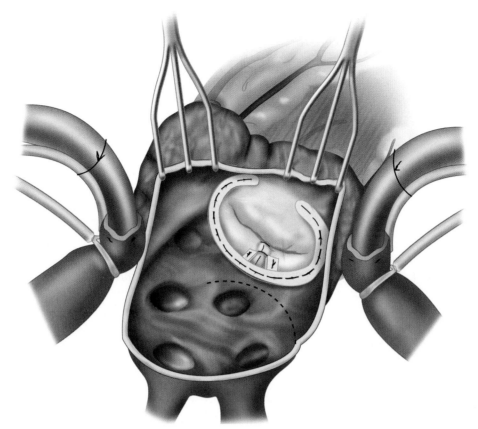

Figure 24-1

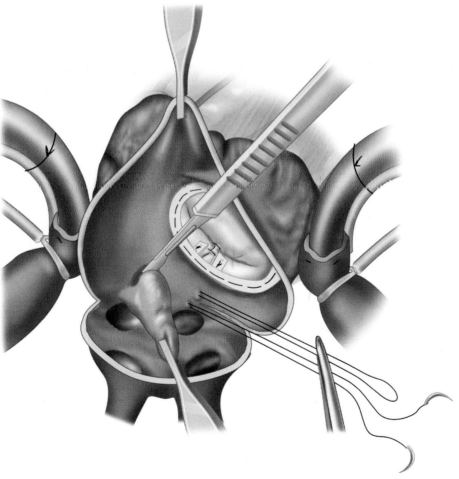

Figure 24-2

- A portion of the pulmonary vein–encircling incision is closed, and an incision is carried up to the mitral annulus at the P2 to P3 level: the coronary sinus is visualized (Fig. 24-3). A cryolesion is created at the coronary sinus and mitral annulus. The left-sided incisions are then closed (Fig. 24-4). The incision in the atrial septum, a component of the original Cox-Maze III procedure, was used to aid exposure and is usually not necessary.
- There are three right atrial incisions: (1) an incision from the superior vena cava to the inferior vena cava, (2) an incision in the right atrial appendage, and (3) an incision in the body of the atrium directed toward the interatrial septum (Fig. 24-5). After making these incisions, cryolesions are created at the tricuspid annulus at the 10 o'clock and 2 o'clock positions as viewed by the surgeon. Right atrial lesions may be created with the heart arrested or beating, although it is easier and quicker to do so on an arrested heart. After the right atrial incisions are closed, the patient is weaned from cardiopulmonary bypass.

2. Concomitant Procedures: Alternative Energy Sources

- All of the lesions created in the Cox-Maze III procedure can be replicated using alternative energy sources, which include radiofrequency, laser, high-intensity focused ultrasound (HIFU), and cryothermia. Each of these is effective on the arrested heart, but there is some concern over their ability to create transmural lesions on a beating heart that is filled with blood. A potential advantage to bipolar radiofrequency devices is that they can be used to perform pulmonary vein isolation on the beating heart; this is followed by assessment of acute exit block (Fig. 24-6). However, lesions to the mitral and tricuspid annulus are difficult to produce with bipolar energy sources.

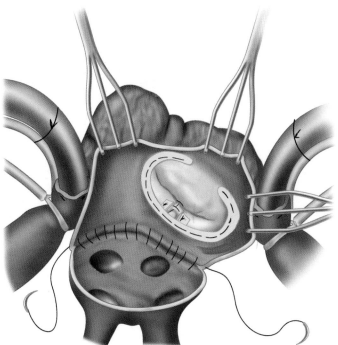

Figure 24-3

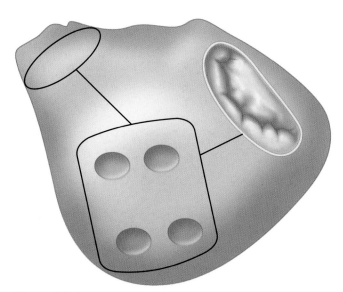

Figure 24-4

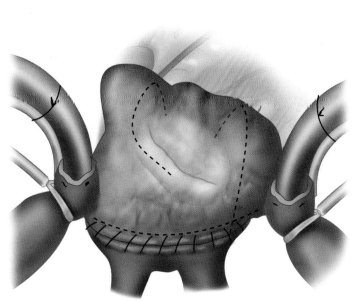

Figure 24-5

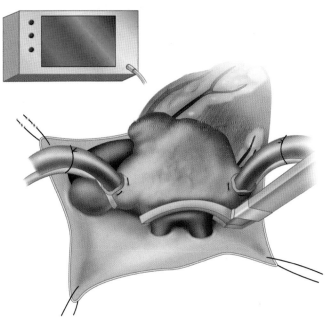

Figure 24-6

♦ Although some favor creation of limited lesion sets when using alternative energy sources, we believe that best results are obtained with a biatrial lesion set. The left atrial lesion set should be that of the Cox-Maze III procedure. In the right atrium, the most effective lesion set is not clear; some have advocated a simple right atrial isthmus lesion (Fig. 24-7).

3. Stand-Alone Therapy

♦ When the surgeon performs ablation of atrial fibrillation as a stand-alone procedure, options range from the Cox-Maze III to a variety of minimally invasive procedures. Minimally invasive procedures may include unilateral or bilateral thoracoscopic approaches using unipolar energy sources or unilateral or bilateral minithoracotomies.

♦ A full Cox-Maze III lesion set can be created through a 6-cm right thoracotomy (Fig. 24-8) with the heart arrested after establishing cardiopulmonary bypass through peripheral bicaval cannulation (Fig. 24-9). The approach is endocardial and biatrial and may use one of several different alternative energy sources.

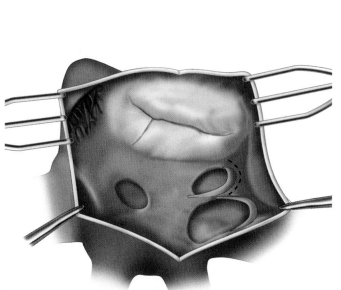

Figure 24-7

Figure 24-8

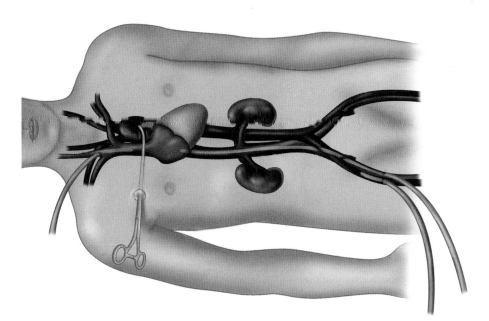

Figure 24-9

◆ There is particular interest in the application of bipolar radiofrequency technology through an approach that includes bilateral minithoracotomies. The incisions are made in the third intercostal space, and each set of pulmonary veins is dissected using specially constructed dissecting instruments. The bipolar device is used to isolate the pulmonary veins, and lesion integrity is confirmed by electrophysiologic testing (Fig. 24-10A and B). On the left side, the left atrial appendage is excised or excluded with a stapling instrument (Fig. 24-11A and B). With this approach, additional left atrial connecting lesions can be created, and autonomic ganglia can be identified and ablated.

Step 4. Postoperative Care

◆ Common early postoperative arrhythmias include atrial fibrillation, atrial flutter, and junctional bradycardia. When atrial fibrillation or flutter develops, an in-hospital trial of antiarrhythmic agents or electrical cardioversion is indicated.
◆ Permanent pacemakers should not be placed for bradycardia until at least 1 week after ablation because return of sinus node function may take several days.
◆ Warfarin anticoagulation with an ideal international normalized ratio of 2.0 to 3.0 is indicated for all patients for 3 months. If Holter monitoring indicates no atrial fibrillation or flutter at 3-month follow-up, discontinuation of anticoagulation may be considered.

Step 5. Pearls and Pitfalls

◆ A biatrial lesion set has the greatest probability of successfully ablating atrial fibrillation.
◆ The left atrial appendage should be removed or carefully excluded in all patients undergoing surgical ablation.
◆ Early postoperative arrhythmias are common and do not indicate failure.
◆ It is prudent to perform a left atrial reduction if the maximum left atrial dimension exceeds 6 cm.

Bibliography

Gillinov AM: Advances in surgical treatment of atrial fibrillation [review]. Stroke 2007;38(2 Suppl):618-623.
Gillinov AM: Choice of surgical lesion set: Answers from the data [review]. Ann Thorac Surg 2007;84:1786-1792.
Gillinov AM, Bakaeen F, McCarthy PM, et al: Surgery for paroxysmal atrial fibrillation in the setting of mitral valve disease: A role for pulmonary vein isolation? Ann Thorac Surg 2006;81:19-26.
Gillinov AM, Bhavani S, Blackstone EH, et al: Surgery for permanent atrial fibrillation: Impact of patient factors and lesion set. Ann Thorac Surg 2006;82:502-513.
Gillinov AM, Saltman AE: Ablation of atrial fibrillation with concomitant cardiac surgery [review]. Semin Thorac Cardiovasc Surg 2007;19:25-32.
Shemin R, Cox JL, Gillinov AM, et al: Guidelines for reporting data and outcomes for the surgical treatment of atrial fibrillation. Ann Thorac Surg 2007;83:1225-1230.

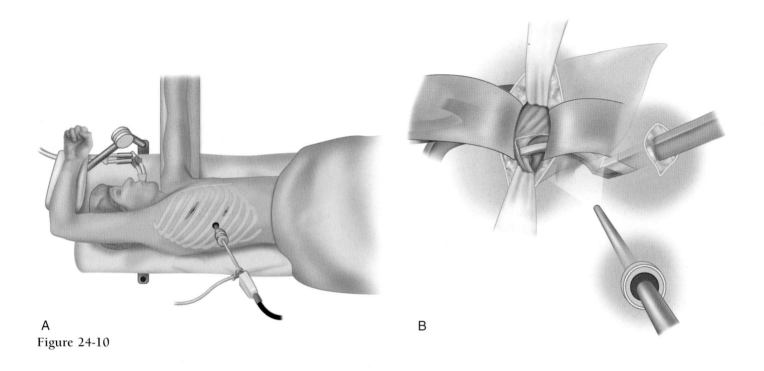

A

Figure 24-10

B

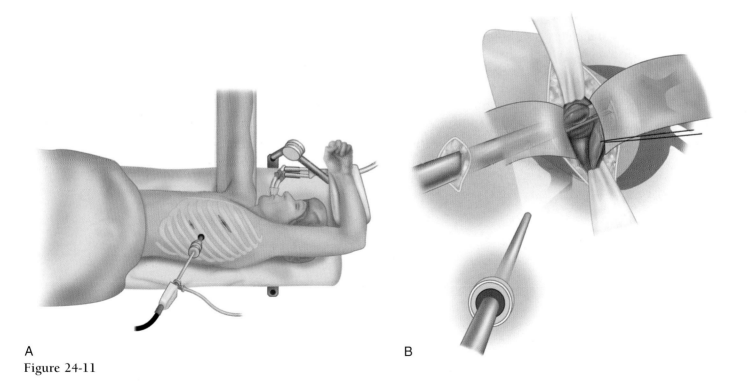

A

Figure 24-11

B

CHAPTER 25

SURGERY FOR LEFT VENTRICULAR ANEURYSM AND REMODELING

Lynn M. Fedoruk and Irving L. Kron

Step 1. Surgical Anatomy

- Thin-walled dyskinetic aneurysms from full-thickness scars are an end result of myocardial infarction. In nontransmural infarction, the epicardial layer is salvaged but necrosis at the endocardial level results in a variable-thickness scar that remains stiff and akinetic. This results in loss of regional contraction and alterations in ventricular geometry, causing the ventricle to take on a more spherical shape—a process known as *ventricular remodeling*. This causes deterioration of the heart's global systolic function and results in heart failure.
- Anatomic considerations in procedures to address left ventricular remodeling include the location of major coronary arteries (left anterior descending artery [LAD] and diagonal arteries) relative to the proposed ventriculotomy (Fig. 25-1; *arrow* indicates LAD).
- Location of the akinetic or dyskinetic segment during intraoperative examination is demonstrated by the characteristic dimpling or flattening of the anterior wall after the aortic crossclamp is applied and the left ventricular vent is on (Fig. 25-2A and B).

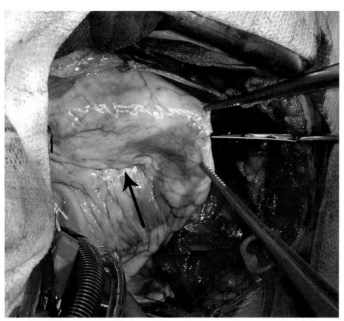

Figure 25-1

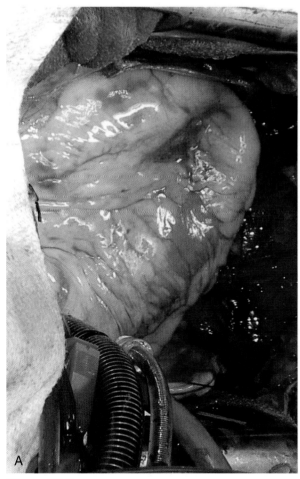

A

Figure 25-2

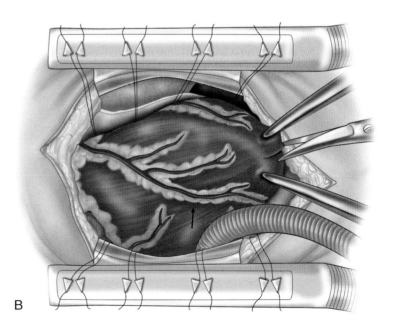

B

Step 2. Preoperative Considerations

- Indications for operation include
  - ▲ Congestive heart failure
  - ▲ Asymptomatic large aneurysm with coronary artery disease
  - ▲ Embolism
  - ▲ Arrhythmia
- The size of the ventricle and location of the akinetic or dyskinetic portion are important.
- The degree of mitral regurgitation should be quantified before surgery by echocardiography.
- Coronary artery anatomy and complete revascularization strategy need to be defined preoperatively by cardiac catheterization.

1. Diagnostic Imaging

- Multiple diagnostic imaging modalities can be used to delineate the presence of an aneurysm or akinetic segment in the left ventricle, as well as to define its extent. Although magnetic resonance imaging (MRI) can define not only akinesis but viability, obtaining the appropriate required gated images can be difficult. Thus, other modalities are still considered a mainstay in the diagnosis. As demonstrated in Figure 25-3, an aneurysm is often demonstrated by a left ventriculogram (highlighted by *red arrows*) obtained during cardiac catheterization.
- Figure 25-4 is an MRI of a left ventricular apical infarction. Note the thinning of the anterior wall and apex (*red arrows*), delineating the extent of the aneurysm. Echocardiography can also demonstrate left ventricular aneurysms.
- Figure 25-5 shows an apical aneurysm in the four-chamber view.

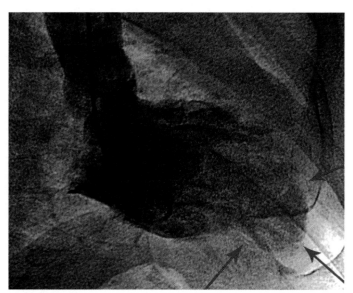

Figure 25-3

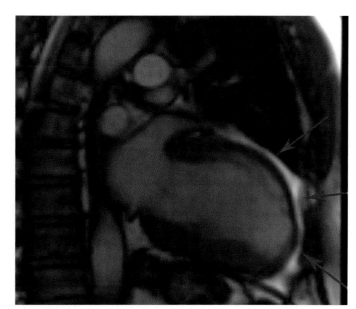

Figure 25-4

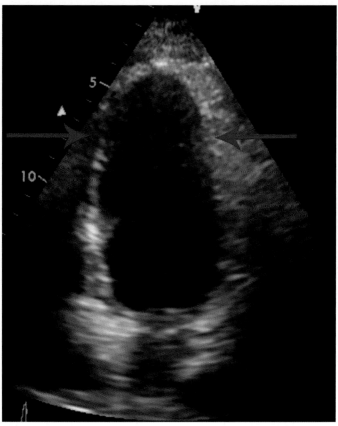

Figure 25-5

Step 3. Operative Steps

- Preoperative transesophageal echocardiography is used routinely to assess mitral valve function, the presence of thrombus in the left ventricle, and regional wall motion abnormalities. To prevent potential embolization from small left ventricular thrombus, care is taken to prevent manipulation of the heart before the cross-clamp is applied.
- The procedure is performed with the aortic cross-clamp applied and total cardiac arrest obtained using cardioplegia. After complete coronary revascularization, including the LAD, the heart is elevated in the pericardial well to allow for visualization.
- The ventricle is opened (Fig. 25-6A and B) with an incision (*dashed line*) approximately 1 to 2 cm lateral to the LAD and in a direction parallel to the LAD (*arrow*). This places the incision parallel to the septum. The myocardial thinning and endocardial scar should be visible through the ventriculotomy.
- After stay sutures are placed, the intraventricular cavity is cleared of thrombus and the anatomy is identified. The scarred region has a white coloration (Fig. 25-7, *yellow arrow*). The papillary muscles are located (*blue arrow*).
- Multiple techniques are used to determine the location of the endoventricular circular (also known as Fontan) suture. Some surgeons suggest placement of an intraventricular balloon (expanded to 50 mL/m^2 body surface area [BSA]) to guide the placement of the Fontan suture and subsequent approximation of the cavity, as demonstrated in Figure 25-8. With the intraventricular balloon in situ, placement of the Fontan suture allows for the ventricular volume to be reduced, primarily in the anterior and septal regions of the left ventricle.
- We use preoperative transesophageal echocardiography to determine heart size and suture placement relative to the ventricular walls and papillary muscles of the mitral valve, aiming for a postoperative ventricular volume of approximately 50 mL/m^2 BSA. An alternative technique involves identifying the transition zone between viable myocardium and scar tissue by grasping the ventricular wall between thumb and forefinger and identifying where the transition point occurs, indicated by the thinning of the ventricle between the finger and thumb.

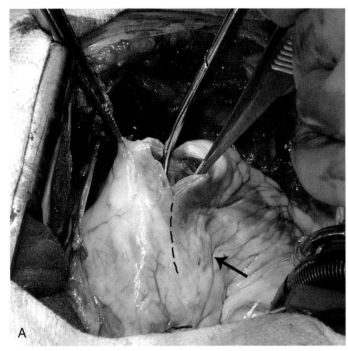

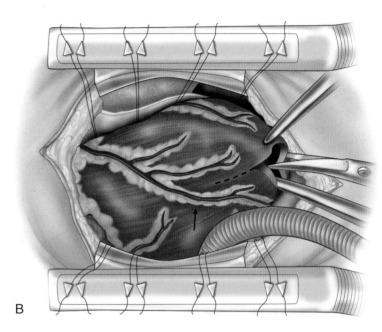

Figure 25-6

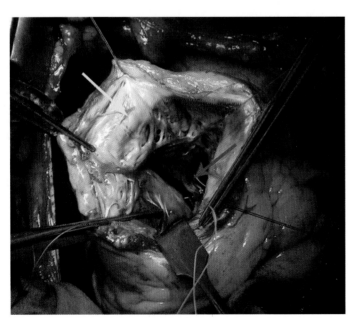

Figure 25-7

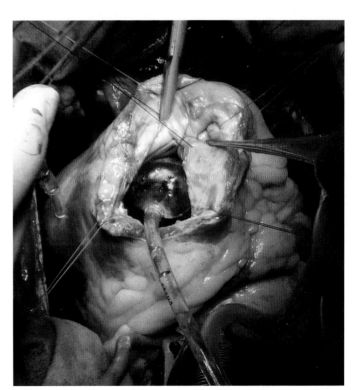

Figure 25-8

◆ A 2-0 polypropylene monofilament suture is passed through the endocardium at the transition between the scarred and the normal myocardium in a circular fashion (Fontan stitch). Care is taken not to include the papillary muscles in this circular suture (Figs. 25-9A and B and 25-10A and B).

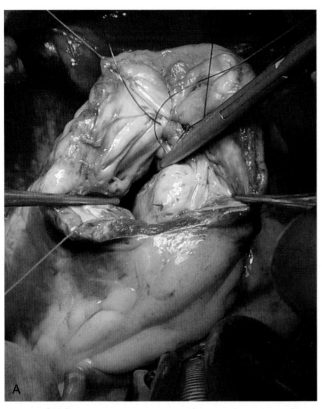

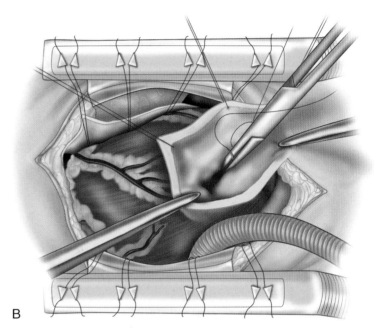

Figure 25-9

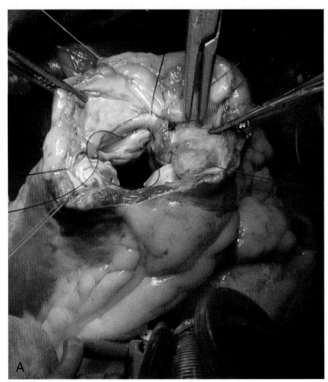

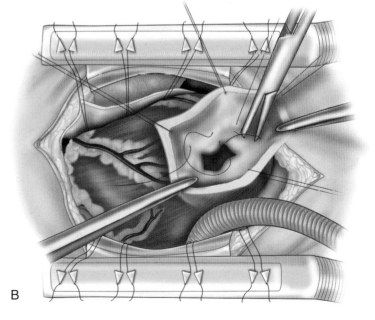

Figure 25-10

- In cinching the Fontan suture (Fig. 25-11), care is taken to tighten the suture to define the new wall, not to close the opening. This reduces the ventricular cavity volume.
- A Dacron patch is then fashioned to close the opening; care is taken to make the patch large enough that it can be readily sutured over the defect. If the residual opening is less than 1 cm wide, the defect may be closed primarily with a second suture line of 2-0 or running 3-0 polypropylene monofilament suture (Fig. 25-12A and B).

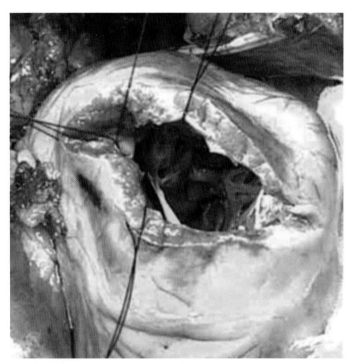

Figure 25-11

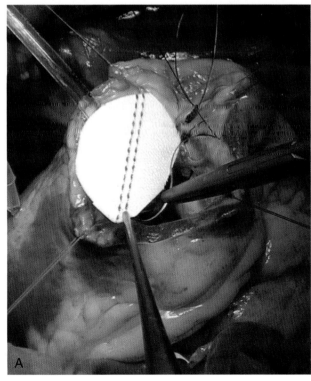

A

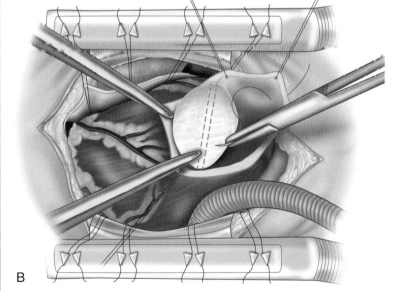

B

Figure 25-12

- The patch is sutured into place with a running 3-0 polypropylene monofilament suture (Fig. 25-13A and B).
- Once the patch is placed, the ventriculotomy is closed in a two-layer fashion, using first a horizontal mattress suture and then a running over-and-over type closure (Fig. 25-14).
- Some surgeons prefer to reinforce the ventriculotomy closure with Teflon strips, as demonstrated; however, this may conceal sources of residual hemorrhage (Fig. 25-15).
- If severe mitral regurgitation is present, the mitral valve must be repaired. Usually the mitral leaflet morphology is normal and the mechanism of regurgitation is secondary to papillary muscle displacement or annular enlargement from a dilated ventricle. These mechanisms are addressed by placement of an annuloplasty ring. The repair is performed through a standard left atrial incision. Interrupted braided 2-0 sutures are placed in a horizontal mattress fashion around the annulus, and the annuloplasty ring is seated to these.
- Inferior aneurysms are treated using the same principles; however, the defect is often smaller.

Step 4. Postoperative Care

- Standard postoperative care is provided.
- Patients may require intra-aortic balloon counterpulsation in the initial postoperative period, especially if there is an element of right ventricular dysfunction or a poor preoperative left ventricular ejection fraction (<25%).

Step 5. Pearls and Pitfalls

- Incomplete revascularization, especially of the septum, prevents optimal contractility and recovery of function.
- Embolism from ventricular thrombus secondary to ventricular manipulation before placement of the aortic cross-clamp can occur.
- Lack of regional basal contraction of the left ventricle portends a poor outcome and should be considered a relative contraindication.
- The residual ventricular cavity may be too small, resulting in inadequate stroke volume and cardiac output.
- Severe right ventricular dysfunction is a relative contraindication to the procedure.
- Significant residual mitral regurgitation portends a poor outcome.
- Areas of ventricular calcification must be removed.
- Ejection fraction should be evaluated at 3 months and the need for an automated implantable cardioverter–defibrillator assessed based on recognized guidelines.
- The use of carbon dioxide should be considered to decrease the amount of air introduced into the ventricular cavity and decrease residual air bubbles after the cross-clamp is removed.

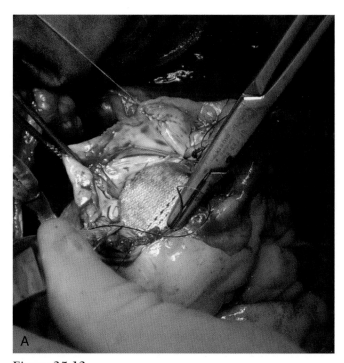

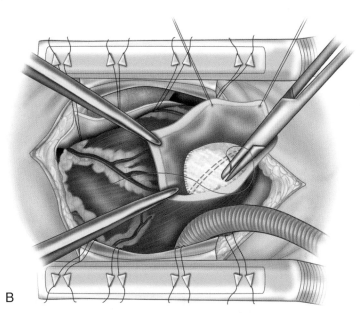

Figure 25-13

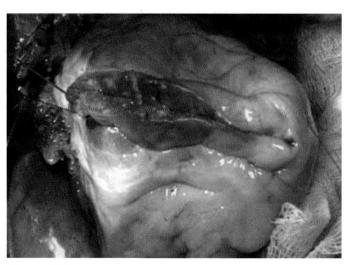

Figure 25-14

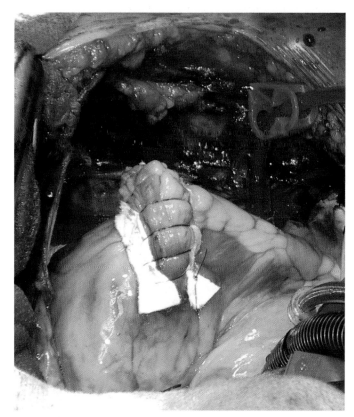

Figure 25-15

Bibliography

Athanasuleas CL, Buckberg GD, Stanley AW, et al, RESTORE Group: Surgical ventricular restoration in the treatment of congestive heart failure due to post-infarction ventricular dilation. J Am Coll Cardiol 2004;44:1439-1445.

Athanasuleas CL, Stanley AW Jr, Buckberg GD, et al: Surgical anterior ventricular endocardial restoration (SAVER) in the dilated remodeled ventricle after anterior myocardial infarction. RESTORE Group. Reconstructive Endoventricular Surgery, returning Torsion Original Radius Elliptical Shape to the LV. J Am Coll Cardiol 2001;37:1199-1209.

Athanasuleas CL, Stanley AW Jr, Buckberg GD, et al, the RESTORE Group: Surgical anterior ventricular endocardial restoration (SAVER) for dilated ischemic cardiomyopathy. Semin Thorac Cardiovasc Surg 2001;13:448-458.

Bolling SF, Smolens IA, Pagani FD: Surgical alternatives for heart failure. J Heart Lung Transplant 2001;20:729-733.

Buckberg GD: Defining the relationship between akinesia and dyskinesia and the cause of left ventricular failure after anterior infarction and reversal of remodeling to restoration. J Thorac Cardiovasc Surg 1998;116:47-49.

Lundblad R, Abdelnoor M, Svennevig JL: Surgery for left ventricular aneurysm: Early and late survival after simple linear repair and endoventricular patch plasty. J Thorac Cardiovasc Surg 2004;128:449-456.

Menicanti L, Di Donato M: The Dor procedure: What has changed after fifteen years of clinical practice? J Thorac Cardiovasc Surg 2002;124:886-890.

Mickleborough LL, Merchant N, Ivanov J, et al: Left ventricular reconstruction: Early and late results. J Thorac Cardiovasc Surg 2004;128:27-37.

Migrino RQ, Young JB, Ellis SG, et al: End systolic volume index at 90 to 180 minutes into reperfusion therapy for acute myocardial infarction is a strong predictor of early and late mortality: The Global Utilization of Streptokinase and t-PA for Occluded Coronary Arteries (GUSTO-I) Angiographic Investigators. Circulation 1997;96:116-121.

White HD, Norris RM, Brown MA, et al: Left ventricular end-systolic volume as the major determinant of survival after recovery from myocardial infarction. Circulation 1987;76:44-51.

CHAPTER 26

PULSATILE AND AXIAL VENTRICULAR SUPPORT

O. H. Frazier, Igor D. Gregoric, and William E. Cohn

- In 1976 and 1980, the National Heart, Lung, and Blood Institute of the National Institutes of Health (NIH) funded programs for the development of an implantable long-term left ventricular assist device (LVAD). The original goal of the LVAD program was to produce a device that would be the ultimate therapy for patients in the final stages of cardiac failure. The LVADs produced as a result of this funding were first used clinically as bridges to transplantation in patients with end-stage heart failure.

- As waiting times for transplantation lengthened, clinical experience was gained with the devices both for short- and long-term support. Today, pulsatile and nonpulsatile mechanical circulatory support devices are increasingly being used as bridges to transplantation and as destination therapy. This chapter describes the surgical techniques used at the Texas Heart Institute to implant the most commonly used devices.

Step 1. Surgical Anatomy

- The anatomy of pump insertion is similar for all devices discussed in this chapter. The inlet cannula of both externally and internally placed LVADs is usually implanted in the left ventricular apex. We have also used the diaphragmatic surface of the left ventricle between the ventricular septum and the origin of the papillary muscles for the inlet cannula or pump (Fig. 26-1). This convenient flat space is particularly suited for implantation of small centrifugal-force pumps and intra-abdominally placed axial flow pumps.

Step 2. Preoperative Considerations

1. Indications for Use of Various Left Ventricular Assist Devices

- LVADs are used to support the failing left ventricle. When temporary support is needed, especially after failure to wean from cardiopulmonary bypass (CPB), we usually use the CentriMag (Levitronix LLC, Waltham, Mass) or the AB5000 (ABIOMED, Inc., Danvers, Mass). We use a pulsatile-flow device on the right side because we have seen alveolar membrane injury when there is too much continuous flow on the right side. To avoid this possibility, we prefer to use the pulsatile AB5000 or the Thoratec intraperitoneal IVAD (Thoratec Corp., Pleasanton, Calif) for right-sided support.
- Only the HeartMate XVE (Thoratec Corp.) is currently approved for long-term support by the U.S. Food and Drug Administration. However, the newer, smaller continuous-flow pumps have the same indications as the implantable XVE (i.e., chronic heart failure unresponsive to conventional medical therapy).

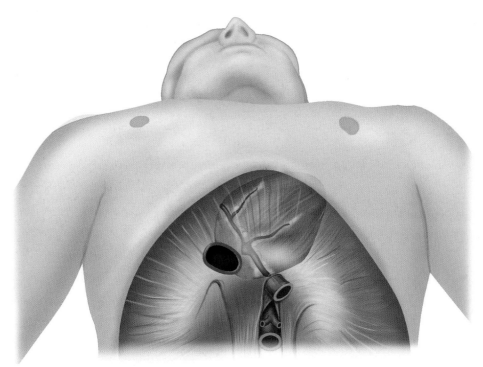

Figure 26-1

Step 3. Operative Steps

1. External Devices

AB5000 (ABIOMED, Inc.)

- The inlet cannula and outflow graft for the AB5000 are implanted through a median sternotomy. The exit site of the inlet cannula should be positioned before the exit site of the outlet cannula because there is little leeway with positioning for the inlet exit site. The apex of the left ventricle is elevated, and two circumferential pursestring sutures of 2-0 Teflon pledget–reinforced polypropylene are placed. In general, a site should be chosen that will center the cannula tip coaxial to and in the center of the left ventricular cavity. The size of the AB5000 inlet cannula (32, 36, or 42) is chosen based on ventricular (and patient) size. Because it can be bent into a suitable angle, a malleable wire-reinforced cannula with a "light-house" tip is ideal. The cannula should extend obliquely from the apical insertion site to the cutaneous exit site in the right upper quadrant, which will allow the heart to drop back into the pericardium without torque on the cannula or insertion site. The cannula tip is inserted into the left ventricle through a cruciate incision and secured by tying the pursestring sutures to the cannulae. We no longer use tourniquets and prefer to place additional sutures for apical control at the time of cannula removal. Securing the inlet cannula in position is critical to prevent cannula dislodgment, which can result in bleeding and catastrophic air embolus during pumping. Transesophageal echocardiography (TEE) is used to confirm acceptable inlet cannula position.
- Once the inlet cannula is tunneled and inserted, an appropriate cutaneous exit site is selected for the outflow graft. This is usually inferior to the inflow graft exit site and crosses internally, posterior to the inflow graft. We use the 12-mm outflow graft routinely to minimize hemolysis. The anastomosis is performed to the ascending aorta with a partial occlusion clamp using 3-0 or 4-0 polypropylene suture.
- If right ventricular assist is needed, the flexible inlet cannula of the pump is placed through the right atrium, secured with 2-0 Teflon-reinforced polypropylene sutures, and bent so that it is directed toward the inferior vena cava. The inlet cannula is brought out to the left of the midline in the anterior subcostal region. The outflow graft is anastomosed to the pulmonary artery with a partial occluding clamp. If access to the pulmonary artery is difficult and pump support is needed urgently, a pursestring suture of 2-0 Teflon-reinforced polypropylene can be placed on the acute margin of the right ventricle and a 28F or 32F cannula inserted through it, directed into the pulmonary artery (Fig. 26-2). With the pursestring suture placed at the acute margin, where there is less tension, the cannula can be safely removed if the patient is successfully weaned and the pump removed. This maneuver avoids catastrophic right ventricular injury. The pulmonary valve usually coapts around the outflow cannula and prevents pulmonary regurgitation. Cannula position can be determined by palpation and confirmed with TEE. Depending on the cannula used, an adapter and a short segment of 0.5-inch tubing may be required to attach the cannula to the AB5000.

Levitronix CentriMag (Levitronix LLC)

- The CentriMag continuous-flow pump can be implanted quickly and is useful for short-term left- and right-sided support (Fig. 26-3). Because of its size and simplicity and the ease of cannula placement, this pump is widely used for temporary right-sided support after implantation of a long-term LVAD becomes necessary. In this case, it is technically simpler, safer, and more effective to place a pulmonary artery cannula than a pulmonary graft. Placing and securing the cannula for this centrifugal pump is identical to the procedure described for the pulsatile AB5000. Device removal may be facilitated at the bedside by placing the inlet cannula through

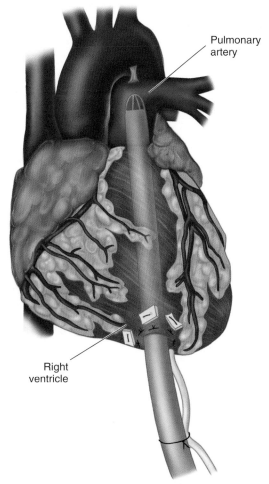

Pulmonary artery

Right ventricle

Figure 26-2

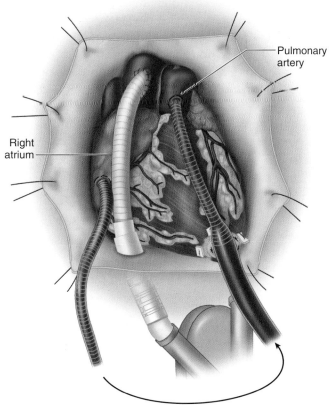

Pulmonary artery

Right atrium

Figure 26-3

a Dacron graft and anastomosing the outflow graft as described. Both grafts are oversewn after device removal (Figs. 26-4 and 26-5).

2. Internal Pulsatile Pumps

HeartMate XVE (Thoratec Corp.)

- The HeartMate XVE is implanted through a median sternotomy with the patient supported by CPB. A cylindrical blade is used to excise a circular plug of myocardium from the ventricular apex anteriorly and approximately 2 cm lateral to the left anterior descending coronary artery for placement of the inlet cannula. Circumferential 2-0 Ethibond sutures (Ethicon, Inc., Somerville, NJ) are used to secure the HeartMate sewing ring to the margins of the opening. The ventricular cavity should be inspected digitally and visually to ensure that no ventricular muscle or clot could embolize or interfere with device placement.
- An incision is made through the lateral anterior diaphragm, juxtaposed to the inlet cannula site. The diaphragmatic incision should be positioned to facilitate an acceptable pump orientation that minimizes torsion on the inlet cannula and should be as small as possible to decrease the likelihood of postoperative herniation of abdominal viscera. The inlet cannula is inserted into the left ventricle through the Silastic sewing ring and secured in place with appropriate heavy sutures (1-0 or 0) or umbilical or sterilized electrician's tape.

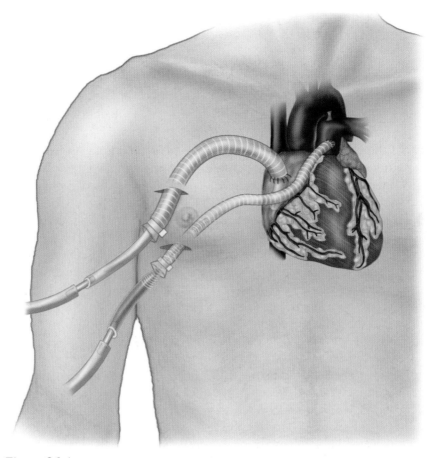

Figure 26-4

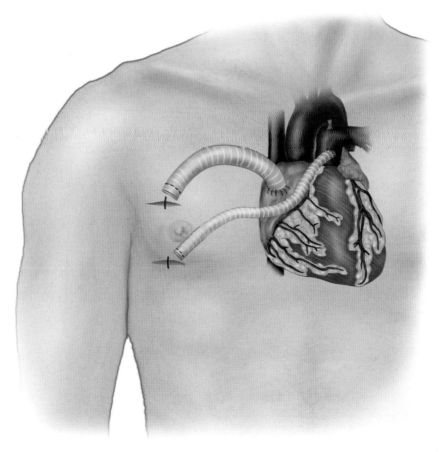

Figure 26-5

- The body of the pump can be placed in either an intraperitoneal or extraperitoneal position. We prefer intraperitoneal placement because there is less of a contained pocket with surrounding surgical hematoma, which we believe decreases the incidence of pump pocket infection (Fig. 26-6). Extraperitoneal placement is also more likely to result in kinking of the inflow graft by forcing the pump to be displaced medially, which impairs filling and risks pannus formation by inducing turbulence.
- The outflow graft is attached to the pump and sutured to the ascending aorta with 3-0 or 4-0 polypropylene sutures and positioned lateral to the right atrium, outside the pericardium. The falciform ligament of the liver is detached so that the outflow graft can be angled smoothly (without kinking) from the pump to the ascending aorta. The right mediastinal pleura is also detached so that the graft goes slightly into the right chest. Measuring and dividing the outflow graft while it is pressurized facilitates obtaining proper length.
- We usually wean patients from CPB as we are performing the aortic anastomosis. If the Heart-Mate XVE needs to be actuated before CPB is discontinued, extreme care must be exercised to avoid air entrainment because recoil of the pusher-plate can generate 10 to 20 cm of negative pressure in this device. Close observation with TEE is essential. The pump should be started in the automatic fill mode to decrease the risk of air entrainment. In closing the abdomen, care should be taken to avoid adherence of the outflow graft to the liver. This can be done either by placing the greater omentum between the graft and the liver or by suturing a sheet of antibacterial-impregnated Gore-Tex (W. L. Gore & Associates, Inc., Flagstaff, Ariz) to the abdominal wall, placing it under the pump and the outflow graft.

3 Axial Flow Pumps

HeartMate II (Thoratec Corp.)

- The HeartMate II has a short, flexible inlet cannula. This pump is usually implanted beneath the diaphragm through a median sternotomy (Fig. 26-7). The inlet cannula and sewing ring of the HeartMate II are identical to those of the HeartMate XVE (Fig. 26-8) and are placed as previously described. Similarly, the outflow graft is pressurized before measuring and dividing to ensure a tension-free, nonkinking graft lie.
- Anastomoses subjected to continuous flow and constant pressure are more prone to leak than anastomoses subjected to pulsatile flow, so we usually perform the aortic anastomosis with 5-0 polypropylene suture reinforced with Teflon or a biologic glue to minimize suture leaks.

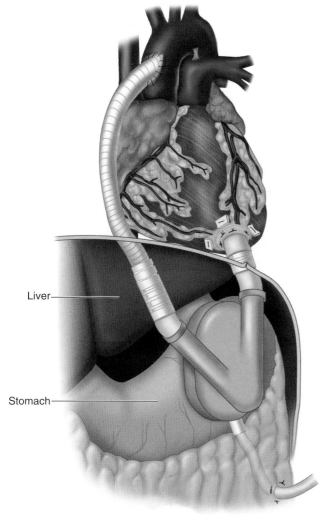

Figure 26-6

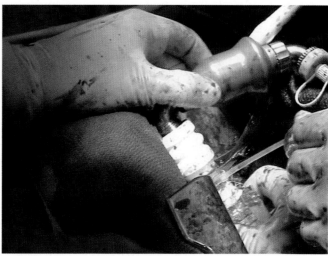

Figure 26-7

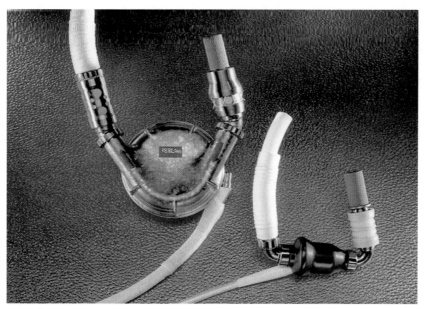

Figure 26-8

- The driveline of the HeartMate II is smaller than that of the HeartMate XVE; however, the driveline connector is larger than the driveline (Fig. 26-9). This results in dead space around the driveline tunnel, which can predispose to infection. To eliminate excessive dead space, we usually have the driveline course in the preperitoneal space until it is directly beneath the cutaneous exit site, at which point we bring it straight through all layers of the body wall (Fig. 26-10A and B).
- The left ventricle should be well filled before pump flow is initiated. The pump is started at 6000 rpm, and the speed is gradually increased until a suitable cardiac output is obtained, usually at 9000 to 10,000 rpm.
- The HeartMate II can also be placed through a left subcostal incision. Before the inlet cannula is inserted, we cannulate the femoral artery for CPB. To ensure safety, CPB should be initiated if patients become unstable in any way during pump placement. Although the HeartMate II can usually be placed without CPB in patients with smaller hearts, we use temporary partial CPB for most patients during placement of the inlet cannula. The inlet cannula can be placed into the apex of the ventricle after the diaphragm is detached, or the cannula can be inserted in the diaphragmatic surface by splitting the diaphragmatic fibers in a manner similar to that done for extrathoracic placement of a Jarvik Heart (Jarvik Heart, Inc., New York, NY). By placing the inlet cannula in the diaphragmatic surface, the outlet graft is more optimally oriented.
- Once the pump is placed subcostally, the aortic outflow graft can be tunneled under the sternum without requiring a more invasive median sternotomy. The aortic anastomosis is performed by making a small incision through the right third intercostal space; the costal cartilage is removed and the mammary vessels are ligated. This incision facilitates exposure of the ascending aorta. A side-biting clamp can be placed on the aorta, and the previously placed Dacron outflow graft attached by a running polypropylene suture. Alternatively, the outflow graft can be initially sewn to the ascending aorta before tunneling through the infrasternal space. Graft length must be estimated before attachment if this approach is used. After aortic anastomosis, the graft is simply tunneled under the sternum and attached to the previously placed outlet of the Heart-Mate II pump (Fig. 26-11).

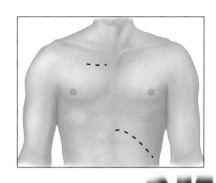

Figure 26-9

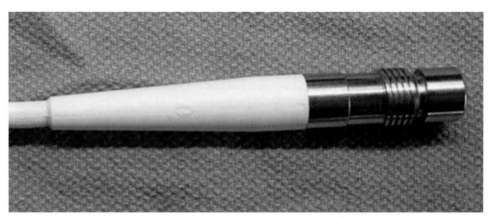

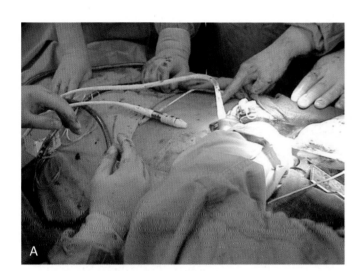

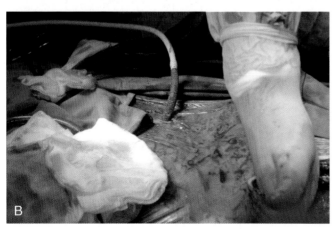

Figure 26-10

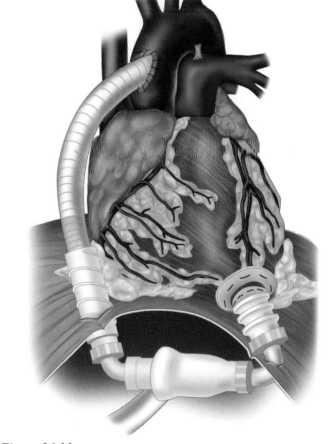

Figure 26-11

Jarvik Heart

- The Jarvik Heart can be implanted through a median sternotomy incision (Fig. 26-12A), a left sixth interspace incision (Fig. 26-12B), or a left subcostal incision (Fig. 26-12C). The outflow graft can be anastomosed to the ascending aorta, the supraceliac aorta, or the descending thoracic aorta (see Fig. 26-12). The femoral vessels are exposed for temporary CPB. The power cable is usually tunneled to exit the right subcostal area 2 to 3 cm below the costal margin at the anterior axillary line. This exit site is common to all of the alternative insertion sites. Before CPB is instituted, an end-to-side anastomosis of the 16-mm outflow graft to the aorta is performed. If the descending thoracic aorta or supraceliac aorta is the site of graft placement, care must be taken to ensure pulses distal to the clamp placement. The anastomosis is made with 4-0 polypropylene suture on a V-6 needle with felt strip reinforcement (see Fig. 26-12).
- If the pump is placed through the left thoracotomy incision, the pericardium is incised parallel to the phrenic nerve anteriorly and posteriorly to ensure pericardial drainage. The position of the sewing ring is marked with electrocautery. The asymmetric sewing ring is placed slightly lateral to the apex, pointing away from the septum toward the left ventricular outflow tract and attached to the myocardium with deep muscular bites of pledgeted 2-0 Ethibond sutures on atraumatic V-7 or MH needles. CPB is initiated, and the heart is fibrillated.
- The Jarvik coring knife is inserted through a cruciate incision. After the myocardial core is removed, the Jarvik Heart is inserted into the left ventricular cavity and secured to the ring. The device is oriented to avoid impingement of the rib cage or diaphragm on the outflow graft. Obstruction to outflow graft flow will result in hemolysis or dysfunction and impair proper functioning of the Jarvik pump. It is particularly important to avoid any kinking of the outflow graft against the rib cage or diaphragm.
- After the heart is defibrillated, it is allowed to fill slowly with blood. During this time, the patient's head is lowered, and the outflow graft is vented continuously. The Jarvik Heart is then started. After complete de-airing is confirmed by TEE, CPB is terminated and heparin reversed.

Jarvik Heart Extrathoracic Off-Pump Implantation

- We have found a suitable location for placement of the pump cannula to be on the diaphragmatic surface posterolateral to the posterior descending coronary artery, approximately halfway between the apex and base of the left ventricle. This position should place the inlet in the flat space between the ventricular septum and insertion of the papillary muscles; having a large enough space is important for large, cardiomyopathic hearts (see Fig. 26-12C). An extended subcostal incision also provides access to the retroperitoneal supraceliac aorta for outflow graft attachment. Each of these approaches, left subcostal and left thoracotomy, obviates the need for repeat sternotomy. Wrapping the outflow graft with externally supported Teflon helps prevent graft kinking.
- The sewing ring is sutured to the epicardial surface of the heart with circumferential pledgeted sutures. Care must be exercised in tying the sutures because the myocardium may be friable in patients with cardiomyopathy. After placement of the sewing ring, a cruciate transmural incision is made in the myocardium within the sewing ring. Gently curved clamps are used to grasp the edge of the sewing ring at three or four points around the circumference to facilitate rapid pump insertion once the apical core is removed. We prefer the Jarvik Heart coring device because the integral conical anvil, when used correctly, ensures that all excised heart tissue is captured and removed. The patient is heparinized, and the femoral artery and vein are cannulated to allow rapid return of shed blood and to allow institution of CPB, if necessary.
- The process of core removal and pump insertion requires the rapid and coordinated actions of two surgeons. The coring device is inserted and actuated by the assistant, after which it is rapidly removed, which allows the surgeon to insert a finger through the ring. If done smoothly and quickly, this procedure is associated with acceptable blood loss and allows the surgeon to assess the geometry of the apex and ensure that the core is removed in its entirety. The surgeon then

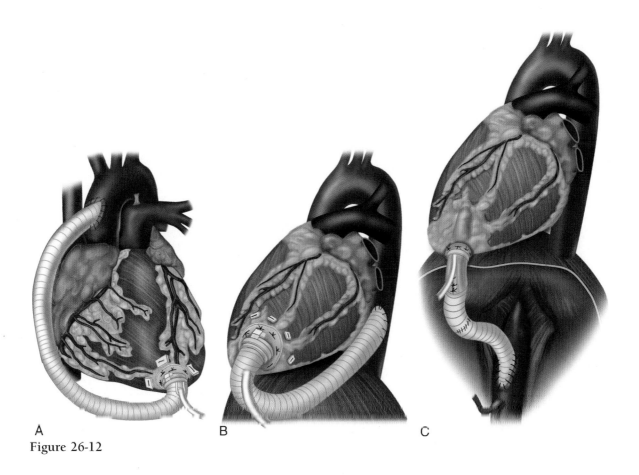

Figure 26-12

rapidly removes his or her finger and replaces it with the pump, again moving quickly to minimize blood loss. Inserting the pump is facilitated by retracting the sewing ring lip with the gently curved clamps.

♦ Depending on the approach used, the pump inlet may be inserted before or after constructing the anastomosis between the outlet graft and the aorta. Regardless of the order, the outlet graft is clamped during pump insertion to allow aggressive de-airing before instituting LVAD support.

5. Explant Procedures for Cardiac Transplantation

HeartMate XVE and HeartMate II

♦ We usually remove only the inlet cannula, perform the heart transplantation, and leave the pump in place, closing only the skin. After bleeding is controlled (usually 24 to 48 hours after implantation), the pump is removed and the incision closed. The intrathoracic portion of the graft to the ascending aorta should also be excised and the point of attachment to the pump removed. The aortic anastomosis should be made distal to the aortic valve, thereby removing the entire aortic graft with the removed recipient ascending aorta. This may shorten the space for the recipient aorta, so the femoral or subclavian artery should be used for cannulation.

Jarvik Heart

♦ Because the Jarvik Heart is inside the ventricle, it is best to remove the pump with the excised heart. Before CPB is instituted, the origin of the graft from the left ventricle should be clamped, if feasible. The graft is excised from its connection to the pump. We usually oversew the graft (5-0 or 4-0 polypropylene suture), but it can be stapled with a rotating-head staple applier. We do not excise the graft from its intrathoracic position because the hazards of bleeding engendered by its removal greatly exceed any possible benefit.

6. Removal after Improvement of Native Ventricular Function

♦ We remove the HeartMate XVE and the HeartMate II through a subcostal incision with the aid of CPB. The inlet cannula is exposed through a subdiaphragmatic incision, and the outlet graft is clamped just before it goes under the right costochondral junction. After the pump and inlet cannula are removed, the open space in the sewing cuff is replaced by a previously fashioned plug of rolled Teflon (Figs. 26-13 and 26-14) fitted at the surgical table to an identical sewing cuff. The outflow graft is oversewn at the costochondral junction. This approach has greatly simplified device removal and has significantly minimized the risk of pump explant.

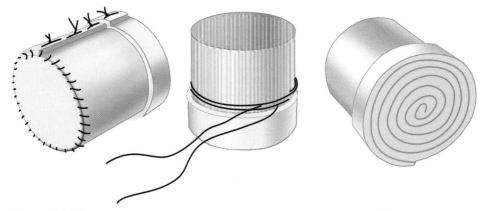

Figure 26-13

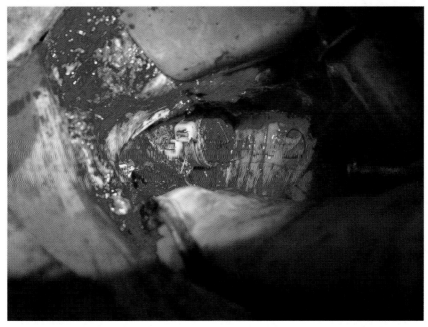

Figure 26-14

Step 4. Postoperative Care

1. Extracorporeal Left Ventricular Assist Devices

♦ Bleeding often occurs in the immediate postoperative period, particularly when CPB has been used. In most cases, we close the skin only when coagulation parameters are normalized and bleeding is minimized. This decreases the chance of cardiac tamponade and device malfunction and allows us to remove blood clots, which can serve as a medium for bacterial growth, before final closure.

♦ No anticoagulant should be given while a patient is bleeding; however, when operative bleeding decreases to less than 200 mL/hr, we give patients low–molecular-weight dextran (10 mL/hr). Once the patients are stable, we close the chest and give low-dose intravenous heparin to maintain the prothrombin time between 60 and 70 seconds. If patients are taking oral alimentation before pump removal or transplantation, they may be given oral warfarin to maintain an international normalized ratio between 2 and 3.

2. HeartMate XVE

♦ Because late infection is a frequent complication after HeartMate XVE implantation, we wait 48 to 72 hours before final closure. At this point, copious antibacterial irrigation should be used to remove blood remaining in the thoracic cavity and around this large, pulsatile pump. We have found such irrigation helpful in decreasing the incidence of subsequent infection.

3. Jarvik Heart

♦ The pump should be run at the lowest speed to allow for aortic valve opening and a satisfactory cardiac index (usually, 9000 to 10,000 rpm). Once ambulatory, patients are the best sources for determining the pump speed needed for their various activities.

♦ Because of the potential for clot formation in the aortic root and the intraventricular area around the pump, anticoagulation with low–molecular-weight dextran is recommended in the immediate postoperative period, progressing to warfarin. Aspirin and dipyridamole (Persantine) can be given to toleration (usually 325 mg of aspirin and 150 mg of dipyridamole daily). The international normalized ratio should be maintained between 2 and 3.

4. HeartMate II

♦ The HeartMate II LVAD is associated with less clot formation in the aortic root and the ventricle because of its extracardiac placement and because of the ascending aortic anastomosis. Implantation of the pump also preserves the correct anatomic position of the interventricular septum. Care should be taken to avoid overdriving this pump and excessively unloading the ventricle in the postoperative period, which can induce ventricular arrhythmias.

Step 5. Pearls and Pitfalls

- Most pearls and pitfalls were described in the sections to which they pertained. A few additional cautions are worth mentioning.

1. AB5000

- Placing the right ventricular outlet cannula through the acute margin of the right ventricle and into the pulmonary valve allows the assistant, using his or her thumb and index finger, to take the tension off the insertion site, minimizing blood loss and facilitating cannula removal when the patient is weaned.
- Circle and securely tie the 2-0 polypropylene sutures around the inlet cannula to ensure that the inlet cannula cannot migrate, which could cause the catastrophic complications of air embolus or bleeding.

2. HeartMate XVE

- If the pneumatic drive console is available, it can be used because it allows a minimal rate of 20, in contrast to the electrical actuator, which has a minimal rate of 50, further reducing the potential for air embolism.
- The diaphragmatic incision should be positioned to facilitate an acceptable pump orientation that minimizes torsion on the inlet cannula and should be as small as possible to decrease the likelihood of postoperative herniation of abdominal viscera.

3. Continuous-Flow Pumps

- We commonly perform the aortic anastomosis without heparin and release the partial occluding clamp with the graft clamped as close to the anastomosis as possible. Once bleeding points have been eliminated by additional sutures or application of topical hemostatics, heparin can be administered for the remainder of the procedure. We have found the aortic anastomoses and graft anastomoses for continuous-flow pumps particularly likely to bleed. The needle point for de-airing must also be carefully closed because this can serve as a site of postoperative bleeding. The area can be wrapped with Surgicel (Johnson & Johnson, Somerville, NJ) or with a circumferential graft.

- If cross-clamping is required for short periods, we administer cardioplegia through the coronary sinus. This is important so that the heart, even in its weakened state, will have sufficient residual function to allow weaning from CPB before pump flow is initiated. This is usually possible and is also the best method for de-airing the pump—that is, allowing the native heart to pump the air out under positive pressure—because initiation of pump flow, with either a pulsatile or a nonpulsatile pump, can result in negative pressure along the apical suture line, which can suck air into the ventricle. In any case, bypass flow should be at the lowest possible level before pump flow is initiated. Clamping and unclamping the graft can also cause cavitation and entrainment and should therefore be avoided.

4. Explant

- When either the HeartMate XVE or HeartMate II is removed, the pump should be stopped at the time of institution of CPB, or the low pressure in the ventricle may allow the pump to entrain air.

Bibliography

Cohn WE, Frazier OH: Off-pump insertion of an extracorporeal LVAD through a left upper-quadrant incision. Tex Heart Inst J 2006;33:48-50.

Cohn WE, Gregoric ID, Frazier OH: A felt plug simplifies left ventricular assist device removal after successful bridge to recovery. J Heart Lung Tx 2007;26:1209-1211.

Cohn WE, Gregoric ID, Frazier OH: Reinforcement of left ventricular assist device outflow grafts to prevent kinking. Ann Thorac Surg 2007;84:301-302.

Frazier OH: Mechanical cardiac assistance: Historical perspectives. Semin Thorac Cardiovasc Surg 2000;12:207-219.

Frazier OH: Implantation of the Jarvik 2000 left ventricular assist device without the use of cardiopulmonary bypass. Ann Thorac Surg 2003;75:1028-1030.

Frazier OH: Ventricular assist devices and total artificial hearts: A historical perspective. Cardiol Clin 2003;21:1-13.

Frazier OH, Benedict CR, Radovancevic B, et al: Improved left ventricular function after chronic left ventricular unloading. Ann Thorac Surg 1996;62:675-682.

Frazier OH, Delgado RM, Kar B, et al: First clinical use of the redesigned HeartMate II left ventricular assist system in the United States: A case report. Tex Heart Inst J 2004;31:157-159.

Frazier OH, Forrester MD, Gemmato G, Gregoric ID: Urgent pump exchange for stroke resulting from a distorted HeartMate XVE inflow conduit. J Heart Lung Transplant 2007;26:646-648.

Frazier OH, Gregoric ID, Cohn WE: Initial experience with non-thoracic, extraperitoneal, off-pump insertion of the Jarvik 2000 Heart in patients with previous median sternotomy. J Heart Lung Transplant 2006;25:499-503.

Frazier OH, Myers TJ, Gregoric I: Biventricular assistance with the Jarvik FlowMaker: A case report. J Thorac Cardiovasc Surg 2004;128:625-626.

Frazier OH, Myers TJ, Gregoric ID, et al: Initial clinical experience with the Jarvik 2000 implantable axial-flow left ventricular assist system. Circulation 2002;105:2855-2860.

Frazier OH, Myers TJ, Westaby S, Gregoric ID: Clinical experience with an implantable, intracardiac, continuous flow circulatory support device: Physiologic implications and their relationship to patient selection. Ann Thorac Surg 2004;77:133-142.

Frazier OH, Shah N, Myers TJ, et al: Use of the FlowMaker (Jarvik 2000) left ventricular assist device for destination therapy and bridging to transplantation. Cardiology 2004;101:111-116.

Gemmato CJ, Forrester MD, Myers TJ, et al: Thirty-five years of mechanical circulatory support at the Texas Heart Institute: An updated overview. Tex Heart Inst J 2005;32:168-177.

Gregoric I, Wadia Y, Radovancevic B, et al: HeartMate vented-electric left ventricular assist system: Technique for intrathoracic or intraperitoneal implantation via a left thoracotomy. J Heart Lung Transplant 2004;23:759-762.

Radovancevic B, Frazier OH, Duncan JM: Implantation technique for the HeartMate left ventricular assist device. J Cardiac Surg 1992;7:203-207.

Rose EA, Gelijns AC, Moskowitz AJ, et al: Long-term mechanical left ventricular assistance for end-stage heart failure. N Engl J Med 2001;345:1435-1443.

CHAPTER 27

HEART TRANSPLANTATION

Daniel Marelli and Scott Silvestry

Donor

Step 1. Surgical Anatomy

- Nine vessels are cut during the retrieval; two caval veins, four pulmonary veins, the aorta, and the two branch pulmonary arteries.
- The superior vena cava lies partly outside the pericardium. It is anterior and to the right of the trachea and its surrounding nodal tissue. The arch of the azygos vein is noted posteriorly as the only branch of the superior vena cava.
- The superior vena cava is dissected along its entire course away from its anterior and posterior attachments to the transverse pericardial sinus, as are the ascending aorta and branch pulmonary arteries. These vessels are severed outside the pericardium. In contrast, the pulmonary veins and inferior vena cava are separated from their attachments to the oblique pericardial sinus but are severed within the pericardium
- After removal of the heart, the transverse pericardial sinus is opened on the back table, and the main and right pulmonary arteries are separated from the dome of the left atrium posterior to the superior vena cava. When the pulmonary artery is divided at its bifurcation (in the case of concomitant lung retrieval), the transverse sinus will be opened in situ.

Step 2. Preoperative Considerations

1. Selection and Management

- Risk matching between donor characteristics and recipient needs ensures maximal utilization of the potential donor pool and minimizes the risk associated with longer waiting lists.[1,2] For example, a heart from a higher risk donor may be used in an older recipient with previous surgery, but not in a younger recipient who is a good candidate for an assist device.
- The average age for a donor is approximately 30 years. Common causes of brain death include trauma and intracranial bleed. Suicide remains a common cause, with the mode of death incorporating both anoxic and traumatic brain injuries.

- Screening for a given recipient begins with confirming blood type compatibility and the approximate size, height, and weight for the patient, as well as sex. Ensuring an appropriate-sized donor (>0.8 recipient size) remains a key component in the selection of donor–recipient matches. The size match formula may be increased if the donor is female and the recipient male. It may be decreased if the donor is a younger male or if there is a shorter anticipated ischemia time. Recipient pulmonary vascular resistance must also be taken into account.
- The female donor older than 35 years of age with an intracranial bleed must be evaluated carefully. This cause of death is frequently associated with hypertensive disease and left ventricular hypertrophy. Left ventricular hypertrophy as assessed by echocardiographic measurement of septal and posterior wall thickness, and electrocardiographic criteria should be judged in the context of the patient's body surface area. The use of hypertrophied hearts can significantly affect graft survival, particularly in the presence of electrocardiographic criteria that reflect a long-standing history.[3]
- The ideal donor should have excellent cardiac function with appropriate filling pressure and normal anatomy. As discussed later, the general rule is inotropic support with dopamine at less than 10 µg/kg/min and a central venous pressure less than 10 mm Hg, with a left ventricular ejection fraction greater than 50%.
- As donor age increases, the depth of evaluation increases as well. With age greater than 45 years or the presence of significant smoking history at a younger age, cardiac catheterization is required. When cardiac catheterization is not available, risk factors should be considered. Hypertension may cause distal coronary artery disease, which may preclude donation.
- The presence of any coronary artery disease is usually a contraindication to utilization for a standard donor.
- Hepatitis C remains a contraindication to heart donation because it may predispose the recipient to liver dysfunction and graft coronary disease. Hepatitis B core antibody immunoglobulin G (IgG)–positive donors may be used for status I recipients if IgM is negative. In such cases, the risk of transmission is considered low (<5% to 10%).[4]

2. Donor Management

- Ideal management would include inotropic support of low-dose dopamine with thyroxine (T_4) infusion, and controlling blood pressure to less than 120 mm Hg systolic. Levophed infusion should be avoided; in its place, low-dose phenylephrine may be used. Short-acting beta blockade may be continued in the setting of hyperdynamic left ventricular function and tachycardia, but long-acting beta blockers should be discontinued as early as possible. Beta blockers should be stopped on arrival to the operating room. Anemia should be corrected because this will cause hypotension. A Pco_2 of 30 to 35 mm Hg should be sought to decrease pulmonary vascular resistance.
- The retrieval team should strive to keep the donor heart relaxed and undistended. Intraoperative management of the donor includes inhaled anesthetic agents for blood pressure control and judicious volume resuscitation to maintain a central venous pressure of 8 to 12 mm Hg. Right ventricular distention or stress is often noted when the systemic blood pressure rises above 110 to 120 mm Hg.

Step 3. Operative Steps

1. Visualization

- On arrival, the retrieval team checks donor blood type against that of the recipient, as well as donor consent, certification of brain death, and other pertinent data.
- Communication between the donor and recipient surgical teams is essential. We use a circulating assistant who travels with the donor team for this purpose. This assistant may be a pump technician or a preservationist specifically trained for heart or liver retrieval.
- Timing and logistics of donor harvest vary from center to center. For local donors (less than 60 to 80 minutes' travel time), we try to have the donor and recipient enter the operating room at the same time.
- A generous median sternotomy is performed. A short retractor is placed with the cross-bar oriented superiorly so as not to disturb exposure for the liver transplantation team.
- A pericardial cradle is created with stay sutures. The lung transplantation team may choose to secure these with clamps so that access to the pleural spaces is maintained.
- The heart is visualized and inspected for adequate function. The right ventricle is readily visible. One should note a relaxed right atrium as well as a relaxed outflow tract. The heart can be picked up gently to assess left ventricular function and to look for a left superior vena cava.
- In older donors, the coronary arteries should be palpated. Usually, a cardiac catheterization study will have been done. Diffuse coronary artery disease may not be obstructive but would still preclude donation. Extensive calcifications, although not necessarily stenotic, also preclude use of the organ. The donor heart is examined for signs of long-standing hypertension such as increased epicardial fat, tortuous coronary arteries, and a shortened ascending aorta with effacement of the sinotubular junction.
- An estimate of heparin/clamp time is determined with the other organ retrieval teams. The timing of recipient and donor operations is individualized secondary to reoperative status, ventricular assist device excision, and anticipated travel times.
- The aorta and pulmonary artery are separated, and the aorta is encircled with a tape for control. This facilitates clamping of the aorta in a busy operative field that will be flooded with blood. Some may choose to separate the inferior vena cava from the diaphragm. It should be kept in mind that the liver team requires an adequate length of the inferior vena cava, including the infradiaphragmatic portion of the vein.
- The superior vena cava is separated from the right pulmonary artery and encircled superior to the azygos vein. If there is no assistant, a stay suture in the adventitia of the aorta may be used to gently retract the ascending aorta leftward. Alternatively, the superior vena cava may be encircled below the azygos and clamped during flush cooling and dissected more completely after flush cooling. The azygos vein can be ligated doubly, but it is not divided until after cross-clamping to prevent risk of bleeding from the stumps.
- A back-table setup is prepared and checked at this time to allow efficient preparation and packaging. The packing plastic bag is prepared in a large basin filled with iced saline slurry. The bag is filled with 1 L of the same solution that is used for flush cooling. This setup keeps the storage solution cold and prevents ice from coming in direct contact with the heart. An aortic cross-clamp is also selected.

2. Organ Recovery

♦ Preparation is made to allow adequate suction and venting into the right chest. The pericardium adjacent to the inferior vena cava is divided to allow drainage into the right chest. This drainage can be collected with a pool suction. Another pool suction is prepared for insertion into the inferior vena cava, which will be incised.

♦ The cardioplegia bag should be kept in a cooler until just before heparin is given. An assistant or preservationist hangs and administers the cardioplegia. Heparin (300 U/kg) is administered intravenously. After 3 minutes, a cardioplegia needle with provision for transducing aortic cardioplegia pressure is secured to the ascending aorta just distal to the fat pad and de-aired and clamped. Measuring cardioplegia pressure is particularly important for pediatric and adolescent donors, in whom the aorta is small and pressure estimation by palpation is unreliable. Flush cooling at supraphysiologic pressures may cause edema of the donor organ, potentially leading to dysfunction. After securing the cardioplegia cannula, the tubing is passed off to be connected to the preservative solution bag. The line is de-aired, clamped, and connected.

♦ In isolated cardiac harvest, the right superior pulmonary vein is vented. Occasionally, there is some aortic insufficiency owing to distortion of the aortic valve. If the lungs are being harvested, care is taken to avoid placing the perfusion cannula too proximal and damaging the pulmonic valve. When the lungs are harvested, the left atrium is vented through the left atrial appendage. In addition, the right pulmonary vein cuff may be initiated for venting. It is important to avoid left ventricular distention by the pulmonary venous effluent.

♦ The flush cooling sequence is initiated by the cardiac team in coordination with the abdominal team. The superior vena cava is ligated and the inferior vena cava is hemisected anteriorly to vent the right heart. A pool suction is placed inside the inferior vena cava and in the right pleural space. This creates an empty beating heart (Fig. 27-1).

♦ The left atrium is vented, and the left ventricle empties. Usually, the operative field is busy and often flooded with blood. The aorta is then clamped on the encircling tape, which is gently retracted. This helps to prevent the clamp blades from distorting the right pulmonary artery, which may be difficult to visualize. Ten to 12 mL/kg of preservative solution is flushed into the aorta while monitoring aortic root pressure, which is kept at 50 to 60 mm Hg. We use University of Wisconsin (Belzer) solution. A prompt arrest should be noted. The heart is then covered in ice slush. Ventilation is turned off and disconnected from the endotracheal tube. If a lung team is present, antegrade pneumoplegia is initiated at this time (after cardiac arrest, so that the aortic valve is closed), and ventilation is maintained.

♦ It usually takes 6 to 8 minutes to flush-cool the heart. During this time, blood is observed clearing from the coronary arteries, and the surgeon ensures that there is no right or left ventricular distention.

♦ Once the cardioplegia is given, the aorta should be transected if pneumoplegia is still being given, as is usually the case. This should help to further vent the left-sided cardiac chambers and to prevent the pneumoplegia from washing out the cardioplegia.

♦ The inferior vena cava is then divided. It is helpful to separate the inferior vena cava from the right inferior pulmonary vein. This is accomplished by dividing the pericardial reflection between these two structures. This will greatly facilitate partitioning the left atrium in the case of concomitant lung harvest. As noted previously, we find it unnecessary to take the infradiaphragmatic portion. The heart is elevated and retracted to the left to expose the right pulmonary veins for division at the pericardial reflection.

♦ The heart is retracted superiorly and to the right to expose the left pulmonary veins, which are divided at the pericardial reflection (Fig. 27-2A and B).

♦ Alternatively, in the setting of lung block harvest, the left atrium is divided posteriorly in the midline and the division continued superiorly around the ostia of the pulmonary veins to create cuffs for the left and right pulmonary veins, respectively. This maneuver is facilitated by looking inside the left atrium while cutting the contour of the cuffs. On the right, the interatrial groove should be developed to facilitate creation of the pulmonary vein cuff (Fig. 27-2C).

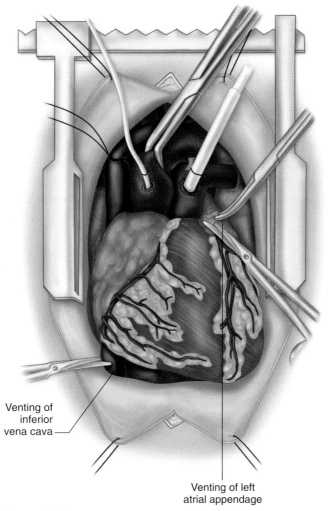

Venting of
inferior
vena cava

Venting of left
atrial appendage

Figure 27-1

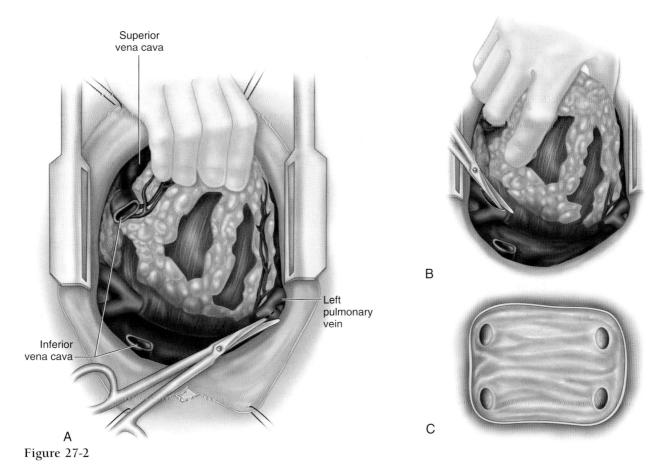

Superior
vena cava

Inferior
vena cava

Left
pulmonary
vein

A

B

C

Figure 27-2

- Caution is needed to avoid damaging the superior vena cava and the sinoatrial node. This is facilitated by avoiding excessive traction on the heart, which would tend to distort the anatomy. The dome of the left atrium is divided along the transverse pericardial sinus.
- The main pulmonary artery is divided distal to the pneumoplegia cannula site at the bifurcation. Again, the surgeon should look inside to follow the contour of the bifurcation and protect the pulmonary valve. It also is necessary to separate the right pulmonary artery from the superior vena cava. We prefer to separate the heart from the lung block in situ (vs. on the back table).
- The left pulmonary artery is then divided. Downward traction is applied to the aorta, and it is divided beyond the clamp site. The azygos vein is divided, as is the superior vena cava and the right pulmonary artery. In cases of simple cardiac retrieval, it is necessary to retract the heart anteriorly to divide the tissue between the pulmonary artery bifurcation anteriorly and the tracheal bifurcation posteriorly, along the transverse pericardial sinus. It may also be necessary to divide the ligamentum arteriosum (Fig. 27-3).
- The heart is then delivered to the back table and placed in the cold preservation solution.

Step 4. Postretrieval Care

- Donor pericardium and paratracheal lymph nodes are harvested at this point, if this was not done previously. The pericardium is packaged with the donor heart. If needed, this can be used for patches or pledgets during the recipient operation. It is treated with glutaraldehyde by the recipient team.
- In case of simultaneous lung block harvest, we retrograde-perfuse the lung block, remove it, and package it before proceeding with the rest of the back-table cardiac preparation. During this time, the donor heart is left submerged in the cold preservation solution bath on the back table. This avoids unnecessary warm lung ischemia time. Lymph nodes are requested from the abdominal team.
- A rapid assessment is performed to assess surgical damage, valve competency, and the presence of a patent foramen ovale, which should be closed. Last, the inferior vena cava and lower right atrium are inspected to ensure that an adequate rim of atrial tissue is present next to the coronary sinus.
- The remaining back table dissection may be performed before packaging. This dissection includes preparing the left atrial cuff for anastomosis by dividing the pulmonary veins from superior to inferior on either side and incising the posterior left atrium. The mitral valve is inspected carefully. The pulmonary artery is splayed open and dissected away from the left atrium and superior vena cava on the right. This will already have been done in situ when a lung retrieval is also planned.
- The pulmonary artery and aorta are then gently separated at the level of the distal ascending aorta. It is unnecessary and dangerous to continue this dissection proximally; such dissection might injure the left main coronary artery, particularly because lighting for the back table is usually poor. Alternatively, these maneuvers may be performed before implantation at the recipient operation (Fig. 27-4).
- A plastic bag containing 700 to 1000 mL cold preservative solution is used to transport the organ and any donor pericardium that is retrieved. The bag is de-aired, closed, and sealed with a tape ligature. Excess plastic is trimmed and the bag is placed in another plastic bag or hard plastic container containing slush. The hard container is particularly useful to protect smaller donor hearts from injury during transport. This container is de-aired and the cap is placed while applying gentle pressure to ensure complete submersion in cold slush solution. A last (third) plastic bag is placed around the two bags or container. This package is labeled and placed into a large cooler completely surrounded by ice.
- At this point, calls are placed to the recipient institution confirming departure from the donor hospital.

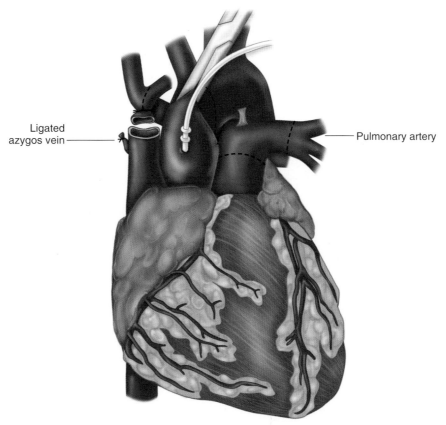

Ligated azygos vein

Pulmonary artery

Figure 27-3

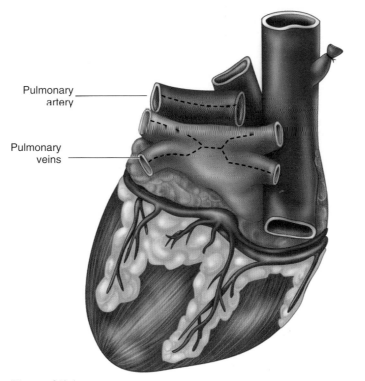

Pulmonary artery

Pulmonary veins

Figure 27-4

- The team should be alert to avoid excess heat exposure during transport, particularly during summer months (e.g., the trunk of a car during a daytime retrieval). When the donor team is about 10 to 20 minutes from arrival, the recipient team is alerted so that cardiopulmonary bypass may be initiated.

Step 5. Pearls and Pitfalls

- Primary graft failure is unusual in the current era. It usually presents as left or biventricular failure. More commonly, we observe right ventricular dysfunction due to recipient factors combined with a donor right ventricle that has not been exposed to the higher, often reactive pulmonary vascular resistance that can occur with heart failure. The importance of a reliable donor procedure cannot be overemphasized.
- Frequent communication is necessary with the recipient team to convey adjustments in time to prevent unnecessarily lengthening the donor ischemic time.
- Donor blood pressure will rise with stimulation. Inhaled anesthetic agents should be used to keep blood pressure at a maximum of 120 mm Hg systolic.
- Focused communication with the lung harvest team is needed to avoid cardiac distention, which can be extremely deleterious to the post-transplantation function of the donor heart. It is important to wait until the left atrial appendage is vented and the heart is arrested before starting lung perfusion. This also prevents the lung perfusate from displacing the cardioplegia solution from the aortic root. If the cardioplegia has finished infusing before the pneumoplegia, the aorta must be transected and a suction carefully advanced toward the aortic valve to prevent the pneumoplegia from washing out the cardioplegia. Pneumoplegia may be toxic to the heart and coronary arteries.
- In severe chest or abdominal trauma, the surgeon must always be alert to the possibility of hematomas around the aorta or innominate vein, which may be a source of important blood loss on opening the chest.
- Excessive manipulation of the donor heart during flush cooling may cause transient aortic valve incompetence with ensuing right and left ventricular distention and therefore should be avoided. Aortic valve regurgitation can be remedied by advancing a blunt-tipped suction from the right superior pulmonary vein toward the left ventricle. This empties it and closes the aortic valve.
- On excision, it is crucial to avoid damage to the coronary sinus during division of the inferior vena cava and left atrium. Suboptimal length of the superior vena cava can lead to sinoatrial node damage.
- Care should be taken in dividing the inferior vena cava to leave adequate length for the liver harvest as well as an adequate cuff on the pulmonary veins for the lung harvest.
- It is prudent to monitor the aortic root pressure to ensure that the aortic perfusion pressure stays between 50 and 70 mm Hg, thus alerting to potentially inadequate preservation solution delivery. Excessive pressure in the flush preservation of organs can lead to endothelial damage and poor short- and long-term function. This is particularly important for pediatric and adolescent donors in whom the ascending aorta usually has a small diameter.
- Suboptimal flush pressure can lead to inadequate preservation, regional discrepancies in cooling, and subsequent wall motion abnormalities on transplantation. We strongly believe that a minimum flush cooling time of 6 to 8 minutes is required to avoid this. In our experience, transporting the organ in a bath of the preservation solution is also important to optimize distribution of the preservation solution.

Adult Recipient

Step 1. Surgical Anatomy

- The recipient's pericardial space is often enlarged, making it prone to postoperative effusions because of the relatively smaller donor heart size.
- The superior vena cava must be mobilized away from the right pulmonary artery posteriorly. It is not always necessary to mobilize it off the pericardial reflection.
- The inferior vena cava is attached to the reflection of the oblique pericardial sinus. Limited mobilization off this attachment can be helpful in selecting a cannulation site and planning for the bicaval anastomosis.
- The right pulmonary artery is often enlarged, thin, and friable owing to heart failure. It is posterior to the aorta and may be injured during aortic clamping or excision of the recipient native heart.

Step 2. Preoperative Considerations

1. Selection

- Adult recipients are on average about 55 years of age. Ninety percent of the time, such recipients have either ischemic or dilated cardiomyopathy, leading to left ventricular enlargement beyond 70 mm in diastole.
- It is important to perform a right heart catheterization preoperatively to verify that the pulmonary vascular resistance is less than 4 Wood units. The absolute value of the pulmonary artery pressure itself can be misleading with regard to pulmonary hypertension because it may be elevated passively secondary to a high left atrial pressure. This assessment is particularly important in the setting of valvular cardiomyopathy or in adults with congenital heart disease.

2. Preparation, Timing, and Coordination with Donor Operation

- Recipients undergo transplantation while hospitalized and waiting (status I) about 80% of the time. When donors are local (transport time less than 60 to 90 minutes), the donor and the recipient procedures are coordinated so that the donor and recipient enter the operating room at the same time.
- If the recipient is anticoagulated, warfarin may be reversed with vitamin K 2 mg given intravenously in slow infusion. The recipient does not undergo anesthesia and line insertion until the donor heart has been found to be satisfactory. A pulmonary artery catheter is inserted but not necessarily advanced because it will be in the operative field.
- Inotropic agent infusions are continued until cardiopulmonary bypass is initiated. Automatic defibrillators are usually turned off.
- Paracorporeal devices must be wrapped in sterile towels and included in the operative field. Cannula exit sites are prepared in sterile fashion.

◆ We usually allow 1 hour from skin incision to arrival of the donor heart in recipients who have not undergone a previous sternotomy. In patients with prior sternotomy, this period is extended to 2 hours to allow adequate time for complete dissection of the native heart before heparin administration. In patients with prior sternotomy, patent internal mammary artery grafts, biventricular failure (with high right ventricular pressure), or assist device, the surgeon may consider exposure of the femoral artery and vein.

◆ Most multiorgan donor procedures require 1 to 2 hours from visualization to cross-clamping. An additional 30 minutes is needed for organ perfusion, excision, and back-table dissection and packaging. It is advisable to err on the side of the recipient team's being ahead of the donor team.

Step 3. Operative Steps

1. Initiation of Cardiopulmonary Bypass and Native Heart Excision

◆ The inferior and superior venae cavae are dissected and prepared for direct cannulation, as is the ascending aorta. The heart is manipulated minimally owing to extreme irritability and possible left ventricle thrombus dislodgement.

◆ For cannulation, we favor pledgets in patients who have previously undergone heart surgery. Felt is avoided on the aorta to minimize the risk of infection and the unusual complication of aortitis and suture line breakdown.[5] Heparin is given when the donor heart is about 45 minutes away. Direct vena cava cannulation is accomplished with low-profile, high-flow cannulae. Cardiopulmonary bypass can be initiated 10 to 20 minutes before the donor heart arrives. Ventricular assist device cannulae and grafts are clamped before cardiopulmonary bypass is initiated. Sometimes it is safer to cannulate the inferior vena cava after initiation of cardiopulmonary bypass. The donor heart is kept in its transport cooler during native heart excision. Carbon dioxide is insufflated into the pericardial well at 4 to 6 L/min. Ultrafiltration is routinely used during cardiopulmonary bypass, and hematocrit is maintained at 28. An insulation pad is used in the pericardium.

◆ The recipient is cooled to 30°C and the aorta is clamped. A small dose of cardioplegia may be given. If an active aortic root vent is used, it is disconnected and used as a third "pump suction" line. The superior vena cava is snared anterior to the right pulmonary artery. If a pulmonary artery catheter has been advanced, it is pulled back out of the surgical field. The inferior vena cava is snared in the usual fashion. Cardiopulmonary bypass flow is maintained at an index of 2.4 L/min/m^2.

◆ The native heart is excised along the atrioventricular groove. Automated implantable cardioverter–defibrillator leads are cut flush with the superior vena cava after gentle traction is applied, so the remnant may retract out of the field. If an assist device pump is present in the abdomen or paracorporeally, it is removed after the transplantation, before chest closure. Inflow and outflow of such pumps are cut so as not to obstruct the operative field. Cardioverter–defibrillator batteries are removed 2 to 3 months after surgery when healing of the pocket will be less affected by immunosuppression.

◆ A small (14F) vent catheter is placed in the right superior pulmonary vein and advanced into the left inferior pulmonary vein to collect the bronchial return. The most proximal opening must be in the most dependent part of the field. This helps exposure and prevents rewarming of the donor heart after completion of the left atrial anastomosis (Fig. 27-5).

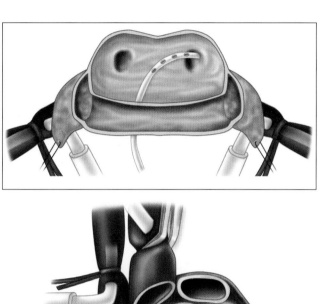

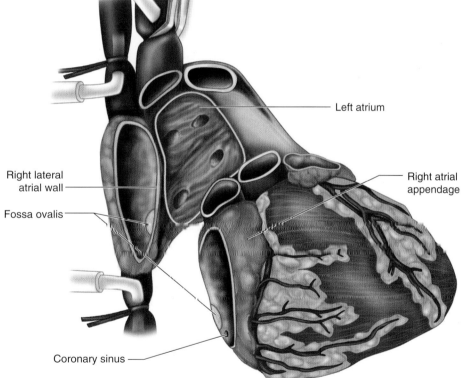

Figure 27-5

- The superior vena cava is transected at its junction with the right atrium. A stay suture is used to mark the anterior edge and to retract it away from the left atrial cuff. The aorta is cut at the sinotubular junction and separated from the right pulmonary artery. The main pulmonary artery is usually divided just distal to the valve. The pulmonary artery should be trimmed carefully before retraction with a stay suture because an untrimmed pulmonary artery can lead to a kinked, obstructive anastomosis. It is unusual to have a shortened pulmonary artery.
- A weighted soft suction catheter can be used to collect the effluent that tends to accumulate in the left branch pulmonary artery. This is best advanced from the left side of the operating field. The branch pulmonary arteries are inspected for thrombus.
- The left atrial cuff is prepared by trimming it back to leave a margin of about 2 cm of tissue around the pulmonary veins. The coronary sinus remnant as well as the appendage are excised. The left atrium is separated from the inferior vena cava with the aid of a C-clamp passed behind the crux of the native heart remnant. If the posterior wall of the inferior vena cava looks as if it will retract excessively toward the cannula, it can be left attached along a short segment of about 1 cm. The remnant of the right atrial portion of the interatrial septum must be checked for a patent foramen ovale and thebesian veins, which need to be oversewn. The edges of the left atrial cuff are cauterized, as is the exposed area of the interatrial septum. Large thebesian veins require suture ligation.
- Preparation of the inferior vena cava cuff can be modified to leave a large flap of right atrial tissue attached anteriorly along 50% to 75% of the circumference. This can then be used to augment the donor right atrial wall in an effort to minimize possible tension on the tricuspid valve, which can lead to regurgitation. A stay suture is used to mark the anterior edge of the inferior vena cava and to retract it away from the left atrial cuff. Additional stay sutures are used to triangulate the left atrial cuff, creating three edges: along the dome, adjacent to the right pulmonary veins, and inferiorly from the base of the appendage to the crux. An insulation pad is placed in the pericardial well.

♦ At this point, the donor heart is removed from the cooler and brought into the operating field. If the donor surgeon has not done so, the pulmonary artery, left atrial, and aortic cuffs are prepared. The atrial septum is inspected for a patent foramen oval, which must be closed to prevent right-to-left shunting in case of transiently elevated pulmonary artery pressures postoperatively.

♦ We usually retrieve donor pericardium and treat it for 2 to 4 minutes in 0.6% glutaraldehyde to make it easier to manipulate. This can be used in lieu of felt strips or pledgets. If needed, it can also be used as patch material to augment the anterior wall of the superior vena cava anastomosis or to reconstruct the pulmonary artery confluence in case of size mismatch or previous Fontan procedure. We do not use secondary cold cardioplegia.

2. Donor Heart Implantation

♦ The atrial connections are more challenging than those of the aorta and pulmonary artery.

Left Atrium Anastomosis

♦ All running anastomoses are constructed using a universal suturing pattern that emphasizes forehand suturing. This helps to make the implant predictable and efficient.

♦ The left atrial anastomosis is started using a long, double-loaded, 3-0 polypropylene suture on an SH or MH needle. The donor heart is wrapped in a large gauze cloth and placed in a small basin filled with slush with the left atrium exposed and oriented superiorly. Additional slush is placed on top of the ventricles to minimize the effects of what is now warm ischemia.

♦ The first needle is passed through base of the native left atrial appendage inside out and placed on a rubber clamp toward the recipient's left shoulder. Half the length of the suture is pulled through. The other half of the suture is now passed through the corresponding point on the donor left atrium, inside out. It is then mounted forehand and passed outside in, inferior to the previous entry on the native atrial cuff. The surgeon must imagine a book closing on itself as the left atrial anastomosis is begun. After three or four passes, the donor heart is partially lowered into the field. The first assistant follows the stitch with the left hand and holds the heart with the right hand, by inserting the second and third fingers through the mitral valve. After several more passes, the heart is completely lowered onto the insulating pad. The first assistant may now follow the suture with the right hand. The inferior wall is sewn from the inside, and the superior wall (dome) is sewn from the outside, both forehand (Fig. 27-6A).

- ◆ As the inferior left atrial suture line progresses, the surgeon must note three things.
    - ▲ First, the suture line should be away from the donor heart circumflex artery. There is a tendency for the donor left atrial cuff to fold back on itself and lie close to the atrioventricular groove.
    - ▲ Second, it is important to observe the alignment of the crux of the donor heart to the recipient's inferior vena cava. Size differences are progressively adjusted along each face of the triangular cuff of the recipient's native left atrium. This maneuver also prevents distortion of the donor mitral and tricuspid valves.
    - ▲ Third, the surgeon should try to exclude the cut edge of the recipient cuff to avoid possible thrombus formation.[6]
- ◆ Once the suture line passes the crux, the stitch is brought out and placed on a rubber clamp. Slush is used to cool the surface of the right ventricle.
- ◆ The other half of the stitch is then sewn forehand along the dome of the left atrium. A stay suture is placed in the donor aorta for retraction, and ice is used to keep the donor right ventricle cold. During construction of this suture line, the surgeon may note that the dome of the native left atrium is enlarged. It is therefore important to use the needle to take deep stitches in the native dome as well as appropriately sized travels to properly align the donor superior vena cava with that of the recipient.
- ◆ The suture line is continued posterior to the superior vena cava to the level of the right superior pulmonary vein. A 12F chest tube or equivalent is advanced into the donor left ventricle, and one additional pass with the suture is used to secure it. Ice-cold Plasmalyte solution is delivered into this tube through sterile intravenous tubing that is passed to the anesthesia station at a rate of 100 to 300 mL/hr. This aids in topical cooling and de-airing of the left ventricle (Fig. 27-6B).
- ◆ The surgeon then rotates 90 degrees clockwise and uses the first stitch forehand to finish the left atrial anastomosis along the interatrial groove. This can also be done by the first assistant. It is important to note the location of the donor sinoatrial node in order to avoid it.
- ◆ Once the suture line reaches the right superior pulmonary vein, the two ends of the suture are placed in a tourniquet to further secure the left ventricular apex catheter. The bronchial return vent is maintained. Additional slush is applied to the right ventricle before starting the next anastomosis.

Pulmonary Artery Anastomosis
- ◆ The donor pulmonary artery is separated from the aorta. The location of the left main coronary artery, which can be seen posteriorly, is noted.
- ◆ The donor pulmonary artery is trimmed so that there is about 1.5 cm of tissue beyond the pulmonary valve. A stay suture is used on the adventitia of the donor pulmonary artery to mark the anteriormost commissure of the pulmonary valve.
- ◆ A double-loaded 4-0 polypropylene suture on an SH or SH-1 needle is used for this anastomosis. It is constructed as described previously. Size mismatch is corrected both posteriorly and anteriorly. A strip of treated pericardium is incorporated into the suture line (Fig. 27-7). As the suture line reaches the 9 o'clock position, it is brought out and placed on a rubber clamp. It can also be passed to the first assistant, who continues the suture line forehand until the 1 o'clock position. The second suture is then sewn forehand from the surgeon's side. The suture may be left untied so that a vent can be inserted into the pulmonary artery to reduce right ventricular afterload when weaning from cardiopulmonary bypass. Additional slush is applied to the right ventricle before starting the next anastomosis. Rewarming to 32°C is started.

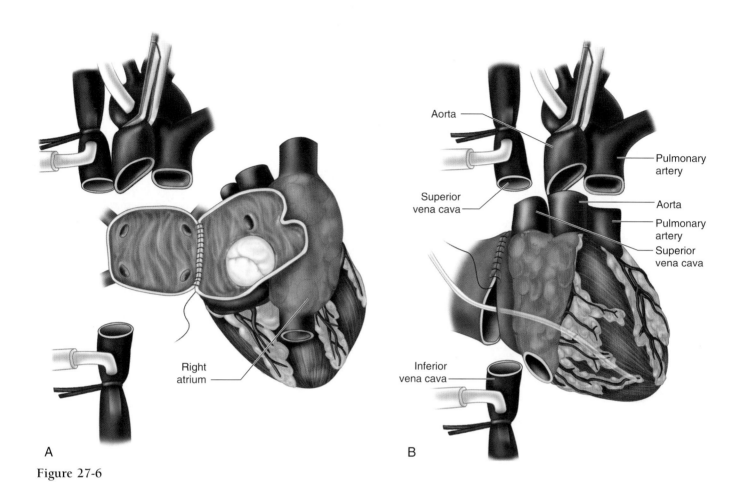

Aorta

Superior
vena cava

Pulmonary
artery

Aorta

Pulmonary
artery

Superior
vena cava

Right
atrium

Inferior
vena cava

A

B

Figure 27-6

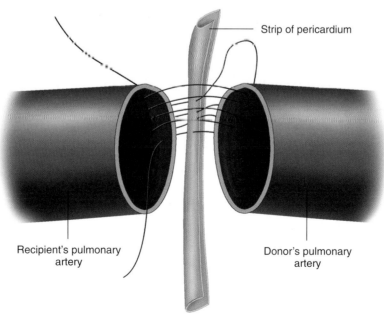

Strip of pericardium

Recipient's pulmonary
artery

Donor's pulmonary
artery

Figure 27-7

Ascending Aorta Anastomosis

- The recipient aorta is trimmed 1 to 1.5 cm proximal to the aortic clamp. This may excise the cardioplegia needle site if one has been inserted. The donor aorta is gently pulled superiorly to the right of the recipient's aorta so that the edges overlap. The donor aorta is usually trimmed distal to the aortic fat pad with an anterior-to-posterior bevel to enlarge the diameter available for the anastomosis. It must be kept in mind that the lesser curve of the aorta is shorter than the greater curve. A 0.5-cm margin is maintained on both the donor and recipient sides to allow for a secure suture line.
- The surgeon must note the location of the left main ostium, this time by looking into the donor aortic root. A 1-cm margin is needed to avoid distortion of the left main coronary artery.
- This suture line is constructed in the same way as that of the pulmonary artery. Size mismatch is corrected mostly anteriorly. Cold Plasmalyte usually is noted coming from the left ventricle.
- On completion of the anastomosis, a cardioplegia catheter is placed in the aortic root, and the Plasmalyte infusion is vented to prevent premature washout of the preservation solution.
- A modified anastomosis technique is considered if the recipient aorta is friable, particularly in older recipients. Two separate sutures are used, and side-by-side everting stitches are placed at the posteriormost point of the anastomosis. The sutures are tied. The anastomosis then proceeds in layers along the right and left aspects of the aorta; the first layer is everting, the second simple running. Rewarming is now extended to 34°C.

Inferior Vena Cava Anastomosis—Bicaval Technique

- The bicaval technique is associated with improved right ventricular function and less tricuspid valve regurgitation.[7] Many surgeons find it easier to perform the inferior vena cava anastomosis immediately after the left atrial anastomosis. This ensures a tension-free connection that remains relaxed as the aorta and pulmonary artery lengths are adjusted accordingly. The biatrial technique is rarely used in our adult practice. It may be required in cases of congenital anomaly, such as persistent left superior vena cava. In such instances, we still attempt to perform a direct superior vena cava anastomosis in addition to a right atrial cuff anastomosis.
- Construction of the inferior vena cava anastomosis requires adequate exposure of the donor inferior vena cava. Two or three stay sutures are used to retract the acute margin of the heart superiorly. The surgeon should note the location of the posterior descending artery when placing these. At this point, the posteriormost aspect of the anastomosis should be clearly visible. Eustachian valve remnants are excised (Fig. 27-8).
- A long, double-loaded 3-0 or 4-0 polypropylene suture on an SH-1 needle is selected. The slightly smaller needle facilitates placement of the "backwall" sutures, which are done from the inside.
- Sometimes it is easier for the person standing on the patient's left to sew this suture line.
- Once the backwall is complete, the recipient is rewarmed to 36°C and methylprednisolone (7 mg/kg) is administered by the perfusionist in anticipation of the controlled reperfusion, which will ensue in a few minutes. The anteriormost portion of the anastomosis is left open so that the coronary sinus effluent from the reperfusion can be collected. The suture line will be completed after the superior vena cava anastomosis. The acute margin is replaced in its normal position. There should be no gradient across this anastomosis because this may cause renal failure and liver and bowel edema.

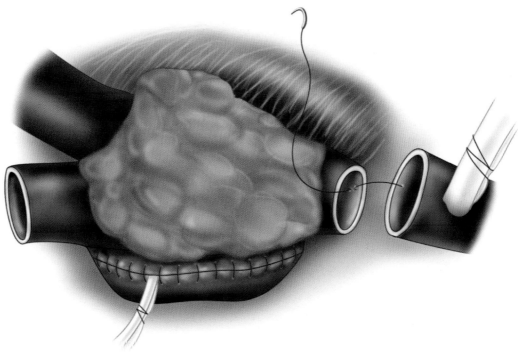

Figure 27-8

Inferior Vena Cava Anastomosis—Modified Technique

- Enlargement of the recipient's native failing heart increases all dimensions of the pericardial space, including the distance between the superior and inferior venae cavae. The traditional left atrial anastomosis affixes the posterior aspect of the right atrium.
- This potentially limits the reach of the donor inferior vena cava to the recipient's, resulting in possible tension on the right atrium of the donor heart, particularly if the aortic anastomosis is performed before the inferior vena cava anastomosis (Fig. 27-9).
- The resulting pull on the anterior wall of the right atrium may distort the tricuspid valve annulus, predisposing the valve to incompetence. This can be remedied with a prophylactic annuloplasty.[8]
- Significant tricuspid valve regurgitation occurs in about 15% of cases despite the bicaval anastomosis. As an alternative to annuloplasty, the inferior vena cava anastomosis may be modified by augmenting it with a triangular flap of recipient right atrial tissue attached to native inferior vena cava remnant anteriorly.[9] This flap is based on at least 65% of the circumference of the recipient's native inferior vena cava. The donor right atrium is incised from the corresponding point on the inferior vena cava anteriorly toward the appendage and away from the sinoatrial node (along the line of a conventional right atrial incision). The flap is then incorporated into the continuous suture line to augment the donor right atrium (Fig. 27-10).

3. Reperfusion

- The left ventricular apex catheter is converted to a vent. The bronchial return vent is removed, which helps to de-air the ventricle.
- The aorta remains clamped. Warm blood is administered in the root through a leukocyte-depleting filter (Pall Corporation, East Hills, NY).[10] We start at a low rate (about 150 mL/min), coming up to 3 mL/kg donor weight and not exceeding a root pressure of 65 to 70 mm Hg, for 10 to 15 minutes. During this time the superior vena cava anastomosis is constructed.
- Electrical activity usually returns to the heart while the clamp is still on. The surgeon observes an empty beating heart. The heart is allowed to fill and the lungs are ventilated a few times to further de-air the left side. Warm blood cardioplegia (Buckberg solution enhanced with glutamate and aspartate) may be used before the blood-only reperfusion.

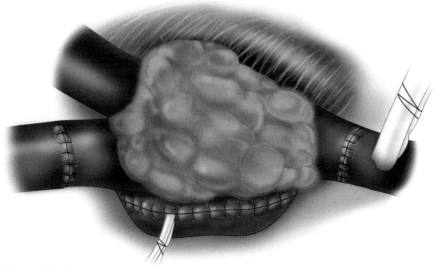

Figure 27-9

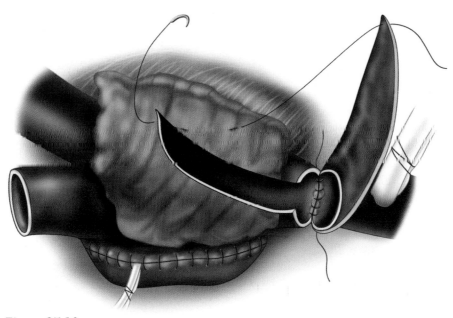

Figure 27-10

4. Superior Vena Cava Anastomosis

- The length of the recipient's native superior vena cava is preserved. Nevertheless, the donor superior vena cava until the azygos branch point is usually required to produce a tension-free anastomosis. This is because the dome of the recipient native left atrium is usually enlarged, causing the donor superior vena cava to be displaced medially after completion of the left atrial anastomosis.
- In extreme cases, the surgeon should not hesitate to augment the anterior (75% circumference) aspect of the anastomosis with a patch of pericardium trimmed in a diamond shape about 1.5 cm at its widest point. The anastomosis is carried out as described previously for the left atrium or pulmonary artery, using a 4-0 polypropylene suture with a small needle. There is no need to reinforce the suture line with pledget material.
- There should be no gradient across this anastomosis because this would cause an acute superior vena cava syndrome. By now, the reperfusion should have been ongoing for about 10 to 15 minutes, and the aortic clamp is released. The aortic root is vented, as is the left ventricular apex. The inferior vena cava anastomosis is rapidly completed, and the caval snares are released (Fig. 27-11).

5. Separating from Cardiopulmonary Bypass

- All surgical sites are checked for bleeding. It is particularly important to pick up the donor heart and expose the left atrial suture line because this cannot be done after weaning from cardiopulmonary bypass. The area near the native coronary sinus remnant should be inspected carefully.
- De-airing includes needle aspiration of the right superior pulmonary vein, the dome of the left atrium, and the left ventricular apex. Transesophageal echocardiography helps guide the de airing.
- A left atrial pressure monitoring line is usually placed so that the transpulmonary gradient, which can be labile, is continuously assessed. This is inserted into the right superior pulmonary vein.
- First-line inotropic support includes low dose dopamine, dobutamine, and nitroglycerin. The heart rate should be over 90. This optimizes cardiac output and decreases the risk of right ventricular overfilling.
- An alternative plan is to replace dopamine with epinephrine and nitroglycerin with milrinone infusion. Venous and pulmonary artery dilators are almost always needed. Low-dose vasopressin (0.02 U/min) or phenylephrine is occasionally used to target a mean blood pressure of 70 mm Hg. This helps to maintain a good coronary perfusion gradient for right ventricular function.
- If the mean blood pressure is greater than 80 mm Hg, arterial dilators are used rather than withdrawal of inotropes, which are needed to stimulate the denervated myocardium. Nitric oxide may be used to target a mean pulmonary artery pressure of less than 25 mm Hg, as the donor right ventricle is not "trained" against higher pulmonary artery pressures. The central venous pressure should not be greater than 12 to 14 mm Hg to avoid right ventricular volume overload. After protamine is given and bleeding has stopped, an additional dose of methylprednisolone is given.

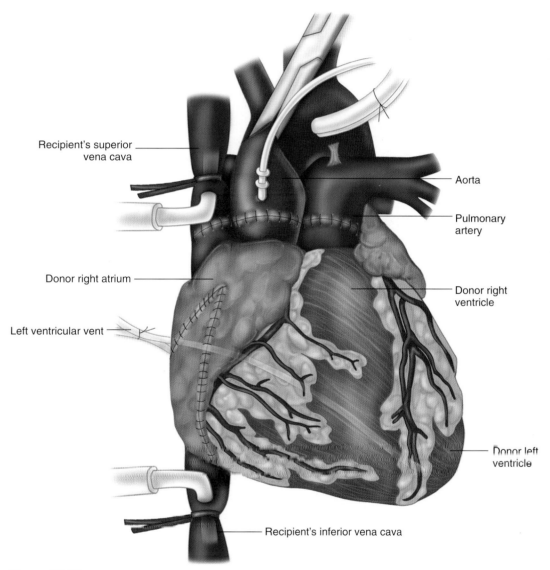

Recipient's superior vena cava

Aorta

Pulmonary artery

Donor right atrium

Donor right ventricle

Left ventricular vent

Donor left ventricle

Recipient's inferior vena cava

Figure 27-11

Separating from Cardiopulmonary Bypass with Anticipated Right Ventricular Dysfunction

- Preexisting pulmonary hypertension and the effects of cardiopulmonary bypass on pulmonary vascular resistance may give rise to perioperative right ventricular dysfunction after heart transplantation.
- To "train" the right ventricle of the donor heart, we use a segmental strategy in weaning off cardiopulmonary bypass. This technique consists of leaving the pulmonary artery anastomosis suture line untied and snared. A small vent line is inserted into the pulmonary artery to suction about 1 to 2 L/min.
- The systemic/right coronary artery pressure is maintained at 70 mm Hg or above by the perfusionist. With the venous drainage tubing partially clamped, the donor heart right ventricle is weaned off cardiopulmonary bypass while its preload is reduced. If the donor right ventricular function remains stable with an acceptable central venous pressure (<14 mm Hg), the preload is slowly increased over 10 to 15 minutes. This segmental weaning protocol may be complemented with inhaled nitric oxide.

6. Closure

- All foreign bodies from assist devices are removed at this time. In the case of paracorporeal devices, the cannulae exit sites are excised and closed primarily. The closure may require retention sutures. In the case of an implantable device, the drive line exit site is similarly closed; the pocket is drained. Peritoneal defects may be repaired with bovine pericardium. All nonbiologic material must be removed.
- The mediastinum is drained with a tube anterior to the heart that is positioned along the right pericardial edge to avoid right ventricular compression. An additional drain is used behind the heart.
- We prefer to open at least the right pleural space widely. Usually, both the right and left spaces are opened. This verifies that there are no preexisting effusions. More important, this window will help drain any pericardial effusions that may accumulate once the mediastinal drains are removed. Such effusions occur because of the enlarged pericardial space. The pleural–pericardial window minimizes the risk of both early and late tamponade.
- The surgeon may take a 15-minute break before chest closure. Even though the procedure may be long, chest closure should be done meticulously to avoid wound complications related to immunosuppression.
- The sternal edges are covered with vancomycin paste to minimize the risk of infection. Typically, for recipients weighing greater than 60 kg, 8 to 12 no. 7 sternal wires are used and the linea alba is closed with interrupted sutures.

Step 4. Postoperative Care

- Triple-drug therapy is used for immunosuppression. Initially, methylprednisolone 125 mg is given intravenously every 8 hours for three doses. Prednisone is then started orally or per nasogastric tube at 1 mg/kg/day in divided doses. This is weaned to 0.3 mg/kg/day over the subsequent 1 to 2 weeks. Further weaning is usually possible over the following months. Tacrolimus or cyclosporine is started per nasogastric tube 12 hours after surgery. Levels are checked daily. Mycophenolate mofetil is started intravenously on arrival at the intensive care unit and converted to oral therapy when appropriate.
- The left atrial line is pulled on postoperative day 1, before the mediastinal tubes are removed. Inotropes are weaned progressively over 48 to 72 hours until only low-dose dobutamine remains. To account for denervation, the final wean is carried out on the telemetry unit once the recipient is ambulatory. Terbutaline may be used to maintain a heart rate above 85 to 90 beats per minute.
- A perioperative rise in serum creatinine may be observed, particularly in older recipients. This usually peaks at 4 to 5 days after surgery and may be associated with oliguria. This rise may require prolonged use of nitroglycerin as a venodilator to relax the central venous pressure and a diuretic to help balance fluids.

Step 5. Pearls and Pitfalls

- The protocol described earlier for organ preservation and reperfusion is highly reliable. We have successfully used it in the setting of 5 to 8 hours of ischemia time.[11] All the steps are important, including transport of the organ in University of Wisconsin solution. Attention to detail is crucial. Occasionally, we have observed bradycardia after reperfusion despite the use of beta agonists. This usually resolves and is treated with temporary pacing. Recently, this risk has been minimized by avoiding warm cardioplegia as part of the reperfusion and using only leukocyte-depleted warm blood for 10 to 15 minutes.
- Implanting the donor heart usually takes about 45 to 80 minutes. This is considered warm ischemia time. The surgeon should be aware of this and use topical ice slush frequently, particularly on the surface of the right ventricle. It is equally important to collect the bronchial return so that it does not warm the left ventricle.
- Right ventricular dysfunction is the most common pitfall because of recipient pulmonary vascular resistance. In addition to the aforementioned treatment plan, one should consider pacing to a rate of 90 to 110 beats per minute. This increases cardiac output and helps prevent overdistention of the right ventricle. The latter causes decreased coronary perfusion and poor function.
- The pulmonary vasculature should always be assessed in terms of resistance. The absolute value of pulmonary artery pressure can be misleading; it may be high secondary to poor left ventricular function, or low owing to poor cardiac output. Nitric oxide is used if the pulmonary artery mean pressure is greater than 25 mm Hg, in the presence of a cardiac normal left atrial pressure and a marginal or low cardiac index.[12]
- Postoperative bleeding is a major concern because extensive transfusions will cause a transient rise in pulmonary vascular resistance and secondary right ventricular dysfunction. Along these lines, cardiopulmonary bypass time should be minimized. In recipients with previous surgery, bypass should be delayed until as much of the dissection as possible is done. This must be weighed against the risk of prolonging cold ischemia time, which may be acceptable.

- Adults with congenital heart disease often present the challenge of pulmonary artery or other great vessel reconstruction at the time of transplantation. This may require use of additional donor conduit or pericardial patches, or polytetrafluoroethylene graft material. Many of these recipients also have a greatly increased bronchial collateral circulation. These recipients may require moderate to deep hypothermia (22°C to 28°C) to reduce this flow and minimize potential warm ischemia of the donor heart. The increased return to the left-sided chambers also requires a larger donor size than usual, usually 20% greater than the recipient.
- When performing transplantation in a recipient who has been bridged with a biventricular assist device, removal of the right ventricular assist device before cannulation for cardiopulmonary bypass should be considered. This is usually well tolerated and allows for a more extensive dissection before anticoagulation.
- The presence of a left superior vena cava without an innominate bridge warrants preservation of the recipient coronary sinus and performance of a biatrial anastomosis. The left superior vena cava must also be cannulated during cardiopulmonary bypass. This can be accomplished by simply everting this edge within the running suture line.
- When performing the left atrial anastomosis, the surgeon should plan the position of the donor inferior and superior venae cavae. Also, as noted earlier, it is important to exclude the recipient cut edge from the suture line posteriorly. Many perform the inferior vena cava anastomosis before the pulmonary and aortic connections so that the exact length can be optimized.
- Two points deserve mention regarding the pulmonary artery anastomosis. First, it is very rare to mistakenly trim the donor and recipient cuffs too short, but making them too long will cause kinking and obstruction.[13] This presents as a marginal cardiac output with low pulmonary vascular resistance and high central venous pressure. A gradient is measured directly using a pressure line and needle on the operative field. Revision is accomplished on cardiopulmonary bypass with a beating heart. Second, because the recipient often has chronically elevated pulmonary artery pressures, the recipient vessel may be enlarged and friable. This can be a source of postoperative bleeding, usually at the junction of the main and right pulmonary arteries. The surgeon should therefore be very careful when separating the aorta from the right pulmonary artery to avoid a tear in this area. Also, it is important to leave a margin of recipient pulmonary artery proximal to the branch bifurcation. Finally, taking many suture bites per centimeter creates a distensible anastomosis that is less likely to bleed with acute swings in pulmonary artery pressure that may occur postoperatively. The suture line should be imagined as an expandable circular coil. Reinforcing the anastomosis with a strip of pericardium also helps to minimize this risk of bleeding.
- Most postoperative surgical bleeding comes from the aorta because of size mismatch and friable recipient tissue. Trimming the donor aorta with a bevel that accentuates the natural curve of the ascending aorta, as described previously, helps to adjust the size mismatch. The surgeon should observe the left main orifice inside the donor aorta to keep at least 1 cm of tissue distal to this on the posterior aspect. There should be a low threshold for performing a double suture line for the aortic anastomosis; it adds very little time to the warm ischemia and provides great benefit with regard to bleeding.

♦ If the donor superior vena cava is unable to reach the recipient's without tension, the surgeon should not hesitate to use a diamond-shaped patch of pericardium, as described above. This augments the anterior aspect of the anastomosis and prevents an hourglass deformity. A stenotic superior vena cava presents as an acute superior vena cava syndrome postoperatively and must be managed urgently. A gradient of 4 to 6 mm Hg should be considered high. Revision is accomplished with anticoagulation but off-pump, using cannulation above the anastomosis and in the right atrium. A temporary shunt such as this allows for an unhurried procedure after clamping. A percutaneous approach is also possible to correct this problem.[14]

References

1. Marelli D, Laks H, Kobashigawa J, et al: Seventeen year experience with 1083 heart transplants at a single institution. Ann Thorac Surg 2002;74:1558-1567.
2. Zaroff JG, Rosengard BR, Armstrong WF, et al: Consensus Conference Report: Maximizing use of organs recovered from the cadaver donor: Cardiac recommendations, March 28-29, 2001, Crystal City, Va. Circulation 2002;106:836-841.
3. Marelli D, Laks H, Fazio D, et al: The use of donor hearts with left ventricular hypertrophy. J Heart Lung Transplant 2000;19:496-503.
4. Marelli D, Bresson J, Laks H, et al: Hepatitis C-positive donors in heart transplantation. Am J Transplant 2002;2:443-447.
5. Viganó M, Rinaldi M, D'Armini AM, et al: The spectrum of aortic complications after heart transplantation. Ann Thorac Surg 1999;68:105-111.
6. Wolfsohn AL, Walley VM, Masters RG, et al: The surgical anastomoses after orthotopic heart transplantation: Clinical complications and morphologic observations. J Heart Lung Transplant 1994;13:455-465.
7. Aziz T, Burgess M, Khafagy R, et al: Bicaval and standard techniques in orthotopic heart transplantation: Medium-term experience in cardiac performance and survival. J Thorac Cardiovasc Surg 1999;118:115-122.
8. Jeevanandam V, Russell H, Mather P, et al: A one-year comparison of prophylactic donor tricuspid annuloplasty in heart transplantation. Ann Thorac Surg 2004;78:759-766.
9. Marelli D, Silvestry S, Zwas D, et al: Modified inferior vena cava anastomosis to reduce tricuspid valve regurgitation after heart transplantation. Tex Heart Inst J 2007;34:30-35.
10. Breda MA, Hall TS, Stuart RS, et al: Twenty-four hour lung preservation by hypothermia and leukocyte depletion. J Heart Transplant 1985;4:325-329.
11. Mitropoulos FA, Odim J, Marelli D, et al: Outcome of hearts with cold ischemic time greater than 300 minutes: A case-matched study. Eur J Cardiothorac Surg 2005;28:143-148.
12. Ardehali A, Hughes K, Sadeghi A, et al: Inhaled nitric oxide for pulmonary hypertension after heart transplantation. Transplantation 2001;72:638-641.
13. Dreyfus G, Jebara VA, Couetil JP, Carpentier A: Kinking of the pulmonary artery: A treatable cause of acute right ventricular failure after heart transplantation. J Heart Transplant 1990;9:575-576.
14. Sze DY, Robbins RC, Semba CP, et al: Superior vena cava syndrome after heart transplantation: Percutaneous treatment of a complication of bicaval anastomoses. J Thorac Cardiovasc Surg 1998;116:253-261.

CHAPTER 28

HEART-LUNG
TRANSPLANTATION

Tanveer A. Khan and Hillel Laks

Step 1. Surgical Anatomy

- Uncorrectable congenital heart disease with severe pulmonary hypertension is the leading indication for heart-lung transplantation, followed by primary pulmonary hypertension. The variety of congenital defect combinations with their anatomic nuances as well as prior surgical repairs is extensive.
- A thorough understanding of the recipient's specific anatomy from preoperative studies and previous operative reports is essential. During the donor procedure, it is important to obtain sufficient donor length of superior vena cava with the innominate vein so that necessary modifications are possible during the recipient procedure.
- Most patients with congenital heart disease and pulmonary hypertension have extensive aortopulmonary collaterals. During and after excision of the native organs in the recipient, attention must be given to these collaterals to achieve the excellent hemostasis that is critical in heart-lung transplantation. Moreover, a significant volume of venous return to the left side of the heart from the aortopulmonary collaterals must be addressed with either increased flow or a cooler temperature while the patient is on cardiopulmonary bypass.

Step 2. Preoperative Considerations

1. Donor Evaluation

- The evaluation of heart-lung donors includes history and physical examination, electrocardiography, arterial blood gas, chest radiography, bronchoscopy, sputum analysis, and laboratory and serologic tests. In donors older than 40 years of age or with significant cardiac risk factors, coronary angiography is performed.

◆ Donor selection criteria
  ▲ Age <50 years
  ▲ Smoking history <20 pack-years
  ▲ Pao$_2$ >140 mm Hg on 40% fraction of inspired oxygen (Fio$_2$) or >300 mm Hg on 100% Fio$_2$
  ▲ Normal chest radiograph
  ▲ Normal electrocardiogram
  ▲ Normal echocardiogram
  ▲ Normal coronary angiogram (donor age >40 years)
  ▲ Negative sputum Gram and fungal stains and normal sputum white blood cell count
  ▲ Bronchoscopy without evidence of purulence or aspiration
  ▲ No major thoracic trauma
  ▲ Negative human immunodeficiency virus (HIV) serology
◆ Because of the need for both the heart and lungs from a donor to meet the criteria, the successful procurement of an adequate heart-lung block is difficult; there also are long lists of potential heart transplant and lung transplant recipients waiting for organs, so heart-lung transplantation is not frequently performed.

2. Recipient Selection

◆ Patients identified and selected for heart-lung transplantation have severe, progressive cardiopulmonary disease refractory to maximal medical therapy with the capacity to functionally recover after the procedure.
◆ In the current era of heart-lung transplantation, most recipients have congenital heart disease not amenable to surgical repair with severe pulmonary vascular disease, also known as Eisenmenger syndrome. The next most common diagnosis is end-stage primary pulmonary hypertension. These two indications together account for more than half of all heart-lung transplants. Cystic fibrosis follows next in frequency, with other diagnoses less often treated with heart-lung transplantation.
◆ In general, patients older than 60 years of age are not selected, nor are those with significant comorbid disease, including renal failure, liver dysfunction, active malignancy, cachexia, obesity, or infection with HIV, hepatitis B, or hepatitis C. Prior thoracic surgical procedures and mechanical ventilation also are relative contraindications.
◆ Given that the pool of listed patients waiting for organs includes critically ill patients needing heart transplants or lung transplants, the number of organs allocated to heart-lung transplantation is limited.

Step 3. Operative Steps

1. **Donor Procedure**

- In the supine position, a median sternotomy is performed and the left and right pleural spaces are opened. The chest and lungs are examined for hemorrhage, contusion, and atelectasis. The heart is inspected with attention to right and left ventricular function, and the coronary arteries are palpated. The lungs are deflated to expose the inferior pulmonary ligaments, which are divided with electrocautery. The aorta, superior vena cava (SVC), and inferior vena cava (IVC) are dissected and controlled with umbilical tapes (Fig. 28-1A). The pericardium is removed, sacrificing the phrenic nerves, back to the hilum of the lung bilaterally. The azygos vein is ligated, and the innominate vein is ligated and divided to expose the distal ascending aorta and trachea. The pericardium overlying the trachea is divided and an umbilical tape is placed around the trachea.

- Intravenous heparin is administered at a dose of 300 U/kg. The main pulmonary artery is cannulated for infusion of pneumoplegia solution, and the ascending aorta is cannulated for infusion of cardioplegia solution. Prostaglandin E_1 500 μg is infused in the main pulmonary artery. Ventilation is continued at normal physiologic tidal volume with 40% oxygen. The SVC is clamped superior to the azygos vein, and the anterior wall of the IVC is divided to drain the heart. Once the heart is emptied, an aortic cross-clamp is placed on the ascending aorta just proximal to the innominate artery, and 10 mL/kg of cardioplegia is administered in the aortic root. The tip of the atrial appendage is excised to vent the heart and prevent distention, and pneumoplegia is infused in the main pulmonary artery at 15 mL/kg/min for 5 minutes. After the cardioplegia infusion is complete, the aortic cross-clamp may be removed, and the ascending aorta may be incised distally for additional venting of the left ventricle and aortic root. Saline ice slush is placed on the heart and lungs, which are ventilated with room air at half-normal tidal volumes. After the pneumoplegia solution is completely infused, the lungs are deflated.

- The aorta is divided as distally as possible. The posterior IVC is divided, and the heart-lung block is dissected from the posterior mediastinum, using caution to stay close to the esophagus and avoid injuring the trachea. The posterior hilar attachments are divided. The SVC is divided, and the innominate vein may be included if additional length is required for the recipient anatomy. The trachea is exposed to the right of the aorta, and the lungs are inflated to functional residual capacity, approximately 20 cm H_2O airway pressure. The trachea is stapled with a TA stapler at five tracheal rings above the carina. The trachea is divided and the heart-lung block is removed from the chest and taken to the back table for further dissection (Fig. 28-1B). The heart is inspected for a patent foramen ovale, which, if present, is closed with a running stitch using 4-0 polypropylene suture. The cannulation sites in the aorta and pulmonary artery as well as the remnant of the left atrial appendage are closed with 4-0 polypropylene suture, and the heart-lung block is packaged in sterile fashion for transport at 4° C in a cooler.

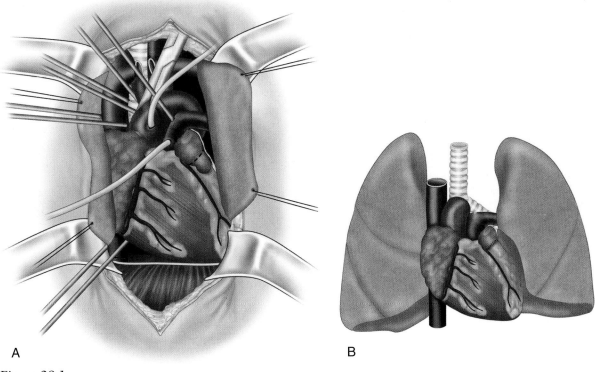

A

B

Figure 28-1

2. Recipient Procedure

◆ Cardiothoracic anesthesia includes a standard endotracheal tube; monitoring of the electrocardiogram, arterial pressure, pulse oximetry, core temperature, and urine output; and transesophageal echocardiography. Under adequate general anesthesia in the supine position, a median sternotomy is performed. The left and right pleural spaces and pericardium are opened. The inferior pulmonary ligaments and any pleural adhesions are divided with electrocautery. The lung hila are dissected, and the pulmonary arteries and veins are encircled with vessel loops and umbilical tapes, respectively. As much of the heart and lung dissection that can be done safely should be done before heparinization, although cardiopulmonary bypass should be initiated for any hemodynamic instability. The aorta, SVC, and IVC are dissected and encircled with umbilical tapes, and snares are placed loosely around the SVC and IVC (Fig. 28-2A). Heparin is administered, and pursestring stitches are placed in the distal ascending aorta, SVC, and IVC, followed by standard cannulation.

◆ The transesophageal echocardiography probe is removed to prevent injury to the esophagus during dissection. An antegrade cardioplegia cannula is placed in the ascending aorta. The patient is then placed on cardiopulmonary bypass and the blood cooled to 24° C. The ascending aorta is cross-clamped, cardioplegia is administered to achieve arrest, and the snares are tightened around the SVC and IVC. The heart is then excised, beginning with the right atrium at the atrioventricular groove, followed by division of the atrial septum. The aorta and pulmonary artery are divided, and the heart excision is completed by dividing the left atrium at the atrioventricular groove. SVC and IVC cuffs are prepared, with excision of the remaining right atrium (Fig. 28-2B). The right pulmonary artery, pulmonary veins, and mainstem bronchus are divided with a TA stapler, and the right lung is removed (Fig. 28-3A). The left lung is removed in similar fashion. The left atrium is divided vertically between the pulmonary vein remnants, and in turn each side is retracted anteriorly, dissected from the posterior mediastinum, and excised. The dissection is kept close to the left atrium and pulmonary vein remnants to prevent injury to the vagus nerve, which lies posteriorly on the esophagus (Fig. 28-3B).

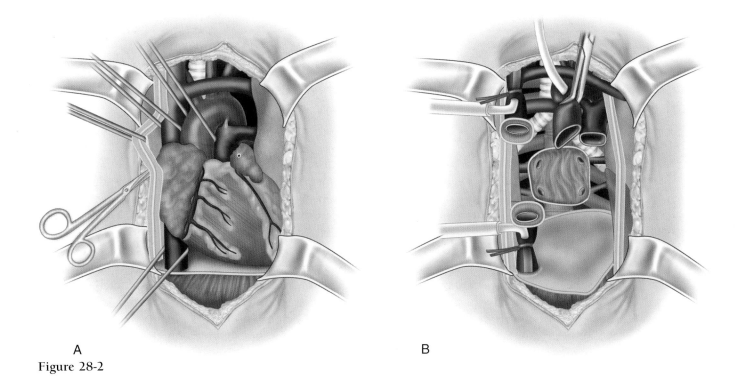

A

Figure 28-2

B

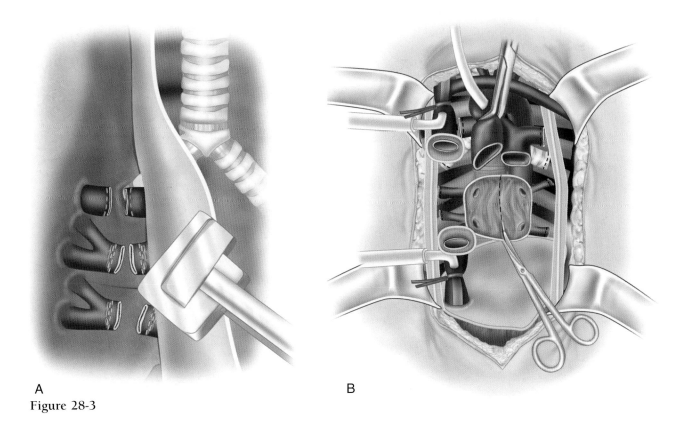

A

Figure 28-3

B

- Complete hemostasis then is achieved in both chest cavities and the mediastinum, with particular attention to control of collateral vessels in the mediastinal and peribronchial tissue. The phrenic nerves are dissected, leaving a 3-cm margin of pericardium on each side of the nerve to create a pedicle, from the diaphragm to just inferior to the subclavian vessels. The right phrenic nerve usually lies closer to the hilum (Fig. 28-4A). Next, the bronchial remnants are dissected with electrocautery back to the trachea. Excision of the pulmonary artery remnants facilitates the exposure. A button of left pulmonary artery around the ligamentum arteriosum at the aortic arch is left intact to prevent injury to the left recurrent laryngeal nerve. The trachea is exposed and divided two rings above the carina, and the bronchial remnants are removed. A culture swab is taken from the airway. Again, perfect hemostasis must be achieved at this point before implanting the heart-lung graft, which will obscure exposure of the posterior mediastinum.
- The graft is prepared on the back table with attention to the presence of a patent foramen ovale or any pulmonary contusions. The aorta is dissected away from the pulmonary artery to allow for a tension-free anastomosis. The trachea is divided one ring above the carina, and the airway is saline lavaged and suctioned for secretions. Adequate peritracheal tissue and posterior membranous tissue must be preserved to allow for a well-vascularized and tension-free anastomosis. A swab of the airway is sent for culture. A strip of mediastinal fat or pericardium is prepared to buttress the tracheal anastomosis.
- The heart-lung graft is then placed in the chest with the lungs posterior to the phrenic nerve pedicles (Fig. 28-4B). Another technique has been described in which the lungs are placed anterior to the phrenic pedicles, which allows for easier rotation of the graft and exposure of the posterior mediastinum to check for bleeding after cardiopulmonary bypass. Ice wrapped in sponges is placed on the heart and lungs for topical cooling, and insulating pads are used posteriorly to protect the heart and lungs from warming. A cannula is placed through the amputated left atrial appendage and secured with a pursestring suture. Cold crystalloid solution is infused

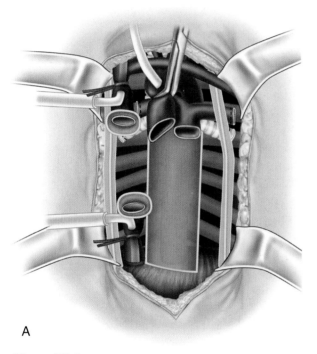

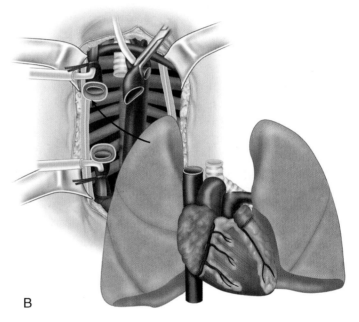

A

B

Figure 28-4

through the cannula for additional topical cooling. The tracheal anastomosis is performed first, and traction stitches of 4-0 polypropylene are placed in the corners where the cartilaginous and membranous portions of the trachea meet to line up the posterior membranous trachea. The posterior membranous tracheal anastomosis is done in a running fashion with 4-0 polypropylene suture, followed by the anterior portion of the anastomosis, which is completed with interrupted stitches of 4-0 polypropylene. Peribronchial tissue is used to cover the anastomosis (Fig. 28-5A).

♦ The aortic anastomosis is done next in a running fashion with 4-0 polypropylene suture, reinforced with glutaraldehyde-treated donor pericardial strips. All vascular anastomoses are performed similarly, with the posterior wall sewn from the inside and the anterior wall completed from the outside. Rewarming of the patient is started, and the IVC anastomosis is performed in a running fashion with 4-0 polypropylene suture. The last anastomosis to be completed is the SVC, again done in running fashion with 4-0 polypropylene suture. Modified blood reperfusion of the heart is initiated through the antegrade cardioplegia cannula. The main pulmonary artery is cannulated and modified blood reperfusion of the lungs is started while the lungs are ventilated with room air. The cannula through the left atrial appendage is now converted to a vent, and the SVC and IVC snares are released. After approximately 10 minutes of modified reperfusion and adequate de-airing of the heart, the cross-clamp is removed.

♦ Venting is done through the antegrade cardioplegia cannula in the ascending aorta and a cannula in the main pulmonary artery. The left atrial appendage vent is removed after a stable rhythm is achieved, and the appendage is oversewn. A left atrial pressure monitoring line is placed in the right superior pulmonary vein. The vascular anastomoses are examined for optimal hemostasis. The patient is then slowly weaned from cardiopulmonary bypass while the lungs are ventilated with an Fio_2 of 50% that is adjusted according to oxygen saturation. Once off cardiopulmonary bypass, venting is continued for 3 minutes, after which the antegrade cardioplegia, main pulmonary artery, and venous cannulae are removed. Protamine is administered and the aorta is decannulated. Intravenous methylprednisolone 500 mg is given. All cannulation sites are doubly secured (Fig. 28-5B). Pacing wires and chest tubes are placed, and the chest is closed in standard fashion. Fiberoptic bronchoscopy is performed to examine the tracheal anastomosis, and cardiac function is examined by transesophageal echocardiography.

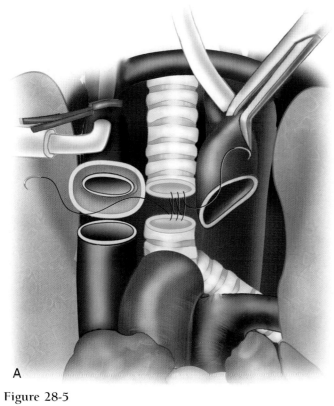

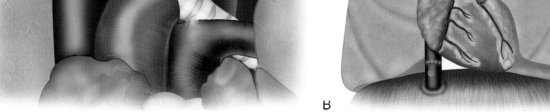

Figure 28-5

Step 4. Postoperative Care

1. Early Postoperative Critical Care

- In the heart-lung transplant recipient, the postoperative care in the cardiothoracic intensive care unit involves attention to ventilator, hemodynamic, and fluid management. Generally, once patients are awake and stable, they are weaned to extubate, which usually is possible within 24 hours. Gentle endotracheal suctioning may be done to remove secretions and prevent atelectasis. Early graft dysfunction associated with reperfusion injury occurs in up to 15% of patients and presents with progressive hypoxia and diffuse infiltrates on chest radiography. Patients are supported with mechanical ventilation while minimizing barotrauma and are treated with diuresis and pulmonary vasodilators such as nitric oxide or inhaled prostacyclin (prostaglandin I_2). Severe cases refractory to intervention may require support with extracorporeal membrane oxygenation. Relisting for transplantation in accordance with United Network for Organ Sharing guidelines also may be appropriate in severe cases.
- Myocardial dysfunction after heart-lung transplantation has been associated with long ischemic times or suboptimal preservation techniques. Inotropic support may be required for several days, during which a pulmonary artery catheter is helpful to guide the therapy. Sinus node dysfunction is usually transient and may be treated with temporary cardiac pacing or isoproterenol. Intravenous fluids should be monitored closely and administered cautiously according to cardiac filling pressures, myocardial function, and tissue perfusion. Accordingly, diuresis is initiated as early as indicated to maintain an appropriate fluid balance and prevent pulmonary edema.

2. Immunosuppression

- Our current immunosuppression protocol consists of quadruple therapy and includes (1) corticosteroids; (2) a calcineurin inhibitor, tacrolimus (Prograf); (3) an antiproliferative agent, mycophenolate mofetil (Cellcept); and (4) antithymocyte globulin. Methylprednisolone is started at 125 mg intravenously every 8 hours for the first 24 hours, then reduced to 1 mg/kg/day or the equivalent dose of oral prednisone. The prednisone taper commences at 1 week after the initial dose and is decreased by 0.1 mg/kg/wk to reach a maintenance dose of 0.1 mg/kg/day. Tacrolimus is administered orally at 0.1 mg/kg every 12 hours and adjusted to achieve whole-blood drug levels of 10 to 20 ng/mL. Mycophenolate mofetil is given at a dose of 1000 to 1500 mg orally every 12 hours. Rabbit antithymocyte globulin (Thymoglobulin) is dosed at 1.5 mg/kg/day intravenously for the first 3 days. These protocols are modified with acute or chronic rejection, serious infection, post-transplantation lymphoproliferative disease (PTLD), or significant drug-related adverse reactions.

3. Infection Prophylaxis

◆ Patients are treated with vancomycin and ceftriaxone for perioperative bacterial prophylaxis. Ceftriaxone is often continued for a full course to treat bacterial pathogens from bronchial cultures. Aerosolized amphotericin B is administered for prevention of *Aspergillus* infection, and caspofungin is used for general fungal prophylaxis. Patients living in endemic areas for fungus may be discharged on voriconazole. Cytomegalovirus (CMV)–positive patients are treated with ganciclovir prophylaxis and discharged on valganciclovir for 1 year. CMV-negative patients receiving a CMV-positive donor graft are treated with ganciclovir and CMV intravenous immunoglobulin and are continued on valganciclovir for life. Trimethoprim-sulfamethoxazole or aerosolized pentamidine are used for *Pneumocystis jiroveci* (previously *P. carinii*) prophylaxis. Prevention of mucosal candidal infection is achieved with oral clotrimazole. *Toxoplasma*-negative recipients who receive a *Toxoplasma*-positive donor graft are treated with pyrimethamine prophylaxis for 6 months.

4. Complications

◆ The most common causes of early (<1 year) mortality after heart-lung transplantation are technical complications, graft failure, and infection, whereas late (>1 year) mortality is due to chronic rejection related to obliterative bronchiolitis and graft failure. Postoperative hemorrhage is a significant source of morbidity and mortality as well, particularly with respect to excessive blood product administration and, in severe cases, multisystem organ failure.

◆ Infection in the early postoperative period is more commonly due to bacterial pathogens, particularly gram-negative bacteria, whereas late infections more often involve opportunistic viral, fungal, and protozoan pathogens. CMV, the most common viral pathogen, usually is responsive to treatment with ganciclovir and hyperimmune globulin. CMV infection has been associated with chronic rejection.

◆ Acute rejection usually occurs in the first year after heart-lung transplantation but very rarely leads to graft failure. Rejection is more likely to involve the lungs than the heart. The diagnosis is made clinically based on lung dysfunction and confirmed by transbronchial biopsy showing perivascular and interstitial mononuclear infiltrate. The mainstay treatment of acute rejection is based on steroids, with resistant cases treated with antilymphocyte therapies.

◆ Chronic rejection manifested as obliterative bronchiolitis is a major source of late mortality with progressive deterioration of graft function. Again, the diagnosis is confirmed by transbronchial biopsy showing a submucosal mononuclear infiltrate and scarring with small airway obliteration. The treatment involves optimization of immunosuppression and maximizing the patient's quality of life while minimizing infectious complications.

◆ Graft coronary artery disease is a relatively uncommon chronic complication that leads to decreased long-term survival. Patients manifest clinical deterioration of cardiac function, and the diagnosis is made by coronary angiography showing a diffuse pattern of atherosclerosis. Percutaneous and surgical revascularization has been effective in some patients, and retransplantation may be necessary in selected cases.

- Airway complications after heart-lung transplantation have a reported incidence of less than 5%. Both tracheal dehiscence and stenosis are rare and appear to be unrelated to steroid use or rejection. Tracheal complications are diagnosed by bronchoscopy and may require bronchoscopic or surgical intervention.
- The more common malignancies associated with transplantation and immunosuppression are PTLD and skin cancers. Early PTLD diagnosed less than 1 year after transplantation is typically benign and responds to a reduction in immunosuppression, whereas late PTLD is a more malignant form that is resistant to treatment and has a high mortality rate.
- Overall, the 1-, 5-, and 10-year survival rates of heart-lung transplant recipients have been reported at approximately 65%, 50%, and 30%, respectively.

5. Graft Surveillance

- Heart-lung transplant recipients are followed closely and regularly to monitor their immunosuppression and check serial arterial blood gases and pulmonary function test results. Patients are also scheduled for routine bronchoscopy with transbronchial biopsies. Endomyocardial biopsies may be performed routinely as well but are not essential given that cardiac rejection is very rare without lung rejection. The early detection of complications, including infection and rejection, allows for prompt treatment.

Step 5. Pearls and Pitfalls

1. Hemostasis

- Perform as much of the recipient heart and lung dissection that can be safely done before the administration of heparin, especially in redo procedures commonly seen in congenital heart disease.
- Particularly important is absolute hemostasis in the posterior mediastinum and pleural spaces before heart-lung implantation because exposure of these areas is extremely difficult after the graft is in the chest.

2. Phrenic and Vagus Nerve Injury

- Avoid injury to the phrenic and vagus nerves during hilar and posterior mediastinal dissection, lung excision, and hemostasis with cautery.
- Vagus nerves are vulnerable to injury during dissection posterior to the carina, resulting in a high vagotomy and postoperative gastroparesis.

3. Recurrent Nerve Injury

- A portion of the left pulmonary artery is left intact, in situ adjacent to the aortic arch, in the recipient to avoid dissection around the left recurrent laryngeal nerve.

4. Airway Anastomosis

- Minimize tracheal dissection to preserve the blood supply.
- Avoid excessive traction down on the membranous trachea before dividing it to prevent unnecessary shortening and removal of tissue needed for the posterior part of the tracheal anastomosis.
- Perform a tension-free anastomosis, and avoid telescoping if possible.

5. Atrial versus Bicaval Anastomosis

- Separate bicaval anastomoses tend to preserve the geometry of the heart, decrease the incidence of tricuspid regurgitation, and reduce postoperative arrhythmias.
- In children younger than 1 year of age, atrial anastomoses may be used to avoid pursestringing very small caval suture lines.

Bibliography

Banner NR, Khaghani A, Yacoub MH: Heart-lung transplantation. In Kapoor AS, Laks H, Schroeder JS, Yacoub MH (eds): Cardiomyopathies and Heart-Lung Transplantation. New York, McGraw-Hill, 1991, p 415.

Jamieson SW, Stinson EB, Oyer PE, et al: Operative technique for heart-lung transplantation. J Thorac Cardiovasc Surg 1984;87:930-935.

Moffatt-Bruce SD, Reitz BA: Heart-lung transplantation: Is it a viable option in the 21st century? In Lynch JP and Ross DJ (eds): Lung and Heart-Lung Transplantation. New York, Taylor & Francis, 2006, pp 217-269.

Perricone A, Jamieson SW: Operative procedure for heart-lung transplantation. In Kapoor AS, Laks H (eds): Atlas of Heart-Lung Transplantation. New York, McGraw-Hill, 1994, p 103.

Reitz BA, Wallwork JL, Hunt SA, et al: Heart-lung transplantation: Successful therapy for patients with pulmonary vascular disease. N Engl J Med 1982;306:557-564.

Sarris GE, Smith JA, Shumway NE, et al: Long-term results of combined heart-lung transplantation: The Stanford experience. J Heart Lung Transplant 1994;13:940-949.

Trulock EP, Christie JD, Edwards LB, et al: Registry of the International Society for Heart and Lung Transplantation: Twenty-fourth official adult lung and heart-lung transplantation report—2007. J Heart Lung Transplant 2007;26:782-795.

Note: Page numbers followed by the letter f refer to figures; page numbers followed by the letter t refer to tables.